Vascular Access for Hemodialysis—III

Vascular Access for Hemodialysis—III

MITCHELL L. HENRY, M.D.
RONALD M. FERGUSON, M.D., Ph.D.

W.L. Gore & Associates, Inc.
Precept Press, Inc.

©1993 by W.L. Gore & Associates, Inc., and Precept Press, Inc.
All Rights Reserved

Except for appropriate use in critical reviews or works of scholarship, the reproduction or use of this work in any form or by any electronic, mechanical or other means now known or hereafter invented, including photocopying and recording, and in any information storage and retrieval system is forbidden without the written permission of the publisher.

Library of Congress Catalog Card Number:
93-83251

International Standard Book Number:
0-944496-36-9

97 96 95 94 93   5 4 3 2 1

Printed in Hong Kong

GORE-TEX, GORE-TEX *Vascular Graft, and* GORE-TEX *Suture are registered trademarks of W.L. Gore & Associates, Inc.*

CONTENTS

Preface xx

SECTION I
1. **Contribution of Vascular Access-Related Disease to Morbidity of Hemodialysis Patients** 3
   J. Michael Lazarus, M.D., W.H. Huang, N. L. Lew, Edmund G. Lowrie, M.D.

2. **Biologic Mediators of Intimal Hyperplasia** 14
   Mark F. Fillinger, M.D., D. Brent Kerns, M.D.

3. **Pharmacologic Intervention to Prevent Intimal Hyperplasia** 41
   Charles J. Diskin, M.D., Thomas J. Stakes Jr., M.D., Andrew T. Pennell, Pharm.D.

   Panel Discussion 74
   Mitchell L. Henry, M.D., moderator; Charles J. Diskin, M.D., Mark F. Fillinger, M.D., J. Michael Lazarus, M.D.

SECTION II
4. **Color Flow Doppler Physics and Clinical Approaches** 81
   Samuel P. Martin, M.D., Kathleen S. Bubb, R.V.T.

5. **Correlation of Color Flow Doppler and Angiography** 95
   William H. Bay, M.D.

6. **Clinical Use of Color Flow Doppler** 102
   Barry S. Strauch, M.D., Robert S. O'Connell, M.D., Kenneth L. Geoly, M.D., Marietta Grundlehner, M.D., Y. Nabil Yakub, M.D., David P. Teitjen, M.D.

   Panel Discussion 109
   Ronald M. Ferguson, M.D., Ph.D., moderator; William H. Bay, M.D., Samuel P. Martin, M.D., Barry S. Strauch, M.D.

SECTION III—ABSTRACT PRESENTATIONS
7. **Incidence of Vascular Access Thrombosis in Patients Treated with Recombinant Human Erythropoietin** 115
   George Carty, M.D., Daniel Hoheim, M.D.

8. **Treatment of Angioaccess Ischemic Steal by Revascularization** 123
   Harry Schanzer, M.D., Milan Skladany, M.D., Moshe Haimov, M.D.

9. **Early Experience with Adjunctive Angioscopy in Thrombectomy of PTFE A-V Fistula** 128
   D.J. Wright, M.D., R.G. Netzley, M.D., K.G. McAree, M.D.

10. **Preliminary Experience with a new PTFE Graft for Vascular Access** 133
    Ingemar Dawidson, M.D., Ph.D., Denise Melone, R.N.

    Panel Discussion 137
    Mitchell L. Henry, M.D., moderator; George Carty, M.D., Ingemar Dawidson, M.D., Harry Schanzer, M.D., D.J. Wright, M.D.

11. **Use of 6 mm Stretch PTFE Grafts for Early Use in Hemodialysis** 142
    Eugene J. Simoni, M.D., Krishna M. Jain, M.D., John S. Munn, M.D.

12. **Dialysis Access Using PTFE-Coated Woven Grafts** 146
    Ralph Didlake, M.D., Edna Curry, R.N., B.S.N., Ed Rigdon, M.D., Seshadri Raju, M.D., John Bower, M.D.

13. **A Prospective Randomized Comparison of Bovine Heterografts Versus Impra Grafts for Chronic Hemodialysis** 157
    Jeffrey C. Reese, M.D., Robert Esterl, M.D., Lisa Lindsey, P.A.-C., Della Aridge, R.N., M.S.N., Harvey Solomon, M.D., Ralph B. Fairchild, M.D., Paul J. Garvin, M.D.

    Panel Discussion 164
    Ronald M. Ferguson, M.D., Ph.D., moderator; Ralph Didlake, M.D., Jeffrey C. Reese, M.D., Eugene J. Simoni, M.D.

SECTION IV

14. **Salvage Surgery for Arteriovenous Conduits: Does It Make Sense?** 169
    Stephen B. Leapman, M.D., Mark D. Pescovitz, M.D., J. Vincent Thomalla, M.D., Martin Milgrom, M.D., Ronald S. Filo, M.D.

15. **4-7 mm Tapered Expanded PTFE Access Grafts: Techniques of Construction and Preservation of Graft Life** 175
    Leonard H. Hines, M.D., G. Randolph Turner, M.D., William Scott King, M.D., Carter E. McDaniel III, M.D., David J. Dodd, M.D.

16. **Graft Curettage** 186
    John W. Puckett, M.D., Stephen F. Lindsay, M.D.

Panel Discussion 196
Ronald M. Ferguson, M.D., Ph.D., moderator; Leonard H. Hines, M.D., Mark Pescovitz, M.D., John W. Puckett, M.D.

SECTION V

17. **Endovascular Salvage of Failing PTFE Grafts** 201
    Michael J. Verta Jr., M.D.

18. **The Role of Endovascular Stents in Hemodialysis Access** 207
    Jeffrey H. Fair, M.D., Scott O. Trerotola, M.D.

19. **The Role of Angioscopy in Vascular Access Surgery** 210
    Arnold Miller, M.B., Ch.B., Edward J. Marcaccio, M.D., William S. Goodman, M.D., Michael N. Gottlieb, M.D.

20. **Venous Hypertension** 219
    Mark B. Adams, M.D.

    Panel Discussion 225
    Mitchell L. Henry, M.D., moderator; Mark B. Adams, M.D., Jeffrey H. Fair, M.D., Arnold Miller, M.B., Ch.B., F.R.C.S., F.R.C.S.C., F.A.C.S., Michael J. Verta Jr., M.D.

    Index 229

ACKNOWLEDGMENTS

Drs. Mitchell L. Henry and Ronald M. Ferguson wish to thank the Medical Products Division of W.L. Gore and Associates, Inc., for their substantial support and help in organizing the Symposium on Dialysis Access. Their ongoing support has been essential to make possible this unique gathering of individuals interested in vascular access. W.L. Gore also made a substantial contribution toward underwriting the publication cost of this book, which is a direct result of the two-day symposium. The authors would also like to thank Teri Bailey and Cindy Narcross for their time and effort in organizing the conference and transcript preparation. A special thanks for the many efforts of Cindy Narcross in final preparation and editing of the manuscripts for this book.

PREFACE

IN A 1978 EDITORIAL, noted nephrologist Carl Kjellstrand described vascular access as the Achilles' heel of the hemodialysis patient. Dialysis access is literally the "lifeblood" of the patient with end-stage renal disease. It is not a glamorous subject, and oftentimes it is an ignored one.

This book is a compilation of presentations and discussions from the third Symposium on Dialysis Access. These ongoing semiannual conferences have been one of the few concentrated efforts to share information and thoughts about vascular access, in an effort to improve outcomes for patients requiring hemodialysis.

This book has required support from many sources. W.L. Gore and Associates has made significant efforts to make it a reality, as also have the individuals who prepared oral and written presentations, the latter of which appear in this volume. Discussions and questions by conference participants also have added to the intrinsic value of the gathering.

Plans are under way for the fourth symposium. It is our hope that we can continue to meet regularly to discuss old problems, as well as new science and technology in order to meet the goal of reducing the morbidity of vascular access in the hemodialysis patient.

Mitchell L. Henry, M.D.
Ronald M. Ferguson, M.D., Ph.D.

SECTION I

1

CONTRIBUTION OF VASCULAR ACCESS-RELATED DISEASE TO MORBIDITY OF HEMODIALYSIS PATIENTS

J. Michael Lazarus, M.D., W. H. Huang, N. L. Lew, and Edmund G. Lowrie, M.D.

DEVELOPMENT OF THE ARTERIOVENOUS SHUNT in the 1960s permitted prolonged hemodialysis in patients with renal failure. Creation of the native vein arteriovenous (A-V) fistula in the 1970s, and, subsequently, prosthetic A-V fistulas, has greatly enhanced our ability to keep patients with renal failure alive on maintenance dialysis. Despite these advances, the A-V fistula remains the "Achilles' heel" of hemodialysis.[1] In recent years, many nephrologists have recognized an increase in the hospitalization rate of dialysis patients for vascular-access–related complications. Although there is much speculation as to the degree of this problem, few data are available concerning the morbidity related to A-V fistulas.

This is a report of such information from National Medical Care, Inc. (NMC), a subsidiary of W.R. Grace, Inc., which operates artificial kidney centers in professional partnership with its affiliated physicians. More than 25,000 patients with end-stage renal disease (ESRD) are treated in 358 National Medical Care dialysis units in the United States. The company maintains a patient statistical profile (PSP) system that captures selected patient-specific data (e.g., birth date, sex, race, renal disease etiology, treatment time and frequency, and other demographics) and important events that occur during the course of treatment (e.g., death, transplantation, and hospitalization, along with the principal cause of hospitalization).

We have reviewed the NMC data base examining morbidity, as measured by hospitalization, related to the diagnosis of vascular access complications (determined by ICD-9 diagnostic codes on discharge from the hospital). It should be appreciated that a large number of access complications (perhaps the majority) are managed without admission to the hospital; therefore, these data will significantly underestimate the problem of access complication and morbidity. Nonetheless, these data provide the most specific and currently available information in a large population of dialysis patients.

Erythropoietin (EPO) has become available to dialysis patients in the last several years.[2] EPO enhances platelet adhesiveness,[3] and, related to the increase in hematocrit, corrects the bleeding time[4] and increases the viscosity of blood.[5] There has been much speculation as to the role of EPO and an increased hematocrit on access clotting.[6,7] Therefore, the effect of EPO on access morbidity and hospitalization was also examined in a subpopulation of patients.

Methods

Hospitalization data were extracted from the PSP system for each quarter during the five years 1986–90. Morbidity was represented by the number of hospital days due to access-related disease per 1,000 days of patient exposure. Home hemodialysis patients and patients treated by peritoneal dialysis were excluded. Selected demographic variables describing the population of patients at the end of each year were collected from the PSP files. The ICD-9 diagnostic codes used were: 996.1 (mechanical complications of vascular device, implant and graft), 996.6 and 996.62 (infection and inflammatory reaction due to internal prosthetic device implant and graft), and 996.73 and 996.74 (other complications of an internal prosthetic device [renal dialysis device] and [other vascular device]). Other causes for hospitalization with the appropriate ICD-9 codes for these admissions were retrieved. A more detailed analysis of discharge diagnoses in the last quarter of 1990 was performed. The company also maintains two other unique patient-specific data bases: a laboratory data base containing test results on patients treated in NMC facilities, and an EPO data base containing data pertinent to patients receiving EPO therapy. The latter data base was implemented in August 1989, coincident with the routine clinical availability of EPO. Data from patients receiving EPO for at least three months during the period Aug. 1, 1989, through Aug. 1, 1990, and those not receiving the drug for the same period were analyzed. Data bases were merged by patient identifiers for the analyses.

All statistical analyses were performed using SAS software. Potential predictors of hematocrit prior to EPO, initial EPO dose, and hematocrit while on EPO were examined using multiple regression and analyses of covariance.[8] Predictors of hospitalization were determined using stepwise logistic regression.[9] Details of this analytical technique were provided in a prior publication.[10]

Table 1-1. All Dialysis Patients

	1986	1987	1988	1989	1990
Number	14,763	17,297	18,935	21,499	26,294
Median age (yr)	59.39	59.52	59.62	59.83	60.35
% Female	49.89	50.04	49.92	49.47	49.64
% White	51.73	51.16	50.70	49.41	49.64
% Diabetic	26.31	27.69	29.69	30.93	34.47

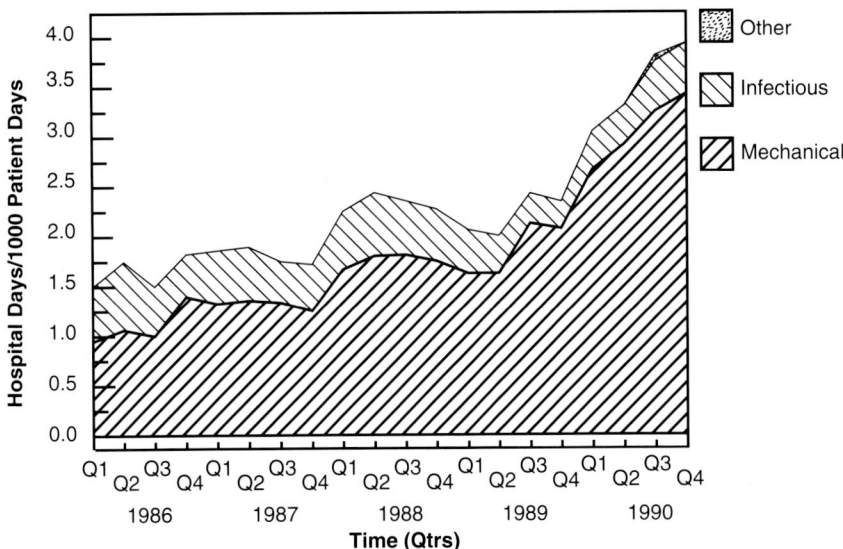

Figure 1-1. Trend of vascular access morbidity due to mechanical, infectious, and other causes. Days hospitalized/1,000 days at risk sum up the Y axis so that morbidity from all causes is shown by the uppermost curve on the graph.

Results

Selected demographic variables describing the population of patients at the end of each year are shown in table 1-1. These characteristics are typical of the ESRD population at large. The time trend for access-related morbidity (dividing hospitalizations into three primary classifications—"mechanical," "infectious," and "other") during the five years 1986–90 is shown in figure 1-1. Mechanical complications as measured by hospital days are by far more severe than infectious causes. Very few causes were classified as "other." Access-related hospitalizations increased from 1.5 days per 1,000 (0.55 days per year) to 2.2 days per 1,000 days at risk (0.80 days per year) between 1986 and early 1989. From early 1989 to the end of 1990, hospitalizations increased from 2.2 days per 1,000 to 4.0 days per 1,000 (1.46 days per year).

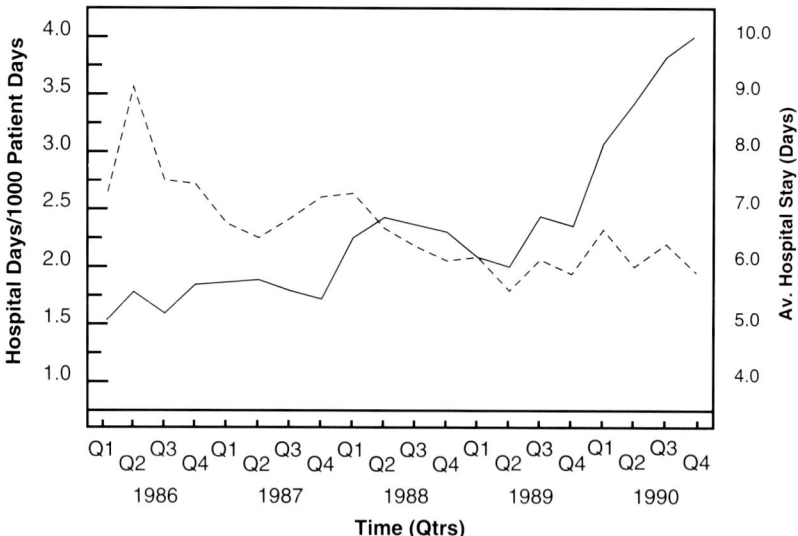

Figure 1-2. Time trend curves for access-related hospital morbidity and average length of hospital stay during access-related hospitalizations.

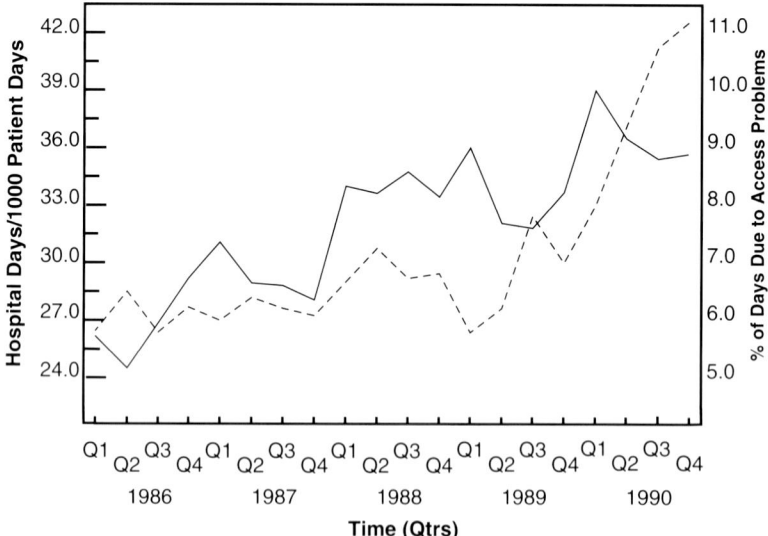

Figure 1-3. Time trend curves for hospitalization days/1,000 days at risk for all causes and the percentage of hospitalization days due to access-related complications.

Figure 1-2 illustrates a superimposition of the time trend for access morbidity (number of days hospitalized/1,000 patient days) and length of hospital stay (days per hospitalization). It can be seen that length of hospital stay has become shorter, whereas the total of hospital days has increased. This observation indicates that the increase in morbidity is related to increased hospitalization rates, not longer hospital stays. This pattern is typical of that

Table 1-2. Leading Causes of Hospitalization

Diagnosis	Hosp. days/ 1,000 days at risk	Days Total	%	Episodes Number	%
Vascular access (mechanical and infectious)	4.0	9,743	11.2	1,649	16.2
Septicemia	1.0	2,546	2.9	218	2.2
G.I. hemorrhage	0.9	2,248	2.6	235	2.3
Renal failure	0.8	2,060	2.4	224	2.2
Pneumonia	0.8	2,035	2.3	214	2.1
Congestive heart failure	0.8	1,913	2.2	243	2.4
Infectious diseases (NOS)	0.7	1,706	2.0	216	2.1
Chest pain	0.7	1,682	2.0	243	2.4
Fluid overload	0.7	1,634	1.9	253	2.5
Peritonitis	0.5	1,317	1.5	148	1.5
All diagnoses	35.8	87,437	100.0	10,148	100.0

for hospitalizations for all other causes in renal patients, probably related to the advent of diagnosis-related groups (DRGs).

To rule out the existence of a similar increasing trend in hospitalization rate in dialysis patients for all causes, the time trend curve for total hospital admissions was compared to that for access problems (figure 1-3). The overall morbidity, as measured by total hospital days/1,000 patient days, increased from about 26 days per 1,000 days of risk in early 1986 to about 36 days per 1,000 days in late 1990. Vascular-access–related morbidity, however, appears to have increased much more rapidly over this time period (e.g., access-related problems contributed to about 6.0% of days admitted in early 1986, but increased to 11% in late 1990). A further comparison of access-related admissions to other causes for hospital admission is illustrated in table 1-2. These data were obtained for hospital admissions from Oct. 1, 1990, through Dec. 31, 1990. Vascular-access–related complications accounted for 11.2% of all days hospitalized and 16.2% of all hospitalization episodes, thereby representing the most frequent discharge diagnosis by a wide margin.

Because access-related morbidity seems to have increased at about the same time (mid-1989) as EPO was introduced in dialysis units, further evaluation of this phenomenon was carried out. The time trend curves of access-related morbidity and the fraction of NMC patients treated with EPO for calendar quarters 1989 through 1990 are shown in figure 1-4. Although the curves appear to be correlated in time, such a finding does not necessarily indicate a cause-and-effect relationship. Hence, the data were further examined in an attempt to reveal an underlying dynamic that would imply cause and effect. Table 1-3 compares patients receiving EPO for at least three months to those patients who never received the drug between Aug. 1, 1989, and Aug. 1, 1990. In this statistical model, which evaluates patients more likely to be selected to receive the drug, it was found that those receiving EPO tended to be older, white, and nondiabetic; a substantially higher proportion were females. Among candidate renal diagnoses, a lesser fraction of patients with cystic renal disease received

Table 1-3. A Comparison of Patients Receiving EPO for at least Three Months to Patients Not Receiving EPO, Aug. 1, 1989 to Aug. 1, 1990

	EPO	No EPO	All patients	P*
Mean age	58.2	56.6		<.001
Median age	61.3	58.4		NA
% Female	53.0	42.5	47.9	<.001
% White	47.5	46.3	47.8	<.001
% Diabetic	32.8	34.8	34.2	<.001
Mean duration of dialysis (yr)	3.03	3.45		<.001
Median duration of dialysis (yr)	1.81	1.98		—
Diagnosis:				
Glomerulonephritis	11.1	12.2	11.8	NS
Pyelonephritis	0.9	1.3	1.1	NS
Cystic disease	2.9	5.9	4.4	<.001

*Multivariate logistic regression analysis
NA = not applicable
NS = not significant

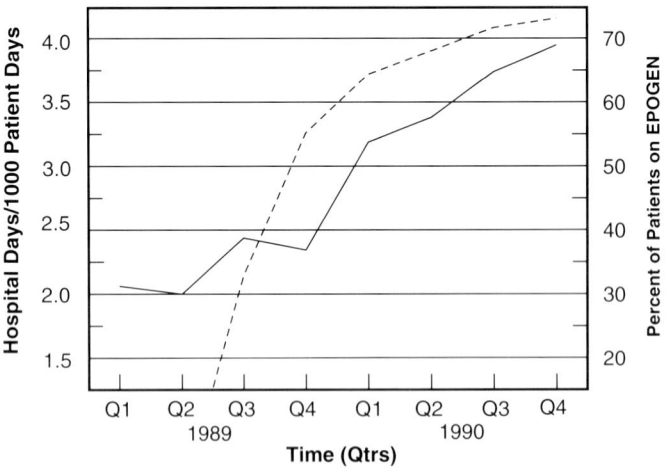

Figure 1-4. Time trend curve for the fraction of patients receiving EPO superimposed on the time trend curve for days hospitalized/1,000 days exposure.

EPO than would be expected by chance alone. This is not surprising, in view of the fact that patients with cystic disease are known to have higher hematocrits without treatment with EPO. Nothing in this analysis suggests a selection factor that would affect access clotting.

Further analyses were performed in a subset of 8,675 patients who had received EPO for at least two full months. Of these patients, 6,057 had received the drug for at least six months, and 1,260 had received it for at least a year. The cumulative distribution of the initial EPO dose factored by body weight in these patients is shown in figure 1-5. Fifty percent of patients received an initial

MORBIDITY OF HEMODIALYSIS PATIENTS   9

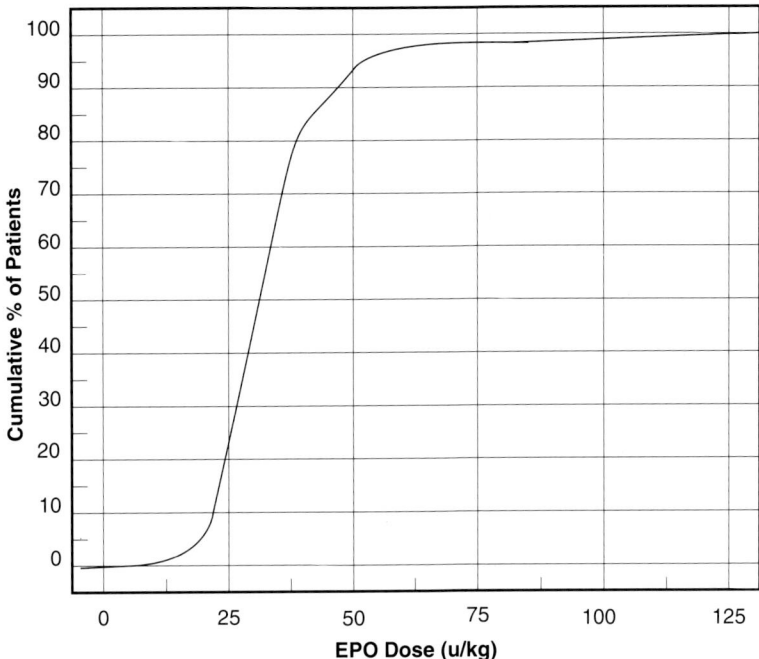

Figure 1-5. Cumulative frequency (%) curve of the initial EPO dose expressed as units per kilogram.

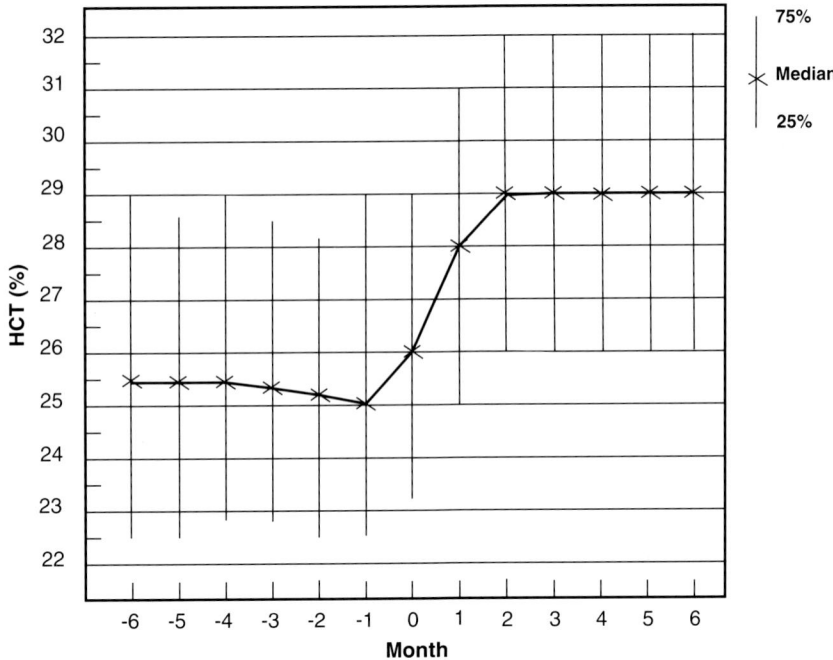

Figure 1-6. The distribution of hematocrit values in all patients before and during EPO therapy. The lower quartile, median, and upper quartile are shown.

Table 1-4. Predictors of Access-Related Hospitalization in Patients on EPO for at least Three Months and Six Months

| | 3 Months ||| 6 Months |||
Variable	β	X²	p	β	X²	p
Age	−0.001	0.1	NS	0.000	0.0	NS
Diabetes	−0.159	1.5	NS	−0.009	0.0	NS
Duration of dialysis	−0.056	7.0	.008	−0.049	7.2	.007
Pre-EPO hospitalization*	2.411	252.0	<.001	1.882	205.1	<.001
Dx = pyelonephritis	−0.560	0.8	NS	0.262	0.4	NS
Dx = cystic disease	−1.770	6.0	.014	−0.302	0.8	NS
Dx = glomerulonephritis	−0.467	4.1	.043	−0.354	3.3	0.071
Diastolic BP	−0.020	11.4	<.001	−0.008	2.7	0.100
Systolic BP	−0.001	0.2	NS	−0.004	1.8	NS
Pre-EPO Hct	0.033	5.0	.025	0.011	0.7	NS
Post-EPO Hct	−0.050	13.2	<.001	0.003	0.1	NS

*Hospitalization within three months (6,633 patients) or six months (5,331 patients) prior to EPO.

dose of about 32 U/kg, about 10% received an initial dose of 50 U/kg, and 25% of patients received an initial dose of 25 U/kg. Thus, these patients received relatively low initial doses. Despite this, a significant increase in hematocrit resulted. The response of hematocrit to EPO (six months before and six months after starting EPO) is shown in figure 1-6. The median hematocrit prior to EPO was 25.5% (lower and upper quartiles were 22% and 29%, respectively); it increased to a median of 29% (lower quartile was 26% and upper quartile was 32%). Figure 1-7 summarizes the transfusion requirements by month for all patients in this sample. Before EPO, the average transfusion for all patients was 0.35 U/patient/month. This was reduced to 0.08 U/patient/month after treatment. In an examination limited to those patients who required transfusions before EPO, this change is more dramatic, decreasing from 0.8 U/patient/month to 0.15 U/patient/month. It is apparent, therefore, that EPO had a significant effect on this large population of patients.

Table 1-4 presents a forward stepwise logistic regression analysis of predictors of hospitalization in patients treated with EPO at three months and at six months.

The β's are numerical estimates of the slope of each independent variable in the model. The slope answers the question: When X (hematocrit in this case) changes by one unit, how does Y (probability of hospitalization) change? The answer is that Y changes by β units. The sign of β indicates whether Y and X change in the same direction, in which case the sign would be positive, or in different directions, in which case the sign would be negative. X^2 (chi-square) is a measure of the relative importance among the independent variables. Large chi-squares have more predictive power in the model. By definition, larger chi-squares will have smaller p values.

Examination of this analysis reveals that age and presence of diabetes were not predictors of access-related hospitalization in this group of patients, at least within six months. Patients who had been on dialysis for longer periods (duration of dialysis) tended to have a lower probability of access-related hospitalization than did patients starting dialysis more recently ($P < 0.01$). Obser-

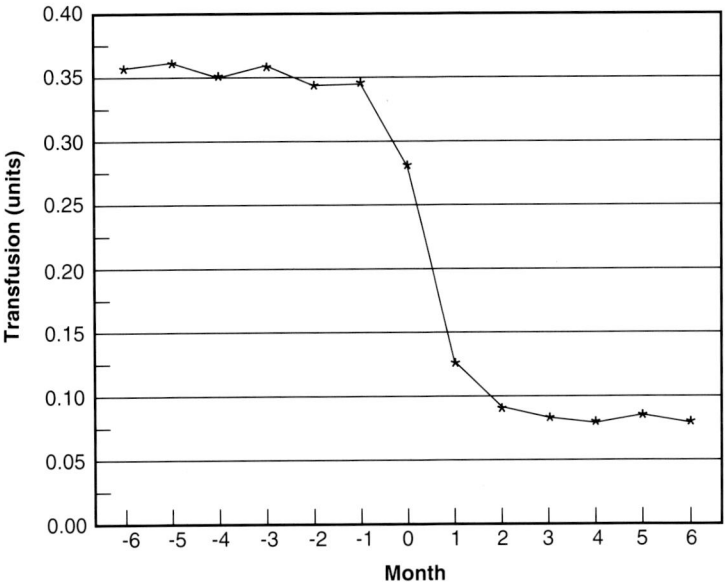

Figure 1-7. Average transfusion requirements are shown for each month before and after starting EPO therapy for all patients.

vation suggests a selection effect, whereby patients who had been on dialysis longer had better accesses, or learned to better care for their accesses. Patients with the renal diagnosis of cystic disease and glomerulonephritis had a lower probability of access-related hospitalization at three months but not at six months. An elevated diastolic pressure was more highly correlated with admission to the hospital in the group at three months, but this was not so at six months. Systolic blood pressure had no effect on the likelihood of access-related hospitalization before or after the use of EPO. There was a very strong correlation between the likelihood of hospitalization prior to the use of EPO and hospitalization after initiation of EPO. This suggests that patients with access problems that frequently required hospitalization continued to have such problems after EPO, whereas patients with few access problems before EPO continued to do well after use of the drug.

Treatment with EPO was *not* a significant predictor of access-related hospitalization among these patients. A higher pre-EPO hematocrit was predictive of access-related hospitalization at three months but not at six months. Low, not high (β is negative), hematocrit *after* the use of EPO was associated with a greater chance of access-related hospitalization at three months. Hematocrit was not predictive of hospitalization at six months. Therefore, there is substantial difficulty in singling out EPO as a cause of increased access-related hospitalization from these data. Eliminating the pre-EPO hematocrit as a control variable made no difference in the analysis. Neither did an analysis substituting the change of hematocrit for the actual hematocrit value. An analysis of the administered dose of EPO likewise showed no significant effect.

Examination of the platelet count and white blood cell count with a statistical analysis similar to that shown in table 1-4 revealed no predictive influence of either of these blood parameters in the three-month EPO-treated group; however, in the six-month group, higher platelet count was weakly associated (p = .034) with a greater probability of access-related hospitalization. Of all the analyses performed, this was the only one suggesting a possible association between EPO and access-related morbidity. In additon to the weak correlation, the analysis was in a small subgroup (only 1,477 of 5,331 patients had platelet counts performed). The role of EPO is suspect here, since the drug is associated with increased platelet adhesiveness, not increased platelet count. In conclusion, we could not demonstrate a relationship between EPO administration and the probability of access-related hospitalization.

Discussion

These data from some 15,000 to 26,000 patients dialyzed in out-of-hospital dialysis facilities over a five-year period reflect a recent and significant increase in the trend of hospitalizations for vascular access morbidity. As indicated earlier, this analysis does not consider those many patients who have access thrombosis and are managed as outpatients. Nonetheless, the data confirm the very significant problem of access-related hospitalizations, which are five to eight times more likely as a cause for hospitalization than other complications in dialysis patients.

Although the increase in hospitalizations for access-related mechanical problems (clotting and stenosis) appears to have occurred at the same time as the use of EPO, logistic regression analyses of the data could not demonstrate a cause-and-effect relationship between the use of EPO, dose of EPO, or level of post-EPO hematocrit and mechanical-access–related admissions. Coumadin and other antiplatelet agents have well-known effects on platelet function.[11-13] The use of such drugs was not examined in this population of patients. Because it is known that EPO has an effect on platelet adhesiveness, further studies should include measurement of platelet adhesion and should include an analysis of the role of antiplatelet agents in preventing a tendency to access clotting. The type of access (i.e., native vein versus polytetrafluoroethylene loop versus straight, upper arm versus lower arm) and a past history of access problems were not examined in this analysis. There might well be a subpopulation of patients with a particular type of access who are at increased risk.[14] Patients with a prior history of elevated venous pressure, increased recirculation, or prior surgery may be at increased risk with EPO therapy. Further analysis of such subgroups is warranted. However, in the overall population of patients on dialysis, at present there is no evidence to warrant modification of the use of EPO or to administer anticoagulant therapy with the drug. The increasing morbidity of access failure does, however, warrant new approaches to this problem. Such approaches are now being assessed.[14-19]

References

1. Lazarus JM, Hakim R. Medical aspects of hemodialysis. In: The kidney. 4th ed. Philadelphia: W.B. Saunders, 1991:2235.
2. Eschbach JW, Abdulhadi MH, Brown JK, et al. Recombinant human erythropoietin in anemic patients with end-stage renal disease. Ann Intern Med 1989; 111:992–1000.
3. Moia M, Vizzotto L, Cattaneo M. Improvement in the haemostatic defect of uraemia after treatment with recombinant human erythropoietin. Lancet Nov. 28, 1987; 1227–29.
4. Vigano G, Benigni A, et al. Recombinant human erythropoietin to correct uremic bleeding. Am J Kidney Dis 1991; 18(1):44–49.
5. Vaziri ND, Brown RP, Atkins K, et al. Effect of erythropoietin administration on blood and plasma viscosity in hemodialysis patients. Trans Am Soc Artif Intern Organs 1989; 35:505–08.
6. Besarab A, Medina F, Musial E, et al. Recombinant human erythropoietin does not increase clotting in vascular access. Trans Am Soc Artif Intern Organs 1990; 36: M749–M753.
7. Paganini EP, Latham D, Abdulhadi M. Practical considerations of recombinant human erythropoietin therapy. Am J Kidney Dis 1989; 14(2 suppl 1):19–25.
8. The GLM Procedure, SAS Institute. SAS user's guide statistics, version 5 ed., Cary, NC:SAS Institute, 1985.
9. Harrell FE. The logist procedure, SAS Institute. SUGI supplemental library user's guide, version 5 ed., Cary, NC: SAS Institute, 1986; 269–93.
10. Lowrie EG, Lew NL. Death risk in hemodialysis patients: the predictive value of commonly measured variables and an evaluation of death rate differences between facilities. Am J Kidney Dis 1990; 15(5):458–82.
11. Kaegi A, Pineo GF, Shimizu A, et al. Arteriovenous-shunt thrombosis: prevention by sulfinpyrazone. N Engl J Med 1974; 290:304–06.
12. Harter HR, Burch JW, Majerus PW, et al. Prevention of thrombosis in patients on hemodialysis by low-dose aspirin. N Engl J Med 1979; 301:577–79.
13. Williams WW. A patient with recurrent thrombosis in polytetrafluoroethylene dialysis grafts. Semin Dialysis 1990; 3:127–31.
14. Palder SB, Kirkman RL, Whittemore AD, et al. Vascular access for hemodialysis: patency rates and results of revision. Ann Surg 1985; 202(2):235–39.
15. Goldberg JP, Contiguglia R, Mishell JL, Klein MH. Intravenous streptokinase for thrombolysis of occluded arterviovenous access. Arch Intern Med 1985; 145:1405–08.
16. Schilling JJ, Eiser AR, Slifkin RF, et al. The role of thrombolysis in hemodialysis access occlusion. Am J Kidney Dis 1987; 10(2):92–97.
17. Schwab SJ, Saeed M, Sussman SK, et al. Transluminal angioplasty of venous stenosis in polytetrafluoroethylene vascular access grafts. Kidney Int 1987; 32:395–98.
18. Rittgers SE, Garcia-Valdez C, McCormick JT, Posner MP. Noninvasive blood flow measurement in expanded polytetrafluoroethylene grafts for hemodialysis access. J Vasc Surg 1986; 3:635–42.
19. Tordoir JHM, Hoeneveld H, Eikelboom BC, Kitslaar P. The correlation between clinical and duplex ultrasound parameters and the development of complications in arterio-venous fistulae for haemodialysis. Eur J Vasc Surg 1990; 4:179–84.

2

BIOLOGIC MEDIATORS OF INTIMAL HYPERPLASIA

Mark F. Fillinger, M.D., and D. Brent Kerns, M.D.

INTIMAL HYPERPLASIA HAS LONG BEEN RECOGNIZED as a common cause of vascular graft failure, especially in arteriovenous (A-V) grafts for hemodialysis access.[1-5] Although the hemodynamic aspects of this problem have been discussed since the first vascular grafts were placed,[6] information about the biologic mediators of intimal hyperplasia has come to the forefront only in the past two decades. More recently, there has been an explosion of literature in this field, primarily a result of advances in molecular biology and immunology. The tools used to study biologic phenomena have increased dramatically in terms of quality and quantity. As more is known about biologic mediators in the vascular system in general, it also appears that there is a surprising amount of overlap in research related to atherosclerosis, intimal hyperplasia, inflammation, immunology, and even oncology. Although the interactions appear increasingly complex, the "pieces of the puzzle" are coming together in a coherent fashion.

Theories regarding biologic mediators of intimal hyperplasia can be divided into three major categories: (1) injury response, (2) immune/inflammatory response, and (3) hemodynamic response. Each theory involves abnormal hemodynamics, mechanical stress, and cellular injury to some degree. In this chapter, we hope to provide a general overview of the proposed biologic responses initiated by these physical stimuli.

Before proceeding further in this discussion, however, one point should be clarified. Intimal hyperplasia and atherosclerosis are *not* one and the same lesion. Certainly, the two processes share many common features. The most important pathologic feature of both lesions is the predominance of smooth muscle cells (SMCs) among the various cellular components (figures 2-1, 2-2). Early stages of both lesions are characterized by the proliferation and migration of SMCs from the media toward the intima. In later stages, both lesions

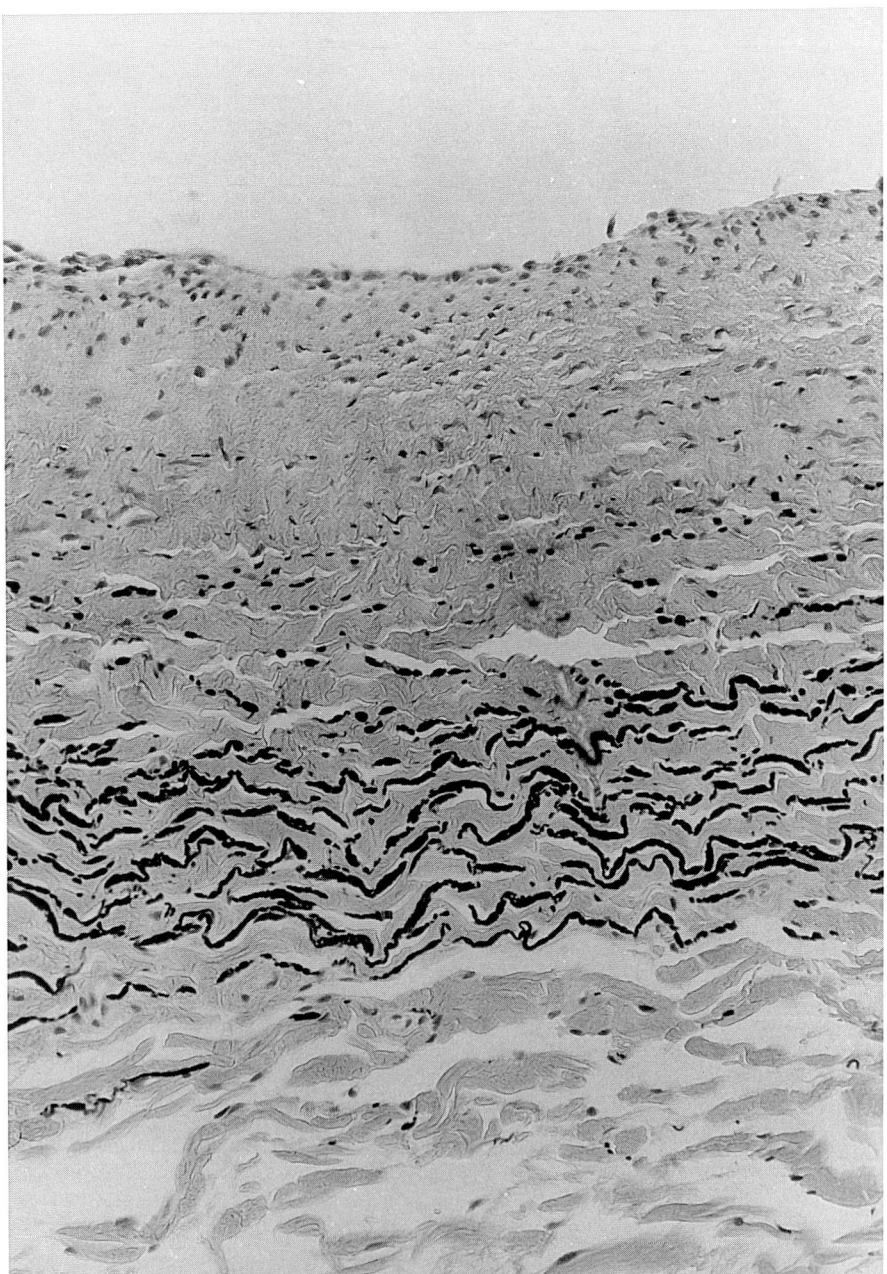

Figure 2-1. Representative histologic section of venous anastomotic hyperplasia in a canine arteriovenous graft model.

contain large quantities of extracellular matrix that further thicken the vascular wall (figures 2-1, 2-2). Atherosclerosis, however, is characterized by lipid droplets and large numbers of macrophages and T lymphocytes.[7-9] Intimal hyperplasia is also associated with lymphocytes and macrophages, but to a lesser extent.[10]

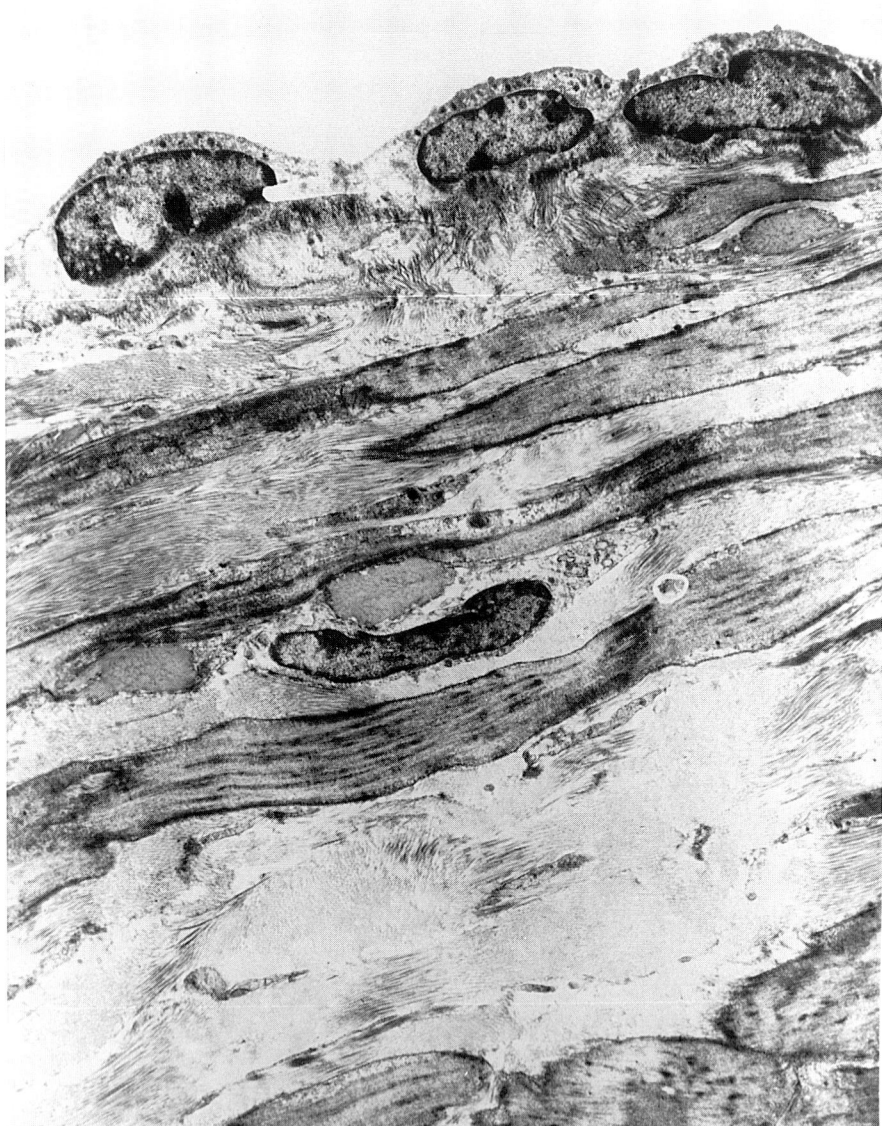

Figure 2-2. Representative transmission electron microcroscopy section from venous anastomotic hyperplasia in a canine arteriovenous graft model. Note intact endothelial cells (top), numerous large smooth muscle cells, and surrounding collagen/extracellular matrix.

Although many investigators have created models of intimal hyperplasia in an effort to study atherosclerosis, most of the literature is directed at the latter phenomenon. To be even more specific, there is much less information on the process of venous hyperplasia, which is most important in the failure of dialysis access grafts. In presenting this brief synopsis of the available data, we will attempt to include only that which seems most pertinent. Last, when discussing venous hyperplasia, it is more "pathologically correct" to describe the process as intimal-medial hyperplasia, since the demarcating internal elastic lamina is often poorly defined in the term *intimal hyperplasia* throughout this chapter.

The 'Response to Injury' Theory

Perhaps the most prominent theory regarding intimal hyperplasia and atherosclerosis, the "Injury Response" theory is based on two major points. First, SMC proliferation has been implicated in the development of both intimal hyperplasia and atherosclerosis.[11-14] Second, it was discovered in 1974 that platelet-derived growth factor (PDGF) is a potent smooth muscle cell mitogen.[15,16] Because intimal hyperplasia occurs after injury, the mechanism of SMC proliferation seems obvious. Similarly, advanced atherosclerotic plaques have areas of endothelial cell denudation and adherent thrombus. Unfortunately, it turns out that this theory was just the beginning of a trial that has been shown to be more complex (and more interesting) than anyone imagined.

The response to injury theory, as championed by Ross and a number of others,[8,11,14,17] has evolved greatly since 1974. Initially, the answers came easily. Injury leads to endothelial denudation, platelet adherence and aggregation, and release of the powerful SMC mitogen PDGF. PDGF then causes the characteristic SMC proliferation and migration associated with hyperplasia and atherosclerosis. An animal model in which a balloon catheter (or other instrument) is used to create an injury of the vascular endothelium will reproducibly result in intimal hyperplasia.[11,18-20] With this amount of information, the theory seems airtight. Unfortunately, further investigation reveals some flaws with this simple theory. It has been shown that a denuding injury to the endothelium associated with platelet adherence and thrombus formation is not sufficient to cause hyperplasia.[21,22] In addition, platelet adherence does not appear to be necessary for initiation of SMC replication.[23] It appears that in the balloon catheter injury model, deeper injury to the underlying vessel wall is necessary to reproduce hyperplastic lesions.[20,24,25] Animal models also have demonstrated that hyperplasia can occur under an intact endothelium,[22] and human models have failed to demonstrate evidence of platelet or thrombus accumulation within hyperplastic lesions.[10] In fact, neointimal hyperplasia within prosthetic grafts occurs only if there is an endothelial lining above the SMCs within the neointima.[12]

How can these various studies be reconciled? First of all, it is now known that PDGF is produced by endothelial cells (ECs) and macrophages (MOs) as well as by SMCs themselves.[26,27] Thus, the potential exists for ECs & MOs to stimulate SMCs in a paracrine fashion or for SMCs to stimulate themselves in an autocrine fashion. Second, it appears that PDGF is truly an important mediator in the process of hyperplasia. A monoclonal antibody to PDGF will blunt the hyperplastic response in an animal model but will not prevent it completely.[28] Interestingly, whereas PDGF stimulates both SMC proliferation and migration in tissue culture, the monoclonal antibody to PDGF inhibits only SMC migration.[28] Although one might question the efficacy of the antibody, it has also been shown that an infusion of PDGF (B chain homodimer, the most common form

Table 2-1. Partial List of Potential Biologic Mediators

Mediator	Source	Target	Role/action	References
PDGF	EC, SMC, MΦ, plts	SMC	↑ SMC migration, ↑ matrix turnover, ↑ PDGF Chemoattractant, leukocyte activation ↑ MHC II antigens, ↑ T cell proliferation, ↑ γ interferon	26, 103–106
bFGF	EC, SMC, MΦ	SMC	↑ SMC proliferation	30, 31, 100
TGFβ	Plts, SMC	SMC	↑ PDGF, ↑ migration, ↑ matrix production	106, 107
TGFα	MΦ	SMC	Enhance SMC/bFGF interaction	39, 40
HBEGF	MΦ, SMC	SMC	Increase SMC proliferation	108
Heparan sulfate	EC, SMC	SMC	Inhibit SMC proliferation	42, 109
Heparanase	MΦ, leukocytes, plts	matrix	Degrade extracellular atrix, allow cell prolif./migration	110, 111
tPA	SMC	SMC	Initiate cascade leading to matrix degradation, SMC prolif.	41, 85
Collagenase	SMC	SMC	Degrade extracellular matrix, allow SMC proliferation	85, 106, 112
Angiotensin II	MΦ, EC via ACE	SMC	Increase SMC proliferation	79, 80
Thrombin	Thrombus	EC	Increase PDGF production	113, 114
Thrombospondin	SMC	SMC	Increase PDGF, SMC mitogen	115
EGF	Plts	EC, SMC	EC, SMC mitogen	8, 116
TNFα	MΦ	SMC	Increase PDGF production	26, 39, 106, 117, 118

EC = endothelial cell; SMC = smooth muscle cell; MΦ = macrophage; plts = platelets; ACE = angiotensin-converting enzyme; ↑ = increase or enhance associated with platelets) is a very weak stimulant of SMC proliferation.[29] This points out that results from tissue culture do not necessarily apply in vivo. It also demonstrates that other mediators must be important in the development of intimal hyperplasia.

As can be seen in table 2-1, a number of potential biologic mediators have been added since the discovery of PDGF (and this is not an exhaustive list). Detailed discussion of each potentially important substance is beyond the scope of this chapter, but some examples are worth noting. One mediator that figures prominently in the injury theory is basic fibroblast growth factor (FGF or bFGF, to distinguish it from acidic FGF). Basic FGF can be produced by ECs, SMCs, and MOs (see table 2-1 references). Although there is no known mechanism by which ECs can secrete bFGF, it is released by these cells in response to injury.[30] Injury may also be an important mechanism in the production/release of FGF by SMCs.[31] It is known to be a potent SMC mitogen in vitro and in vivo,[30,32] and blocking its action with monoclonal antibody inhibits SMC proliferation in vivo.[33] Once again, however, monoclonal antibody to bFGF does not completely inhibit intimal thickening, as SMC migration and extracellular matrix production are not prevented.[33]

Because a large portion of intimal thickening is related to the production of extracellular matrix, any discussion of the injury theory would be incomplete without the inclusion of transforming growth factor beta (TGF_β). Produced by activated platelets and SMCs, this substance is known to increase SMC migration,[34] production of extracellular matrix,[35] and production of PDGF.[36] Curiously, TGF_β can stimulate or inhibit SMC proliferation,[37] suggesting an action that would enhance migration of SMCs to the site of an injury but aid in controlling proliferation upon arrival. SMCs in the "secretory" (as opposed to the "contractile") state are capable of proliferation or matrix production. Because both are likely to be important in healing a vascular injury, TFG_β may be an important mediator. In an arterial injury model, it appears that its primary role is to stimulate SMC proliferation and extracellular matrix production through an autocrine mechanism. In a similar role, transforming growth factor alpha (TGF_α) appears to enhance SMC proliferation via FGF.[39,40]

Now that we have covered potential mediators of SMC proliferation, migration, and extracellular matrix production, it might appear that all of the mediators for the process are covered. However, as can be seen in table 2-1, this is not the case. A number of potential mediators have been discovered with functions similar to those already outlined. Some, such as thrombin, thrombospondin, and tumor necrosis factor alpha (TNFα) are important in increasing local PDGF production from various sources. Others, such as heparin-binding endothelial cell growth factorlike growth factor (HBEGF), are powerful SMC mitogens in their own right. The importance of adding these mediators to the discussion is to demonstrate that there appears to be a great deal of redundancy "built into" the process, as one might expect for an injury response mechanism. Some of these complex interactions are demonstrated schematically in figure 2-3. Although monocytes are known to be part of the thrombus adhering to a vascular injury, the "cytokines" will be discussed along with the immune response theory. The vasoactive mediators and angiotensin II-related phenomena will also be discussed in another section.

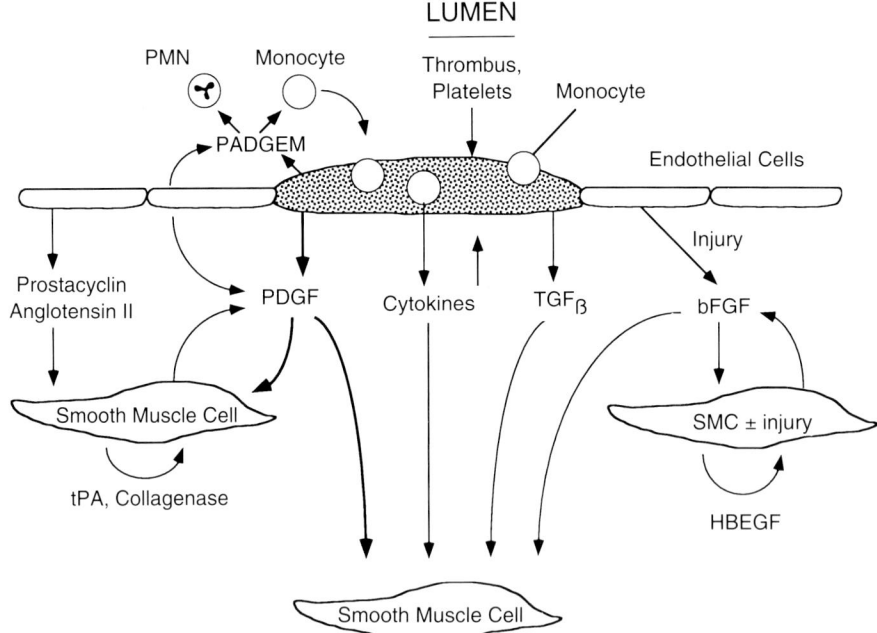

Figure 2-3. Schematic diagram illustrating some of the many potential interactions among biologic mediators in an injury model of initimal hyperplasia. See text and table 2-1.

One other class of mediators deserves mention at this point. Because the mechanism resulting in hyperplasia is so complex and redundant, and because the process revolves around the action of SMCs, perhaps attention should be focused on modifying the process at the SMC level. An important theory regarding hyperplasia is that in order for SMCs to proliferate or migrate, they must digest the extracellular matrix that surrounds them.[41] This theory, championed by Clowes,[41] has a great deal of supporting evidence. It appears that the extracellular matrix (including heparan sulfate) produced by ECs and SMCs can inhibit SMC proliferation and possible migration.[42] Tissue-type plasminogen activator (TPA) is produced by SMCs and is necessary to begin a cascade resulting in degradation of the extracellular matrix by plasmin and collagenase. It now appears that the inhibitory effect of heparin on SMC proliferation and migration is due to inhibition of TPA and collagenase.[43] Although heparin does not completely inhibit intimal hyperplasia, this avenue of research is obviously promising.

No matter how many mediators are added to the "injury" theory, a number of questions are left to be answered. Although platelet activity after a denuding injury is most intense in the first 48 hours, the hyperplastic process continues for a much longer period. In fact, the cells more likely to be associated with a chronic endothelial injury are leukocytes, as seen in figures 2-4A and 2-4B. Also, how does the lesion progress under an intact and apparently "healed" endothelium, or under an endothelium that has never had an overt mechanical injury? Why do cells characteristic of an immune response or "inflammatory

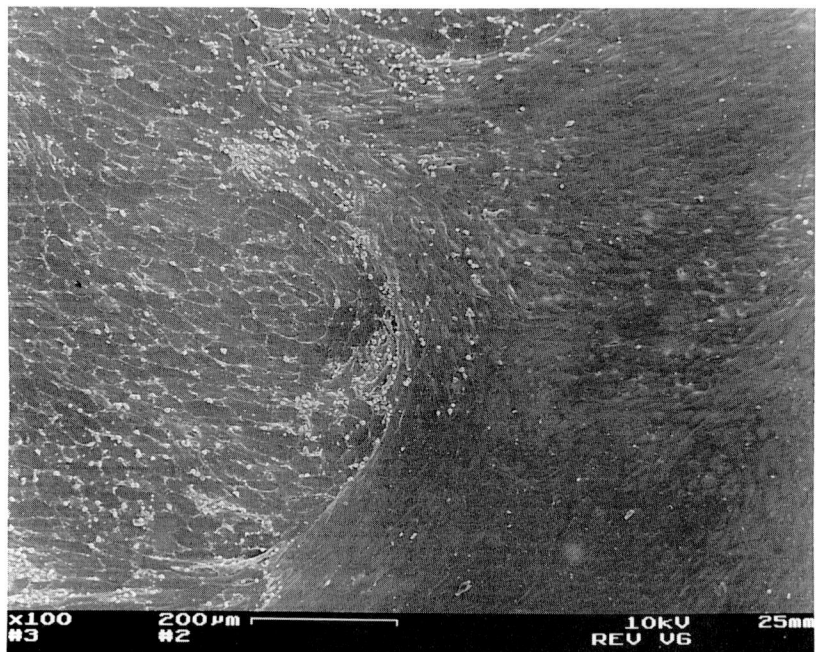

Figure 2-4 A. Demonstration of leukocyte attachment to a vein graft that lacks endothelial coverage four weeks after implant (rabbit arterial bypass model). **A**—Low magnification view demonstrates areas of intact and denuded endothelium.

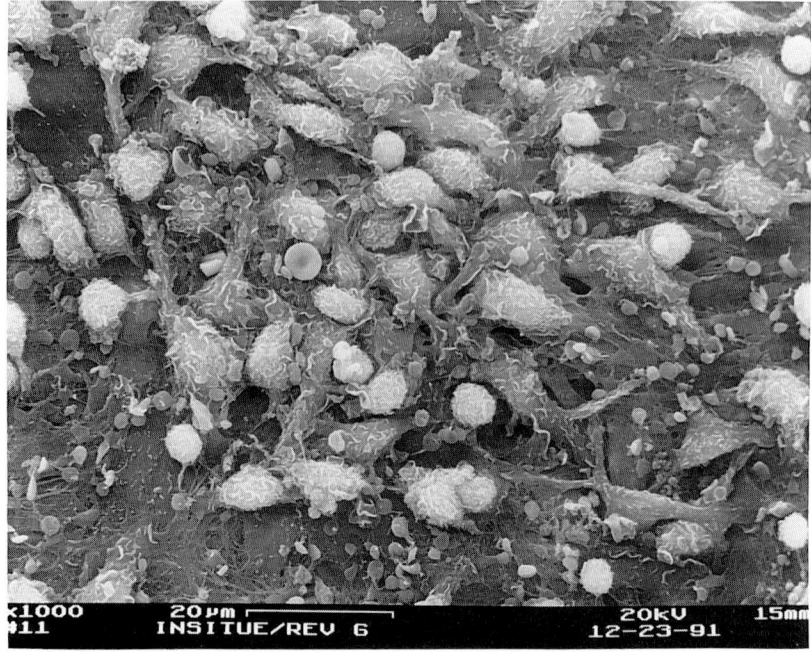

Figure 2-4 B. Higher magnification view reveals a high degree of leukocyte attachment and relatively little platelet aggregation.

mediators" infiltrate the lesion? Are the cytokines produced by these cells important to the lesions of hyperplasia or atherosclerosis? These questions are partially answered by a model that includes a chronic, nondenuding injury to the vascular wall. However, no theory is now complete without addressing the immune system, as recognized by Ross himself in his "update" on the injury theory.[8]

The 'Immune/Inflammatory Response' Theory

In many ways, the "immune response" theory is better expressed as an addendum or update of the injury theory. The processes resulting in hyperplasia clearly involve abnormal hemodynamics, mechanical stress, and cellular injury. However, these physical mediators of hyperplasia can initiate or promote a number of biologic responses that involve not only platelets, endothelial cells, and smooth muscle cells, but leukocytes as well.

It is easy to see why a denuding vascular injury will result in leukocyte adherence. To be complete, however, a proposed etiology of hyperplasia must include a mechanism by which the process can take place under an intact endothelium.[8,22,39,44] It is well known that leukocytes can penetrate an intact endothelial lining. In fact, it appears that it is their "job" to move through the vasculature, locally penetrate at the appropriate site, and migrate through tissue and into the lymphatic system for a return to the bloodstream.[44] Immunohistochemistry has helped demonstrate that atherosclerotic lesions contain a large number of macrophages and lymphocytes.[9] Although these cells are not as prevalent in intimal hyperplasia, they are nonetheless still present.[10] Because the macrophage is a prominent cell in early atherosclerotic lesions, a great deal of recent research revolves around monocytes and monocyte-derived macrophages. The study of cell adhesions phenomena involves how they get there and what controls the process.

Cell Adhesion Phenomena and the Immune Response

In a properly stimulated blood vessel, leukocytes, including monocytes and neutrophils, "roll" on the endothelial cell surface via reversible binding to a class of adhesion molecules known as selectins.[44,45] Rolling, which takes place through a rapid, reversible binding process, is illustrated schematically in figure 2-5A (although we illustrate the process for monocytes, the adhesion molecules involve other leukocytes as well—see table 2-2.)

Upon leukocyte activation by cytokines or chemoattractant peptides, another class of adhesion molecule on the leukocyte surface (an "integrin") is apparently responsible for causing the cell to stop rolling and "stick" to an immunoglobulin-class ligand (e.g., ICAM-1)[45] at a particular location (figure 2-5B). Once it has attached, the leukocyte migrates below the endothelial cell

BIOLOGIC MEDIATORS OF INTIMAL HYPERPLASIA   23

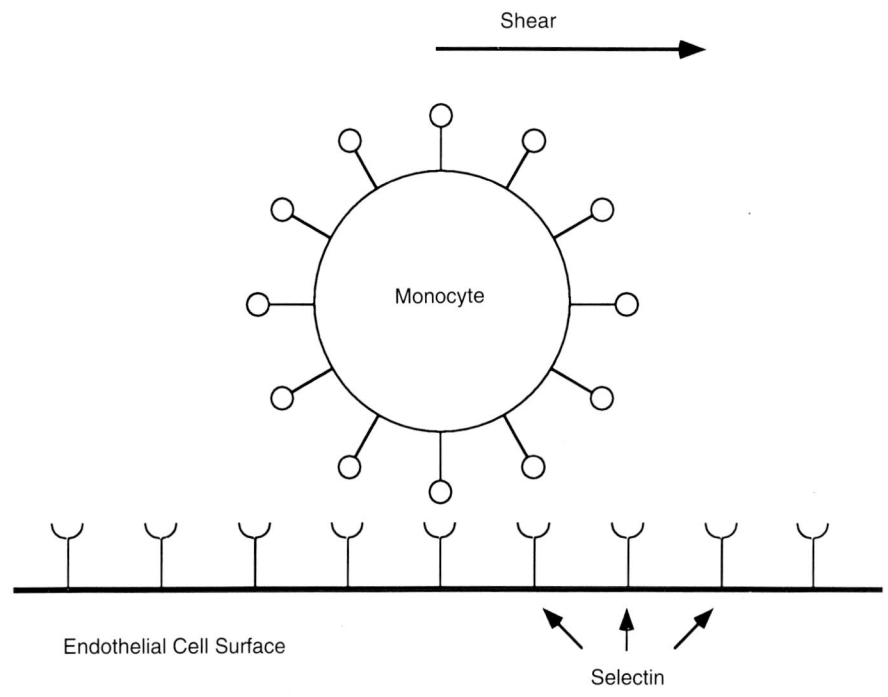

Figure 2-5 A. Schematic illustration of the cell adhesion molecules and their proposed roles (see text and table 2-2): "rolling."

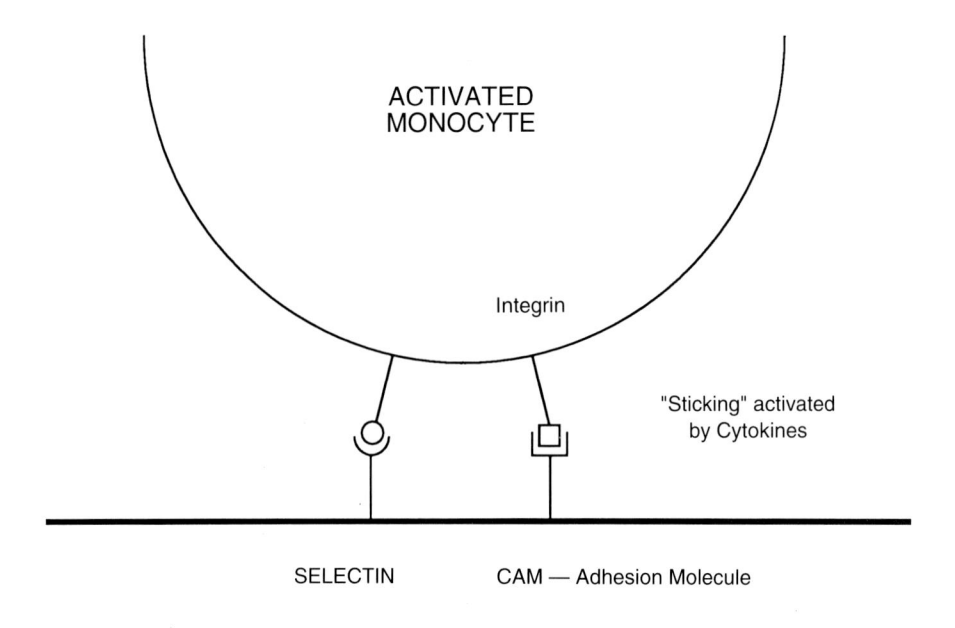

Figure 2-5 B. Schematic illustration of cell adhesion molecules and their proposed roles: "sticking."

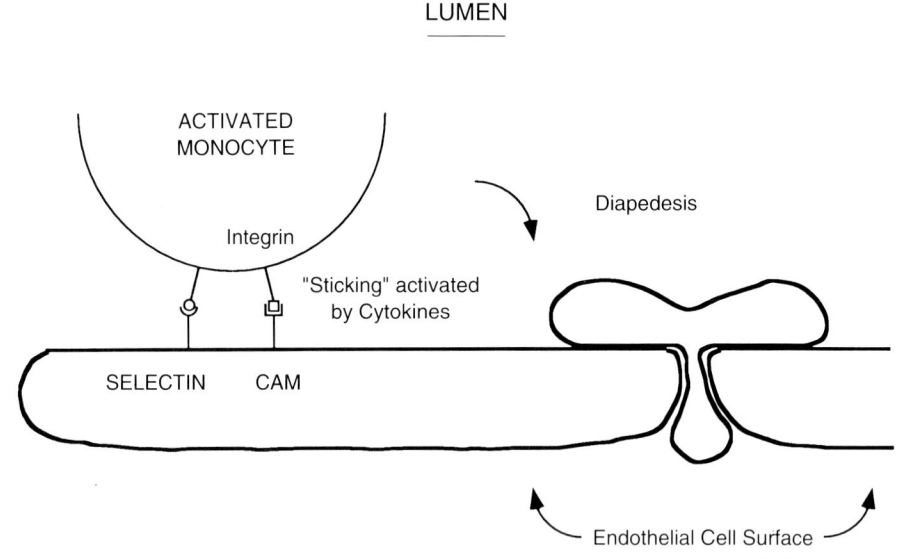

Figure 2-5 C. Schematic illustration of cell adhesion molecules and their proposed roles: diapedesis.

layer and into the evolving lesion (diapedesis, figure 2-5C). Monocytes become activated macrophages, secreting a whole host of biologically active substances that elicit responses from nearby ECs, cells, leukocytes, and SMCs (figure 2-6). These responses, outlined in table 2-3, include the migration and proliferation of SMCs, which leads to hyperplasia. Other responses include an increase in the expression of adhesion molecules and further stimulation of leukocytes (especially monocytes) at the endothelial cell surface. Thus the stimuli-response cycle can be self-perpetuating. In addition, the list of potential cytokine mediators and known responses in table 2-3 could easily be expanded to include almost all of the mediators listed in table 2-1.

As with the mediators in table 2-1, most known actions involve enhancement of the hyperplastic process, and a large amount of redundancy is apparent. Some mediators that have the capability to "down-regulate" the process, such as interleukin-8, also have the capability to up-regulate it. Although evidence suggests that only small numbers of T cells are present in these lesions,[10,46] it appears that the number is sufficient to have important effects.[39,46,47] Thus the balance that will ultimately control the process appears delicate.

Rather than describe the "cytokine" mediators in detail, we refer the interested reader to the references of tables 2-2 and 2-3. It is more important to discuss how the mediators of the immune response may function to promote hyperplasia without the occurrence of overt damage to the vascular wall. It appears that the function of selectins is twofold. First, the adhesive forces keep the "target cell" (the leukocyte) in close proximity to the vascular wall where the important chemoattractants are located. If the effect of chemoattractants at the site of injury were not highly localized, nonspecific adhesion and activation of leukocytes would occur at points remote from the injury. The mild, rapid, and reversible adhesions allow the leukocyte to "roll" slowly in response to local shear forces, which again makes it more likely to be affected by local

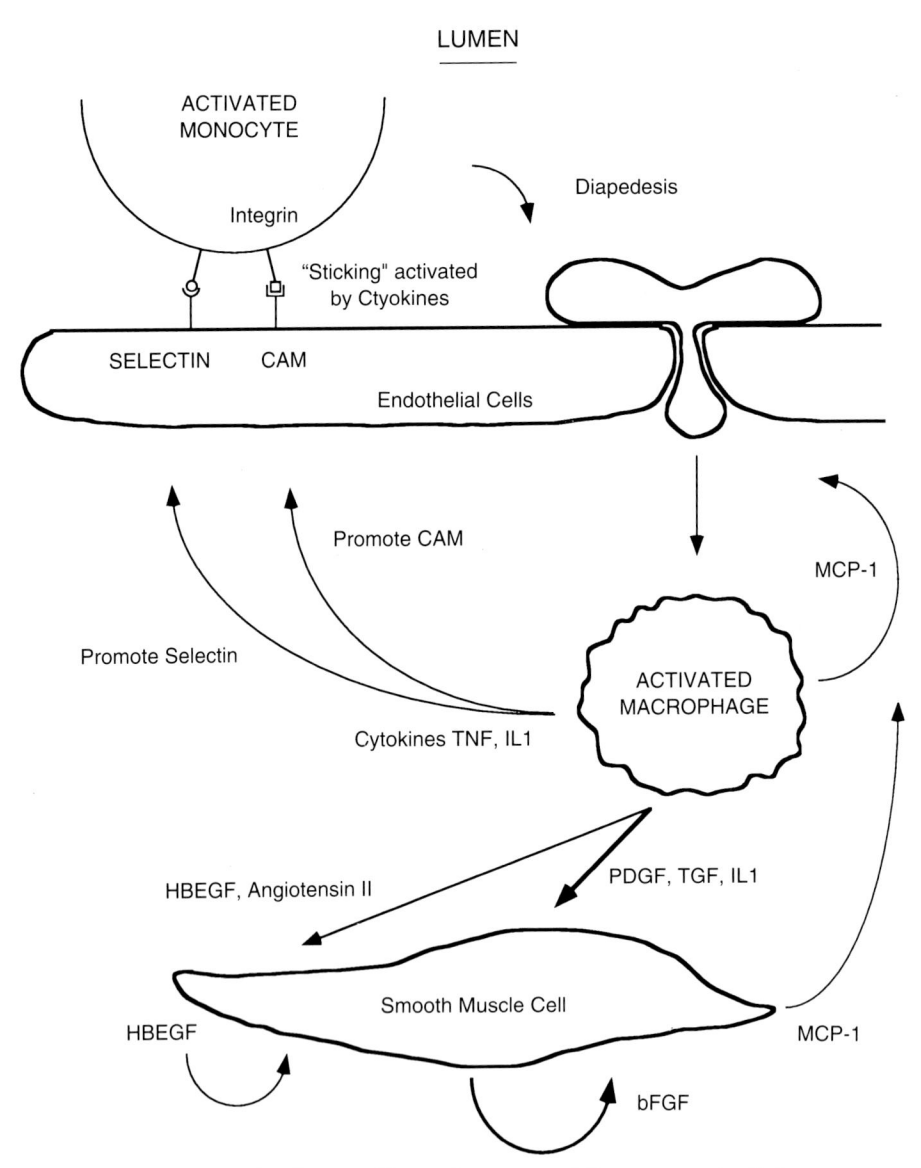

Figure 2-6. Schematic diagram illustrating some of the many potential interactions in an immune/inflammatory response model of intimal hyperplasia. See text and table 2-3.

chemoattractants. Because lower shear rates decrease rolling velocity (and therefore increase the potential for "sticking"), this may help explain the localization of hyperplasia and atherosclerosis to locations of low shear and boundary layer separation. With certain biologic stimuli, the adhesion molecules are expressed in greater density on the endothelial surface. This increased density also causes the leukocyte to roll more slowly and further facilitates activation and "sticking."[45,48,49] The much stronger adhesion associated with sticking also appears to have a role in diapedesis.[44,45,50]

Table 2-2. Mediators Associated with Cell Adhesion

Mediator	Source	Target	Stimulus—Action	References
Selectins				
ELAM-1	EC	Leuk	IL-1, TNF—increase leukocyte adherence to ECs	48, 119, 120
PADGEM	EC, plts	G, M	Thrombin—increases M,G adherence to ECs	45, 121
Athero-ELAM	EC	M	Cytokines, lipids—increase M adherence to ECs	122, 123
Integrins				
LFA-1	B, T, M, G	ICAM-1,2 (EC)	EC, leukocyte activation—"sticking" of B,T,M,G to ECs	45, 50, 124
Mac-1	M, G	Factor X, Fb	EC, leukocyte activation—"sticking" of M,G to ECs	45, 50, 124
p 150,95	M, G	?	EC, leukocyte activation—"sticking" of M,G to ECs	45, 50, 124
VLA-4/LPAM-1	B, T, M	VCAM-1 (EC), Fn	EC, leukocyte activation—"sticking" of B,T,M to ECs	50, 125–127
Ig class integrin ligands				
ICAM-1	EC	Leuk	EC, leukocyte activation—EC ligand for integrins	44, 50
ICAM-2	EC	Leuk	EC, leukocyte activation—EC ligand for integrins	44, 50
VCAM-1	EC	Leuk	EC, leukocyte activation—EC ligand for integrins	44, 50, 126

EC = endothelial cell; B = B lymphocyte; T = T lymphocyte; M = monocyte; G = granulocyte/PMN; Leuk = leukocyte; Fib = fibrinogen

Table 2-3. Biologic Mediators Associated with the Immune Response Theory

Mediator	Source	Target	Role/Action	References
Interleukin-1	EC, SMC, MΦ	All	Increase SMC proliferation, PDGF production	128, 129
			Increase IL-1, IL-6, IL-8, γ-IFN, TNFα, MCP-1	39, 130–132
			Increase leukocyte and EC adhesion	119, 133
			Increase cell surface coagulability	120
Interleukin-2	T cells (activated)	T, MΦ	Activates MΦ and T cells	134
Interleukin-6	EC, SMC, MΦ	T	Amplify, T, B cell activation, adhesion, infiltration	39, 135
Interleukin-8	EC, MΦ	G, ?M	Up- and down-regulation of leukocyte adhesion	136
Leukotriene B4	MΦ, M	Leuk	Chemoattractant, stimulates adhesion	137, 138
TNFα	MΦ	SMC	Increase PDGF production	119, 133
MCP-1	EC, SMC, MΦ	M	Chemoattraction, activation of monocytes	139, 140
Heat shock prot.	EC, SMC, MΦ	T cells	May act as an autoantigen	141, 142
TGFα	MΦ	SMC	Enhance SMC/bFGF interaction	143
PDGF	EC, SMC, MΦ, plts	SMC	See table 2-1	See table 2-1
HBEGF	MΦ, SMC	SMC	Increase SMC proliferation	108
Angiotensin II	MΦ, EC via ACE	SMC	Increase SMC proliferation	79, 80
Heparanase	MΦ, leuk, plts	matrix	Degrade extracellular matrix, allow cell prolif./migration	110, 111
Cell adhesion	EC, T	EC, T	See table 2-2	See table 2-2

Abbreviations are as noted in previous tables

Although this scenario is fascinating, one point must be emphasized. Normal endothelial cells do not express large numbers of cell adhesion molecules on their surface. Although several stimuli are capable of initiating or perpetuating the process (see tables 2-2 and 2-3), the "key" stimulus or stimuli remain unknown at this point. In atherosclerosis, it appears that mildly oxidized low-density lipoprotein results in the production of MCP-1, which could initiate the sequence illustrated above. Candidates for initiating the process in intimal hyperplasia include the production of MCP-1, TNF, HSP, or interleukin-1 (IL-1) as a result of stress of subacute injury.[39] ECs and SMCs are also capable of expressing class II MHC antigens on their surface.[39] This property can be induced by gamma interferon,[51] a product of T lymphocytes (which have been described in hyperplastic lesions from dialysis access grafts).[10] It is also interesting that IL-1 is a prominent component of the dialysate recovered from hemodialysis filters, probably secondary to activated leukocytes attached to the filters.[52] IL-1 has numerous properties that could help stimulate and perpetuate the hyperplastic process (table 2-3). The characteristic lesion of dialysis is unclear. This also brings up the matter of hemodynamic stimuli in intimal or intimal-medial hyperplasia.

The 'Hemodynamic Response' Theory

The processes resulting in hyperplasia have always been associated with abnormal hemodynamics, mechanical stress, and cellular injury.[17,24,53,56-70] Initially, investigators were unable to proceed beyond the study of physical processes, but recent advances have produced a large number of discoveries linking physical stimuli to biologic mediators. It has been demonstrated that hemodynamic stresses such as high shear stress and turbulence can result in cellular injury,[17] and it is known that cell injury can result in intimal hyperplasia. It is also known that abnormally low shear stress (as might be associated with disturbed flow and boundary layer separation) results in a characteristic thickening of the vascular wall.[71] As noted by Glagov and Zarins, this type of hyperplasia is sometimes an appropriate "adaptive" thickening of the vascular wall that may normalize shear stress.[61] Last, it has been shown that the degree of anastomotic turbulence and kinetic energy transfer is strongly correlated with venous anastomotic hyperplasia in a dialysis access graft model.[54,55] For these reasons, it seems important to include hemodynamic stimuli in any proposed theory regarding biologic mediators of intimal hyperplasia.

To reconcile the evidence presented thus far, it seems appropriate to discuss the potential scenarios for the interplay of hemodynamics and biologic mediators. The first scenario involves a simple alteration in shear stress. As shown in table 2-4, numerous biologic responses are associated with even a simple alteration in shear stress on the EC surface. Ion channels in ECs appear to act as sensors or transducers of physical forces such as shear stress and tensile stress.[72,73] Most of the mediators known for their vasoactive properties also promote or inhibit DNA synthesis in SMCs. It cannot be a coincidence that substances that

Table 2-4. Potential Mediators of a Hemodynamic Response

Mediator	Hemodynamic effect	Possible role of mediator	References
K⁺ channels	↑ shear → ↑ K⁺ current	Vasorelaxation	73, 144
Ca⁺⁺ channels	↑ stretch → ↑ Ca⁺⁺ flux	Vasoconstriction	72
PDGF	↑ shear → ↓ PDGF	Remodel vessel wall (SMCs)	145
Prostacyclin	↑ shear → ↑ prostacyclin	Vasoactive, SMC proliferation	74, 146
Endothelin	↑ shear → ↓ endothelin	Vasoactive, SMC proliferation	147
EDRF	↑ shear → ↑ EDRF	Vasoactive, SMC prolifration	148
VCAM-1	↑ shear → ↓ VCAM-1	Leukocyte adhesion	49
MCP-1	↑ shear → ↓ MCP-1	Activate and attract monocytes	49
tPA	↑ shear → ↓ tPA	SMC migration, proliferation	149, 150

↑ = "increased"; ↓ = "decreased"; → = "results in"

cause vasorelaxation, such as prostacyclin and endothelial-derived relaxing factor (EDRF), also inhibit SMC DNA synthesis,[74,76] whereas endothelin, a potent vasoconstrictor, promotes DNA synthesis in SMCs.[77] The dual role of these molecules seems clear. If there is an acute change in blood flow, an acute change in vessel diameter will help to normalize shear stress. If the change is chronic, the increase or decrease in SMC DNA synthesis will result in a more permanent remodeling of the vessel wall. A similar scenario was described by Langille and O'Donnell in a rabbit carotid model of reduced blood flow.[78]

Angiotensin II may function in a similar manner to the other vasoactive mediators, but in this case the mechanism of action includes a "twist." Vascular endothelial cells contain angiotensin converting enzyme (ACE), which converts angiotensin I to angiotensin II. SMCs are known to possess angiotensin II receptors, and the use of ACE inhibitors or an angiotensin II receptor blocker will blunt the hyperplastic process.[79,80] As noted in table 2-1, it also appears that macrophages are capable of producing angiotensin II,[79,80] so the biologic responses involving this potential mediator may be more complex than currently realized.

The simple alteration in the shear stress scenario is important, but our discussion of the potential interaction between hemodynamics and biologic mediators is still incomplete. As noted earlier, hemodynamic stresses such as abnormal shear and turbulence can result in cellular injury,[17] and this represents the other major hemodynamic scenario that may serve to induce hyperplasia. In contrast to an acute mechanical injury, the hemodynamic injury is likely to occur on a chronic basis.[53,61,81] As such, it may be more difficult to ameliorate by repair or remodeling of the vessel wall and therefore more likely to perpetuate the hyperplastic process.

It is easy to envision this scenario in dialysis access grafts. The extremely high flow rates of an A-V communication are desirable because they facilitate the process of hemodialysis and discourage thrombosis. Unfortunately, these flow rates are far beyond the normal physiologic range for vessels of the diameter commonly used for A-V grafts and fistulas. This combination results in extremely unstable flow, to the extent that luminal or anastomotic irregularities may create severe flow disturbances.[53] When these severe disturbances occur, kinetic energy transfer occurs,[54,55] an event that is essentially certain to create stress within the vascular wall, especially at areas of compliance mismatch that serve as "stress risers."[55] Depending on the level of stress created within the vascular wall, this could stimulate any number of biologic mediators (including those related to injury or immune response). This theory is consistent with the finding that areas of hyperplasia in a canine A-V graft model are associated with the presence of bFGF and activated macrophages that are not seen in nearby "normal" vessels (unpublished data). On another level, perianastomotic flow disturbances or boundary layer separation may be perceived as low shear by the venous endothelium, activating the vasoactive and cell adhesion mechanisms previously described (table 2-4). Interestingly, prostacyclin production appears to be suboptimal at the venous anastomosis of a canine A-V graft model (unpublished data).

From the above evidence, it appears that the cascade of events leading to hyperplasia is a response to stresses caused by trauma, hemodynamic abnormalities, or mechanical stimuli. The biologic response involves a complex and interconnected cascade of events that appears to be the cellular equivalent of a feedback control loop. The "goal" of the biologic responses is repair of the vessel and/or correction of the abnormal hemodynamic stress. If the biologic processes are unable to ameliorate these stresses by repairing or remodeling the vessel wall, the hyperplastic process will manifest itself. Hyperplasia or intimal-medial thickening is difficult to control because the biologic mechanisms are grounded in the cellular response to infection, trauma, and stress. Nonetheless, some means of intervention are possible.

Potential Areas of Intervention

Now that we have outlined the potential mediators of intimal hyperplasia, let us briefly review some of the studies directed at pharmacologic modulation of the process. To date, many avenues have been explored: anticoagulants, calcium channel blockers, ACE inhibitors, platelet inhibitors, modulators of the inflammatory and immunologic response, omega-3 fatty acids, and gene therapy. Unfortunately, the flaw that all possess is that the exact etiology of intimal hyperplasia remains unknown. However, with our current level of understanding, the complexity of the pathways leading to this lesion suggest that no one agent will be entirely effective in its elimination. In addition, little experimental work has focused specifically on the inhibition of anastomotic intimal hyperplasia in A-V graft models. As a result, we are left to study data on the pharmacologic manipulation of this lesion in a wide variety of arterial injury, endothelial denudation, bypass graft, atherosclerosis, and in vitro cell culture models in several different species. It is important to note that effective therapies in one model may not be effective in other models or in humans. The following discussion will attempt to formulate recent experimental work into a useful review.

Of all the potential pharmacologic modulators of intimal hyperplasia, heparin has been the most extensively studied. Heparan sulfate is the predominant subendothelial matrix and basement membrane glycosaminoglycan found in the vasculature. Heparin is closely related to heparan sulfate and is a well known inhibitor of SMC mitogenesis and extracellular matrix production in vivo.[82,84] As noted earlier, it has been suggested that the extracellular matrix serves to maintain the vascular wall SMC in a quiescent state and that heparin may inhibit matrix degradation. Clowes et al have demonstrated that intimal hyperplasia can be reduced (but not prevented) following heparin treatment in a rat carotid balloon injury model.[11] The effect persists even when heparin is given as late as 18 hours after injury and is independent of the anticoagulant function of the molecule. The true mechanism of heparin's effect on intimal hyperplasia is unknown, but it is probably related to inhibition of matrix degradation (via TPA).[41,85] Heparin also affects SMC responsiveness to heparin-binding endothelial cell growth factorlike growth factor (HBEGF) mitogens.[84]

Heparin seems to be less effective in suppressing intimal hyperplasia in models where the injury to the vessel wall is less extensive, and EC regeneration and confluence proceed rapidly.[86] Likewise, several groups have demonstrated that heparin has been unsuccessful in inhibiting intimal hyperplasia formation in vein graft models of intimal hyperplasia.[87,88] Postulated reasons for the differences between models include differing nature of injury,[89] populations of arterial and venous SMCs with inherently different susceptibilities to heparin,[88] and the predominance of hemodynamic factors in the formation of hyperplasia in arterialized vein graft models.[70] The ability of heparin to suppress intimal hyperplasia in A-V grafts has not been studied, but if the foregoing suppositions are borne out and hemodynamic stimuli predominate in this setting, then heparin might be ineffective. Obviously, hemodialysis patients receive large quantities of heparin during routine dialysis but continue to be plagued by graft loss from intimal hyperplasia. This could be related to the intermittent administration (dosing) of heparin in dialysis patients, an unrelated stimulus from dialysis (such as IL-1), or the ineffectiveness of heparin in this setting. Nevertheless, heparin possesses significant inhibitory properties and merits continued study.

Another promising avenue for further study includes the ACE inhibitors. Angiotensin II has been demonstrated to stimulate SMC proliferation both in vitro and in vivo.[79,90] Daemen et al. also have shown that neointimal SMCs were more responsive to angiotensin II than were SMCs in the underlying media or SMCs of normal artery.[90] The mechanism of this proliferation is unknown, but recent work has demonstrated reduction of intimal hyperplasia in a rat balloon injury model with the use of cilazapril (a long-acting ACE inhibitor) and with dup 753, an angiotensin II receptor antagonist. Clinical trials are now exploring the efficacy of ACE inhibitors in the inhibition of intimal hyperplasia in coronary angioplasty patients. Although ACE inhibitors are not completely effective in preventing intimal hyperplasia, it appears that they produce an additive inhibitory effect when given in conjunction with heparin.[85]

Another major avenue of research has concentrated on platelet-SMC interactions. The original "response to injury" hypothesis of intimal hyperplasia stimulated a number of clinical and experimental studies that attempted to prevent the formation of this lesion via platelet inhibition. Unfortunately, inhibition of platelet function has been largely unsuccessful when examined in clinical trials of coronary angioplasty and peripheral arterial bypass. These clinical findings agree with experimental work done by Clowes et al. in which a modest reduction in intimal hyperplasia was observed following antiplatelet antibody-induced thrombocytopenia in a rat carotid balloon injury model.[23] The reasons for this remain obscure but may be related to the fact that these agents block platelet aggregation but not adherence, or the fact that platelet aggregation and granule release proceeds via thromboxane-independent pathways in vivo.[91]

As noted previously, several models have demonstrated that SMC proliferation in animal injury models continues long after the overlying endothelium has been regenerated and the stimulus for platelet activation no longer exists.[92] Clinical trials of aortocoronary bypass have demonstrated modest improvement in one-year graft patency from 80% to 90% in patients treated with antiplatelet agent.[93] However, this may be secondary to a reduction in acute thrombosis rather than a reduction in intimal hyperplasia. With these considerations in mind, it seems unlikely that agents that attempt to block platelet adherence, aggregation, and growth factor release will significantly alter the formation of intimal hyperplasia in the clinical setting. Similarly, results from experimental models suggest that calcium channel blockade will significantly reduce intimal hyperplasia formation. Again, however, laboratory successes have not translated into lower re-stenosis rates following coronary angioplasty clinically.[94]

Attempts at pharmacologically reducing the intimal hyperplastic response have also included fish oils (omega-3 fatty acids). Fish oils are long-chain unsaturated fatty acids found in high concentrations in certain species. Research interest was generated when epidemiologic studies of Inuits, whose diet contains large quantities of these fatty acids, were noted to have a low prevalence of atherosclerosis.[95] Arterial injury and vein bypass models have demonstrated a reduction in intimal hyperplasia in animals fed omega-3 fatty acids. Proposed mechanisms for this include decreased platelet aggregation, decreased platelet counts, decreased thromboxane A_2, inhibition of leukotriene B4 production in monocytes, and altered serum lipid profiles.[96,97] Unfortunately, clinical trials in coronary angioplasty patients have shown mixed results, and conclusions about the efficacy of fish oils are difficult to formulate.

Another interesting avenue for the pharmacologic modulation of intimal hyperplasia targets the host's immune system and the immunologic response to vascular injury. Colburn et al. have demonstrated the dose-related suppression of intimal hyperplasia by dexamethasone in a rabbit carotid balloon injury model.[98] Mechanisms for this phenomenon are unknown but might include inhibition of SMC proliferation, prevention of leukocyte adhesion and migration, prevention of leukocyte cytokine production or release, and interruption of cellular messenger signals.[98] The vascular effects of the immunospecific agent cyclosporine A (which blocks interleukin-2–mediated T helper lymphocyte proliferation) are currently under investigation. Ferns et al. found that cyclosporine A inhibited arterial SMC proliferation in vitro, but was associated with increased intimal thickening in a rabbit carotid balloon model.[99] This result may be related to a toxic effect on SMCs.

Delineation of novel injury-mediated and inflammatory cell pathways is progressing at feverish pitch. The role leukocytes play in the initiation and propagation of intimal hyperplasia is a case in point. The discovery of new classes of cellular adhesion molecules continues,[50] and newly refined monoclonal antibody techniques will provide access to an array of very specific targets. Some interesting applications of monoclonal antibodies have also taken place on other fronts. A large number of growth factors have been identified as smooth muscle mitogens in vitro, but until recently, conclusive proof that they play a role in the formation of intimal hyperplasia has been lacking. Linder et al. have made great strides in the study of basic fibroblast growth factor (an SMC mitogen released by injured smooth muscle cells).[33,100] They have demonstrated that proliferation (but not migration) of SMCs is inhibited by a monoclonal antibody against basic fibroblast growth factor in a rat carotid balloon injury model.[32,33] Although this intervention does not prevent intimal thickening, it provides a key piece of data in the effort to understand the pathogenesis of intimal hyperplasia. As noted previously, similar efforts regarding monoclonal antibodies to PDGF have also been informative, but are not ready for clinical application.

Genetic therapy also has enormous potential and may play a future role in the prevention/modulation of intimal hyperplasia. The description of this technique is beyond the scope of this text, but in brief, segments of DNA can be altered, introduced into balloon-occluded arterial segment, incorporated by the ECs, and expressed in a living animal.[101] Technical constraints still limit this tool, but it is hoped that these will be worked out. Interesting preliminary data are already being produced by Nabel and co-workers regarding the effects of PDGF, FGF, and TGF in vivo.

As noted earlier, caution must be used when reviewing the literature on intimal hyperplasia. Results from tissue culture do not necessarily apply in vivo. Similarly, whereas many of the mediators and "modulators" discussed in this chapter are highly conserved from one species to another, any promising research from animal models must be applied to humans before its true impact is known. Unfortunately, the complexity of the process requires all methods (tissue culture, animal models, and human trials) if there is to be any hope of solving the problem.

Hemodynamic Intervention

Obviously, if the biologic process is related to hemodynamic stimuli, the ideal solution would be to create a less "stressful" hemodynamic environment. Unfortunately, the hemodynamic stimuli associated with intimal hyperplasia are nearly as complex as the biologic response. The "key" stimulus is unknown. Although there are many potential hemodynamic stimuli,[17,24,53,57,58,60,64,68-70] it appears that anastomotic turbulence and kinetic energy transfer are strongly and reproducibly associated with intimal hyperplasia in A-V grafts.[54,55] In our animal models, increased flow leads to increased turbulence, kinetic energy loss, and venous hyperplasia. Unfortunately, decreased flow leads to thrombosis and may prevent high-flux dialysis. Thus, there is a delicate balance, just as with biologic mediators. The question is whether it is possible to achieve sufficient flow to permit dialysis and discourage thrombosis without causing venous hyperplasia. Thrombosis is more likely when flow rates are <400 cc/min,[102] and detectable energy loss (which leads to hyperplasia) occurs at flow rates of >400 cc/min (unpublished data). This leaves little or no room for error, especially if one is intentionally creating a critical graft stenosis with banding.[53] A tapered graft configuration may help, but the initial model chosen to test this hypothesis used 6 mm diameter veins and flow rates of 900 cc/min.[54] It is not clear if these results can be extrapolated to lower flow rates or other vessel geometries. It seems, then, that hemodynamic intervention is no closer to the "magic bullet" than is biologic intervention.

Summary

The cascade of events leading to hyperplasia is a response to physical stresses resulting from trauma, hemodynamic abnormalities, or mechanical stimuli. The biologic response involves a complex and interconnected series of events that appears to be the cellular equivalent of a feedback control loop. If the biologic response is unable to ameliorate the abnormal stresses by repairing or remodeling the vessel wall, the hyperplastic process will continue. Hyperplasia, or intimal-medial thickening, is difficult to control because the biologic mediators are grounded in the cellular response to stress, trauma, and infection. There is evidence that the biologic response may be blunted via pharmacology, molecular biology, or genetic therapy, but any conclusions are difficult because of the redundant mechanisms involved. Developing a means to completely inhibit the process may not be possible or even desirable because the mediators are important for appropriate wound healing. Intervening at the hemodynamic level would be ideal, but the anatomic and hemodynamic requirements of dialysis access grafts make a universal solution difficult to achieve. Until methods of intervention improve, hyperplasia will remain a difficult problem and a major cause of graft failure.

References

1. Imparato AM, Bracco A, Kim GE, Zeff R. Intimal and neointimal fibrous proliferation causing failure of arterial reconstructions. Surgery 1972;72:1007-17.
2. Palder SB, Kirkman RL, Whittemore AD, Hakim RM, Lazarus JM, Tinley NL. Vascular access for hemodialysis. Ann Surg 1986;202:235-39.

3. Bell DD, Rosenthal JJ. Arteriovenous graft life in chronic hemodialysis. Arch Surg 1988;123:1169-1172.
4. Hurt AV, Batello-Cruz MB, Skipper BJ, et al. Bovine carotid artery heterografts versus polytetrafluoroethylene grafts. Am J Surg 1983;146:844-47.
5. Tellis VA, Kohlberg W, Bhat DJ, et al. Expanded polytetrafluorethylene graft fistulas for chronic hemodialysis. Ann Surg 1980;189:101-05.
6. Carrel A, Guthrie C. Results of the biterminal transplantation of veins. Am J Med Sci 1906;132:415-22.
7. Gown AM, Tsukada T, Ross R. Human atherosclerosis: II. Immunocytochemical and biochemical characterization. Am J Pathol 1986;126:51-60.
8. Ross R. The pathogenesis of atherosclerosis—an update. N Engl J Med 1986;314:488-500.
9. Jonasson L, Holm J, Skalli O, Bonders G, Hansson GK. Regional accumulations of T cells, macrophages, and smooth muscle cells in the human atherosclerotic plaque. Arteriosclerosis 1986;6:131.
10. Swedberg SH, Brown BG, Sigley R, Wight TN, Gordon D, Nicholls SC. Intimal fibromuscular hyperplasia at the venous anastomosis of PTFE grafts in hemodialysis patients. Circulation 1989;80:1726-36.
11. Clowes AW, Clowes MM. Kinetics of cellular proliferation after arterial injury. IV. Heparin inhibits rat smooth muscle mitogenesis and migration. Circ Res 1984;58:839-45.
12. Clowes AW, Reidy MA. Mechanisms of arterial graft failure: the role of cellular proliferation. Ann N Y Acad Sci 1987;516:673-678.
13. Ross R, Glomset JA. Atherosclerosis and the arterial smooth muscle cell. Science 1973;180:1332-9.
14. Ross R, Glomset JA. The pathogenesis of atherosclerosis. N Engl J Med 1976;295:369-77.
15. Kohler N, Lipton A. Platelets as a source of fibroblast growth-promoting activity. Exp Cell Res 1974;87:297-301.
16. Ross R, Glomset JA, Kariya B, Harker L. A platelet-dependent serum factor that stimulates the proliferation of arterial smooth muscle cells in vitro. Proc Natl Acad Sci USA 1974;71:1207-10.
17. Fry DL. Acute vascular endothelial changes associated with increased blood velocity gradients. Circ Res 1968;22:165-97.
18. Stemerman MB, Ross R. Experimental arteriosclerosis. I. Fibrous plaque formation in primates, an electron microscope study. J Exp Med 1972;136:769.
19. Bjorkerud S, Bondjers G. Arterial repair and atherosclerosis after mechanical injury. Part 2. Tissue response after induction of a total local necrosis (deep longitudinal injury). Atherosclerosis 1971;14:259.
20. Clowes AW, Clowes MM, Fingerle J, Reidy MA. Kinetics of cellular proliferation after arterial injury. V. Role of acute distension in the induction of smooth muscle proliferation. Lab Invest 1989;60:360-364.
21. Reidy MA, Silver M. Endothelial regeneration. VII. Lack of intimal proliferation after defined injury to rat aorta. Am J Pathol 1985;118:173.
22. Schwartz SM, Reidy MA. Common mechanisms of proliferation of smooth muscle in atherosclerosis and hypertension. Hum Pathol 1987;18:240-247.
23. Fingerle J, Johnson R, Clowes AW, Majeski MW, Reidy MA. Role of platelets in smooth muscle cell proliferation and migration after vascular injury in rat carotid artery. Proc Natl Acad Sci USA 1989;86:8412-16.
24. Clowes AW, Reidy MA, Clowes MM. Mechanisms of stenosis after arterial injury. Lab Invest 1983;49:208-15.
25. Fingerle J, Au YPT, Clowes AW, Reidy MA. Intimal lesion formation in rat carotid arteries after endothelial denudation in the absence of medial injury. Arteriosclerosis 1990;10:1082-87.
26. Ross R, Masuda J, Raines EW. Cellular interactions, growth factors, and smooth muscle proliferation in atherogenesis. Ann N Y Acad Sci 1990;598:102-12.
27. Birinyi LK, Warner SJ, Salomon RN, Callow AD, Libby P. Observations on human smooth muscle cell cultures from hyperplastic lesions of prosthetic bypass grafts: production of a platelet-derived growth factor-like mitogen and expression of a gene for a platelet-derived growth factor receptor—a preliminary study. J Vasc Surg 1989;10:157-65.

28. Ferns GA, Raines EW, Sprugel KH, Motani AS, Reidy MA, Ross R. Inhibition of neointimal smooth muscle accumulation after angioplasty by an antibody to PDGF. Science 1991;253:1129–32.
29. Jawien A, Lindner V, Bowen-Pope DF, Schwartz SM, Reidy MA, Clowes AW. Platelet-derived growth factor (PDGF) stimulates arterial smooth muscle cell proliferation in vivo. FASEB J 1990;4:342.
30. McNeil PL, Muthukrishnan L, Warder E, D'Amore PA. Growth factors are released by mechanically wounded endothelial cells. J Cell Biol 1989;109:811–22.
31. Edelman ER, Nugent MA, Smith LT, Karnovsky MJ. Basic fibroblast growth factor enhances the coupling of intimal hyperplasia and proliferation of vasa vasorum in injured rat arteries. J Clin Invest 1992;89:465–73.
32. Lindner V, Lappi DA, Baird A, Majack RA, Reidy MA. Role of basic fibroblast growth factor in vascular lesion formation. Circ Res 1991;68:106–13.
33. Lindner V, Reidy MA. Proliferation of smooth muscle cells after vascular injury is inhibited by an antibody against basic fibroblast growth factor. Proc Natl Acad Sci USA 1991;88:3739–43.
34. Bell L, Madri JA. Effect of platelet factors on migration of cultured bovine aortic endothelial and smooth muscle cells. Circ Res 1989;65:1057–65.
35. Chen JK, Hoshi H, McKeehan WL. Transforming growth factor type-β specifically stimulates synthesis of proteoglycan in human adult arterial smooth muscle cells. Proc Natl Acad Sci USA 1987;84:5287–91.
36. Majack RA, Majesky MW, Goodman LV. Role of PDGF-A expression in the control of vascular smooth muscle cell growth by transforming growth factor-β. J Cell Biol 1990;111:239–47.
37. Battegay EJ, Raines EW, Seifert RA, Bowen-Pope DF, Ross R. TGF-beta induces bimodal proliferation of connective tissue cells via complex control of an autocrine PDGF loop. Cell 1990;63:515–24.
38. Majesky NW, Lindner V, Twardzik DR, Schwartz SM, Reidy MA. Production of transforming growth factor beta 1 during repair of arterial injury. J Clin Invest 1991;88:904–10.
39. Libby P, Hansson GK. Involvement of the immune system in human atherogenesis: current knowledge and unanswered questions. Lab Invest 1991;64:5–15.
40. Madtes DK, Malden LT, Raines EW, Ross R. Induction of transcription and secretion of TGF-alpha by activated human monocytes. Chest 1991;99:79S.
41. Clowes AW, Clowes MM, Au YP, Reidy MA, Belin D. Smooth muscle cells express urokinase during mitogenesis and tissue-type plasminogen activator during migration in injured rat carotid artery. Circ Res 1990;67:61–67.
42. Fritze LMS, Reilly CF, Rosenberg RD. An antiproliferative heparan species produced by postconfluent smooth muscle cells. J Cell Biol 1985;100:1041–9.
43. Au YPT, Clowes AW. Effect of heparin on interstitial collagenase and tissue plasminogen activator expression. J Cell Biol 1990;111:234.
44. Springer TA. The sensation and regulation of interactions with the extracellular environment: the cell biology of lymphocyte adhesion receptors. Annu Rev Cell Biol 1990;6:359–402.
45. Lawrence MB, Springer TA. Leukocytes roll on a selectin at physiologic flow rates: distinction from and prerequisite for adhesion through integrins. Cell 1991;65:859–73.
46. Ferns GA, Reidy MA, Ross R. Balloon catheter de-endothelialization of the nude rat carotid. Response to injury in the absence of functional T lymphocytes. Am J Pathol 1991;138:1045–57.
47. Hansson GK, Jonasson L, Holm J, Cowes MM, Clowes AW. Gamma-interferon regulates vascular smooth muscle proliferation and Ia antigen expression in vivo and in vitro. Cir Res 1988;63:712–19.
48. Gimbrone MA Jr, Bevilacqua MP, Cybulsky MI. Endothelial-dependent mechanisms of leukocyte adhesion in inflammation and atherosclerosis. Ann N Y Acad Sci 1990;598:77–85.
49. Sprague EA, Cayatte AJ, Nerem RM, Schwartz CJ. Time-dependent shear stress modulation of platelet and monocyte adherence to cultured bovine aortic endothelial cells. In: Norman J, ed. Cardiovascular science and technology: basic & applied: II. Louisville: Oxymoron Press, 1990:125–28.
50. Springer TA. Adhesion receptors of the immune system. Nature 1990;346:425–34.
51. Warner SJ, Friedman GB, Libby P. Regulation of major histocompatibility gene expression in human vascular smooth muscle cells. Arteriosclerosis 1989;9:279–88.
52. Port FK, VanDeKerkhove KM, Kunkel SL, Kluger MJ. The role of dialysate in the stimulation of

interleukin-1 production during clinical hemodialysis. Am J Kidney Dis 1987;10:118-122.
53. Fillinger MF, Reinitz ER, Schwartz RA, Resetarits DE, Paskanik AM, Bredenberg CE. Beneficial effects of banding on venous intimal-medial hyperplasia in arteriovenous loop grafts. Am J Surg 1989;158:87-94.
54. Fillinger MF, Reinitz ER, Schwartz RA, et al. Graft geometry and venous intimal-medial hyperplasia in arteriovenous loop grafts. J Vasc Surg 1990;11:556-66.
55. Fillinger MF, Kerns DB, Bruch D, Reinitz ER, Schwartz RA. Does the end-to-end anastomosis offer a functional advantage over the end-to-side venous anastomosis in high-output arteriovenous grafts? J Vasc Surg 1990;12:676-690.
56. Zamora JL, Gao ZR, Weilbaecher DG, et al. Hemodynamic and morphologic features of arteriovenous angioaccess loop grafts. Trans Am Soc Artif Intern Organs 1985;31:119-23.
57. Abbott WM, Megerman J, Hasson JE, L'Italien G, Warnock DF. Effect of compliance mismatch on vascular graft patency. J Vasc Surg 1987;5:376-82.
58. Asakura T, Karino T. Flow patterns and spatial distribution of atherosclerotic lesions in human coronary arteries. Circ Res 1990;66:1045-66.
59. Faulkner SL, Fisher RD, Conkle DM, Page DL, Bender HW. Effect of blood flow rate on subendothelial proliferation in venous autografts used as arterial substitutes. Circulation 1975;51-52:163-72.
60. Imparato AM, Lord JW, Texon M, Helpern M. Experimental atherosclerosis produced by alteration of blood vessel configuration. Surg Forum 1961;12:245-47.
61. Glagov S, Giddens DP, Bassiouny H, White S, Zarins CK. Hemodynamic effects and tissue reactions at graft to vein anastomosis for vascular access. In: Sommer BG, Henry ML, eds. Vascular access for hemodialysis II. Chicago: Precept Press, 1991:3-20.
62. Karayannacos PE, Hostetler JR, Bond MG, et al. Late failure in vein grafts: mediating factors in subendothelial fibromuscular hyperplasia. Ann Surg 1978;187:183-88.
63. Karino T. Goldsmith HL. Disturbed flow in models of branching vessels. Trans Am Soc Artif Intern Organs 1980;26:500-06.
64. LoGerfo FW, Soncrant T, Teel T, Dewey CW Jr. Boundary layer separation in models of side-to-end arterial anastomoses. Arch Surg 1979;114:1369-73.
65. Megerman J, Abbott WM. Compliance in vascular grafts. In: Wright C, ed. Vascular grafting. Littleton, Mass: Wright-PSG, 1983;344-64.
66. Okuhn SP, Connelly DP, Calakos N, Ferrell L, Man-Xiang P, Goldstone J. Does compliance mismatch alone cause neointimal hyperplasia? J Vasc Surg 1989;9:35-45.
67. Sottiurai VS, Yao JST, Flinn WR, Batson RC. Intimal hyperplasia and neointima: an ultrastructural analysis of thrombosed grafts in humans. Surgery 1983;93:809-17.
68. Sumpio BE, Banes AJ, Levin LG, Johnson G. Mechanical stress stimulates aortic endothelial cells to proliferate. J Vasc Surg 1987;6:252-56.
69. Szilagyi DE, Whitcomb JG, Schenker W, Waibel P. The laws of fluid flow and arterial grafting. Surgery 1960;47:55-73.
70. Zwolak RM, Adams MC, Clowes AW. Kinetics of vein graft hyperplasia: association with tangential stress. J Vasc Surg 1987;5:126-36.
71. Zarins CK, Zatina MA, Giddens DP, Ku DN, Glagov S. Shear stress regulation of artery lumen diameter in experimental atherogenesis. J Vasc Surg 1987;5:413-20.
72. Lansman JB, Hallam TJ, Rink TJ. Single stretch-activated ion channels in vascular endothelial cells as mechanotransducers. Nature 1987;325:811-13.
73. Olesen SP, Clapham DE, Davies PF. Haemodynamic shear stress activates a K+ current in vascular endothelial cells. Nature 1988; 331:168-70.
74. Sinzinger H, Zidek T, Fitscha P, O'Grady J, Wagner O, Kaliman J. Prostaglandin I2 reduces activation of human arterial smooth muscle cells in vitro. Prostaglandins 1987;33:915-18.
75. Garg UC, Hassid A. Nitric oxide-generating vasodilators and 8-bromo-cyclic guanosine monophosphate inhibit mitogenesis and proliferation of cultured rat vascular smooth muscle cells. J Clin Invest 1989;83:1774-77.
76. Kariya K, Kawahara Y, Araki S, Fukuzaki H, Takai Y. Antiproliferative action of cyclic GMP-

elevating vasodilators in cultured rabbit aortic smooth muscle cells. Atherosclerosis 1989;80:143-47.
77. Nakaki T, Nakayama M, Yamamoto S, Kato R. Endothelin-mediated stimulation of DNA synthesis in vascular smooth muscle cells. Biochem Biophys Res Commun 1989;158:880-83.
78. Langille BL, O'Donnell F. Reductions in arterial diameter produced by chronic decreases in blood flow are endothelium-dependent. Science 1986;231:405-07.
79. Campbell-Boswell M, Robertson AL Jr. Effects of angiotensin II and vasopressin on human smooth muscle cells in vitro. Exp Mol Pathol 1981;35:265-276.
80. Powell JS, Clozel JP, Muller RKM, et al. Inhibitors of angiotensin-converting enzyme prevent myointimal proliferation after vascular injury. Science 1989;245:186-88.
81. Fillinger MF, Kerns DB, Schwartz RA. Hemodynamics and intimal hyperplasia. In: Sommer BG, Henry ML, eds. Vascular access for hemodialysis II. Chicago: Precept Press, 1991:21-51.
82. Snow AD, Bolender RP, Wight TN, Clowes AW. Heparin modulates the composition of the extracellular matrix domain surrounding arterial smooth muscle cells. Am J Pathol 1990;137:313-30.
83. Clowes AW, Clowes MM, Kocher O, Ropraz P, Chaponnier C, Gabbiani G. Arterial smooth muscle cells in vivo: relationship between actin isoform expression and mitogenesis and their modulation by heparin. J Cell Biol 1988;107:1939-45.
84. Thompson RW, Orlidge A, D'Amore PA. Heparin and growth control of vascular cells. Ann N Y Acad Sci 1989;556:255-67.
85. Clowes AW, Reidy MA. Prevention of stenosis after vascular reconstruction: pharmacologic control of intimal hyperplasia—a review. J Vasc Surg 1991;13:885-91.
86. Majesky MW, Schwartz SM, Clowes MM, Clowes AW. Heparin regulates smooth muscle S phase entry in the injured rat carotid artery. Circ Res 1987;61:296-300.
87. Kohler TR, T K, Clowes AW. Effect of heparin on adaptation of vein grafts to arterial circulation. Arteriosclerosis 1989;9:523-528.
88. Cambria RP, Ivarsson BL, Fallon JT, Abbott WA. Heparin fails to suppress intimal proliferation in experimental vein grafts. Surgery 1992;111:424-29.
89. Graham DJ, Alexander JJ. The effects of thrombin on bovine aortic endothelial and smooth muscle cells. J Vasc Surg 1990;11:307-13.
90. Daemen MJ, Lombardi DM, Bosman FT, Schwartz SM. Angiotensin II induces smooth muscle cell proliferation in the normal and injured rat arterial wall. Circ Res 1991;68:450-56.
91. Clagett GP, Genton E, Salzman EW. Antithrombotic therapy in peripheral vascular disease. Chest 1989;95:128S-39S.
92. Tada T, Reidy MA. Endothelial regeneration. IX. Arterial injury followed by rapid endothelial repair induces smooth-muscle-cell proliferation but not intimal thickening. Am J Pathol 1987;129:429-33.
93. Fanelli C, Aronoff R. Restenosis following coronary angioplasty. Am Heart J 1990;119:357-68.
94. Schlant RC, King SB III. Usefulness of calcium channel blockers during and after percutaneous transluminal coronary artery angioplasty. Circulation 1989;80(suppl IV):88-92.
95. Dyerberg J, Bang HO, Stofferson E, Moncada S, Vane JR. Eicosapentaenoic acid and prevention of thrombosis and atherosclerosis. Lancet 1978;15:117-19.
96. Weiner BH, Ockene IS, Levine PH, et al. Inhibition of atherosclerosis by cod liver oil in a hyperlipidemic swine model. N Engl J Med 1986;315:841-46.
97. Landymore RW, Kinley CE, Cooper JH, MacAuley M, Sheridan B, Cameron C. Cod liver oil in prevention of intimal hyperplasia in autogenous vein grafts used for arterial bypass. J Thorac Cardiovasc Surg 1985;89:351-57.
98. Colburn MD, Moore WS, Gelabert HA, Quinones-Baldrich WJ. Dose responsive suppression of myointimal hyperplasia by dexamethasone. J Vasc Surg 1992;15:510-18.
99. Ferns G, Reidy M, Ross R. Vascular effects of cyclosporine A in vivo and in vitro. Am J Pathol 1990;137:403-13.
100. Lindner V, Majack RA, Reidy MA. Basic fibroblast growth factor stimulates endothelial regrowth and proliferation in denuded arteries. J Clin Invest 1990;85:2004-08.
101. Nabel EG, Plautz G, Nabel GJ. Gene transfer into vascular cells. J Am Coll Cardiol 1991;17:189B-94B.

102. Rittgers SE, Garcia-Valdez C, McCormick JT, Posner MP. Noninvasive blood flow measurement in expanded polytetrafluoroethylene grafts for hemodialysis access. J Vasc Surg 1986;3:635-42.
103. Fox DL, DiCorleto PE. Regulation of production of a platelet-derived growth factor-like protein by cultured bovine aortic endothelial cells. J Cell Physiol 1984;121:298-308.
104. Limanni A, Fleming T, Molina R, et al. Expression of genes for platelet-derived growth factor in adult human venous endothelium: a possible non-platelet-dependent cause of intimal hyperplasia in vein grafts and perianastomotic areas of vascular prostheses. J Vasc Surg 1988;7:10-20.
105. Nilsson J, Stölund M, Palmberg L, et al. Arterial smooth muscle cells in primary culture produce a platelet-derived growth factor like protein. Proc Natl Acad Sci USA 1985;82:4418-22.
106. Ross R, Bowen-Pope DF, Raines EW. Platelet-derived growth factor and its role in health and disease. Philos Trans R Soc Lond [Biol] 1990;327:155-169.
107. Assoian RK, Fleurdelys BE, Stevenson HC, et al. Expression and secretion of type beta transforming growth factor by activated human macrophages. Proc Natl Acad Sci USA 1987;84:6020-24.
108. Klagsbrun M, Marikovsky M, Abraham J, Thompson S, Damm D, Higashiyama S. Heparin-binding EGF-like growth factor, structural and biological properties. J Cell Biochem 1992;Supp 16A:6.
109. Clowes AW, Karnovsky MJ. Supression by heparin of smooth muscle proliferation in injured arteries. Nature 1977;365:625-26.
110. Campbell JH, Campbell GR. Potential role of heparanase in atherosclerosis. News Phys Sci 1989;4:9-12.
111. Matzner Y, Bar-Ner M, Yahalom J, Ishai-Michaeli R, Fuks A, Vlodavsky I. Degradation of heparan sulphate in the subendothelial matrix by a readily released heparanase from human neutrophils. Possible role in invasion through basement membranes. J Clin Invest 1985;76:1306-13.
112. Chua CC, Geiman DE, Keller GH, Ladda RL. Induction of collagenase secretion in human fibroblast cultures by growth promoting factors. J Biol Chem 1985;260:5213-16.
113. Harlan JM, Thompson PJ, Ross R, Bowen-Pope DF. α-thrombin induces release of PDGF-like molecule(s) by cultured human endothelial cells. J Cell Biol 1986;103:1129-33.
114. Gajdusek C, Carbon S, Ross R, Nawroth P, Stern D. Activation of coagulation releases endothelial cell mitogens. J Cell Biol 1986;103:181-90.
115. Majack RA, Cook SC, Bornstein P. Control of smooth muscle cell growth by components of the extracellular matrix: autocrine role for thrombospondin. Proc Natl Acad Sci USA 1986;83:9050-54.
116. Oka Y, Orth DN. Human plasma epidermal growth factor/beta-urogastrone is associated with blood platelets. J Clin Invest 1983;72:249-59.
117. Pober JS, Lapierre LA, Stolpen AH, et al. Activation of cultured human endothelial cells by recombinant lymphotoxin: comparison with tumor necrosis factor and interleukin 1 species. J Immunol 1987;138:3319-24.
118. Hajjar KA, Hajjar DP, Silverstein RL, Nachman RL. Tumor necrosis factor-mediated release of platelet-derived growth factor from cultured endothelial cells. J Exp Med 1987;166:235-45.
119. Bevilacqua MP, Pober JS, Wheeler ME, Cotran RS, Gimbrone MA Jr. Interleukin 1 (IL-1) acts on cultured vascular endothelium to increase the adhesion of polymorphonuclear leukocytes, moncytes and related cell lines. J Clin Invest 1985;76:2003-11.
120. Bevilacqua MP, Wheeler ME, Pober JS, et al. Interleukin 1 (IL-1) activation of human endothelium: Effects on procoagulant activity and leukocyte adhesion. Am J Pathol 1985;121:393-403.
121. Larsen E, Celi A, Gilbert GE, et al. PADGEM protein: A receptor that mediates the interaction of activated platelets with neutrophils and monocytes. Cell 1989;59:305-12.
122. Cybulsky MI, Gimbrone MA Jr. Endotoxin-stimulated monocyte-selective adhesive mechanism in rabbit endothelium. FASEB J 1989;3:A1319.
123. Cybulsky MI, Gimbrone MA Jr. Endothelial expression of a mononuclear leukocyte adhesion molecule during atherogenesis. Science 1991;251:788-91.
124. Kishimoto TK, Larson RS, Corbi AL, Dustin ML, Staunton DE, Springer TA. The leukocyte integrins. Adv Immunol 1989;46:149-82.
125. Dustin ML, Springer TA. Lymphocyte function-associated antigen-1 (LFA-1) interaction with intercellular adhesion moecule-1 (ICAM-1) is one of at least three mechanisms for lymphocyte adhesion to cul-

tured endothelial cells. J Cell Biol 1988;107:321-31.
126. Elices MJ, Osborn L, Takada Y, et al. VCAM-I on activated endothelium interacts with the leukocyte integrin VLA-4 at a site distinct from the VLA-4/fibronectin binding site. Cell 1990;60:577-84.
127. Hemler ME. VLA proteins in the integrin family: structures, functions, and their role on leukocytes. Annu Rev Immunol 1990;8:365-400.
128. Raines EW, Dower SK, Ross R. Interleukin-1 mitogenic activity for fibroblasts and smooth muscle cells is due to PDGF-AA. Science 1989;243:393.
129. Libby P, Warner SJ, Friedman GB. Interleukin 1: a mitogen for human vascular smooth muscle cells that induces the release of growth-inhibitory prostanoids. J Clin Invest 1988;81:487-98.
130. Kurt-Jones EA, Fiers W, Pober JS. Membrane interleukin 1 induction on human endothelial cells and dermal fibroblasts. J Immunol 1987;139:2317.
131. Libby P, Ordovas JM, Auger KR, Robbins H, Birinyi LK. Endotoxin and tumor necrosis factor induce interleukin-1 gene expression in adult vascular endothelial cells. Am J Pathol 1986;124:179.
132. Loppnow H, Libby P. Adult human vascular endothelial cells express the IL6 gene differentially in response to LPS or IL1. Cell Immunol 1989;122:493-503.
133. Dustin ML, Rothlein R, Bhan AK, Dinarello CA, Springer TA. Induction by IL-1 and interferon-gamma: tissue distribution, biochemistry, and function of a natural adherence molecule (ICAM-1). J Immunol 1986;137:245.
134. Dinarello CA, Mier JW. Lymphokines. N Engl J Med 1987;317:940.
135. Balkwill FR, Burke F. The cytokine network. Immunol Today 1989;10:299.
136. Gimbrone MA Jr, Obin MS, Brock AF, et al. Endothelial interleukin-8: a novel inhibitor of leukocyte-endothelial interactions. Science 1989;246:1601.
137. Gimbrone MA Jr, Brock AF, Schafer AI. Leukotriene B$_4$ stimulates polymorphonuclear leukocyte adhesion to cultured vascular endothelial cells. J Clin Invest 1984;74:1552.
138. Martin TR, Altman LC, Albert RK, Henderson WA. Leukotriene B, production by the human alveolar macrophage: a potential mechanism for amplifying inflammation in the lung. Am Rev Respir Dis 1984;129:106.
139. Berliner JA, Territo M, Almada L, Carter A, Shafonsky E, Fogelman AM. Monocyte chemotactic factor produced by large vessel endothelial cells in vitro. Arteriosclerosis 1986;6:254.
140. Valente AJ, Fowler SR, Sprague EA, Kelley JL, Suenram CA, Schwartz CJ. Initial characterization of a peripheral blood mononuclear cell chemoattractant derived from cultured arterial smooth muscle cells. Am J Pathol 1984;117:409.
141. Minota S, Cameron B, Welch WJ, Winfield JB. Autoantibodies to the constitutive 73-kD member of the hsp70 family of heat shock proteins in systemic lupus erythematosus. J Exp Med 1988;168:1475.
142. Kaufman SH. Heat shock proteins and the immune reponse. Immunol Today 1990;11:129.
143. Madtes DK, Raines EW, Sakariassen KS, et al. Induction of transforming growth factor-alpha in activated human alveolar macrophages. Cell 1988;53:285.
144. Davies PF. Biology of disease. Vascular cell interactions with special reference to the pathogenesis of atherosclerosis. Lab Invest 1986;55:5-24.
145. Hsieh H-J, Li N-Q, Frangos JA. Shear stress increases endothelial platelet-derived growth factor mRNA levels. Am J Physiol 1991;260:H642-46.
146. Koller A, Kaley G. Prostaglandins mediate arteriolar dilation to increased blood flow velocity in skeletal muscle microcirculation. Circ Res 1990;67:529-34.
147. Sharefkin JB, Diamond SL, Eskin SG, McIntire LV, Dieffenbach CW. Fluid flow decreases preproendothelin mRNA levels and suppresses endothelin-1 peptide release in cultured human endothelial cell. J Vasc Surg 1991;14:1-9.
148. Cooke JP, Stamler J, Andon N, Davies PF, McKinley G, Loscalzo J. Flow stimulates endothelial cells to release a nitrovasodilator that is potentiated by reduced thiol. Am J Physiol 1990;259:H804-12.
149. Diamond SL, Sharefkin JB, Dieffenbach C, Frasier-Scott K, McIntire LV, Eskin SG. Tissue plasminogen activator messenger RNA levels increase in cultured endothelial cells exposed to laminar shear stress. J Cell Physiol 1990;143:364-71.
150. Diamond SL, Eskin SG, McIntire LV. Fluid flow stimulates tissue plasminogen activator secretion by cultured human endothelial cells. Science 1989;243:1483-05.

3

PHARMACOLOGIC INTERVENTION TO PREVENT INTIMAL HYPERPLASIA

Charles J. Diskin, M.D., Thomas J. Stakes Jr., M.D., and Andrew T. Pennell, Pharm.D.

Historical Attempts

ATTEMPTS AT PHARMACOLOGIC PREVENTION of access thrombosis began with the use of warfarin in the days of Scribner shunts.[1] The annals of medicine are filled less with reports of success than with their tragic complications before they were abandoned.[2-5] At that point, investigators began to recognize that thrombosis involved more than enzymes cascading down the clotting pathway toward coagulation. By 1978, the Canadian Cooperative Study Group found that aspirin was successful in stroke and TIA prevention when agents affecting the clotting cascade had not been.[6]

In a landmark study in 1980, Harter proposed the use of low-dose aspirin to irreversibly inhibit platelet cylooxygenase without affecting the synthesis of vascular prostacyclin to prevent access thrombosis in hemodialysis patients.[7] Forty-two patients scheduled to receive a Scribner shunt were randomized to receive either placebo or 160 mg of aspirin a day. Thrombosis occurred in 72% of the placebo group but only 32% of the aspirin group. Although intimal hyperplasia develops in Scribner shunts,[8] these results were particularly difficult to extrapolate to arteriovenous (A-V) fistulas or polytetrafluoroethylene (PTFE) grafts, since histologic evidence of intimal hyperplasia was not specifically examined. Nevertheless, the theory was launched. Shortly thereafter, intimal hyperplasia became recognized as the most common cause of long-term access thrombosis[9] and predictably, aspirin and dipyridamole were enthusiastically investigated to produce a similar decrease in thrombosis, as well as prevent the in-

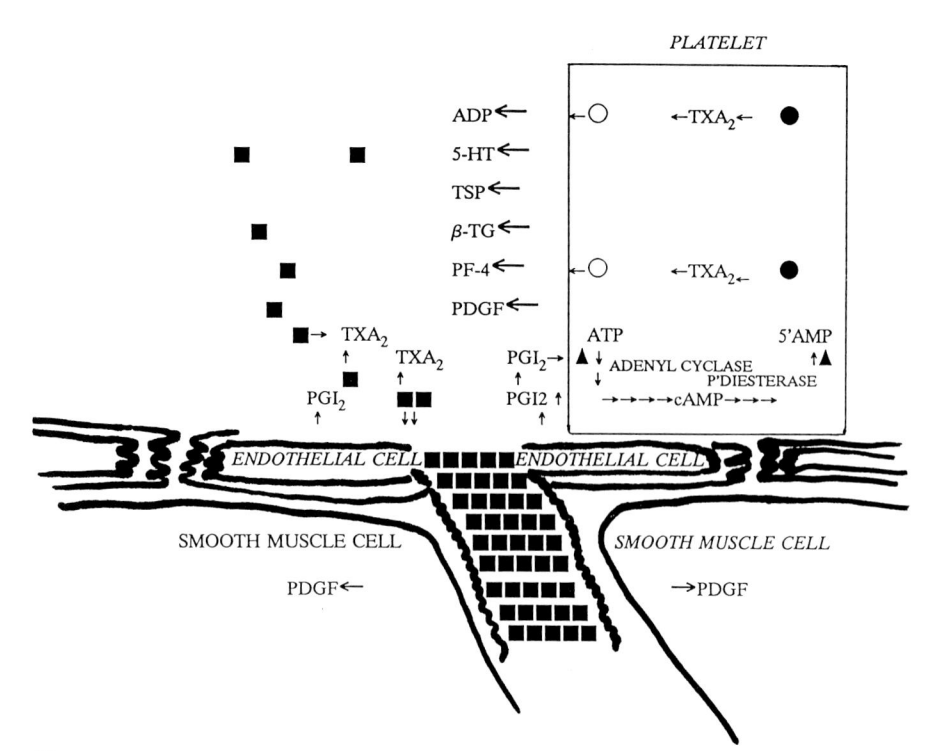

Figure 3-1. Prostacyclin/thromboxane balance. The former promotes and the latter inhibits granule release and platelet aggregation.

timal hyperplasia itself. The results were encouraging through the early 1980s.[10-12] Furthermore, the results were easy to accept because they fit well with newly developed concepts of the roles of a platelet-endothelial balance to maintain vascular flow and hemostasis. In 1977, Friedman had shown that experimental thrombocytopenia prevented intimal hyperplasia in rabbits[13] at about the same time that prostacyclin was discovered.[14] The attraction of the experimental benefits of aspirin and dipyridamole, combined with the use of newly discovered prostaglandins incorporated into the theory, was irresistible.

Cyclooxygenase Inhibitors

Prostacyclin (PGI_2), made by endothelial cells, stops clot propagation and is a vasodilator (figure 3-1). Thromboxane A2 (TXA_2), generated by platelets, induces platelet aggregation and vasoconstriction. The dynamic interplay of the eicosanoids was supposed to allow hemostasis and platelet plugging at areas of injury such as along a needle track. However, clot propagation would stop when the lumen of the blood vessel was reached by the production of prostacyclin. Both $PGI2$ and $TXA2$ are products of the enzyme cylooxygenase. Aspirin irreversibly inhibits cyclooxygenase by acetylation of a serine residue in its active site (figure 3-2).[15] Endothelial cells (ECs) continously produce cyclooxygenase and recover the ability to produce $PGI2$ within hours, but the nonnucleated platelets lose their ability to produce TXA_2 for the life of the platelet. Low-dose

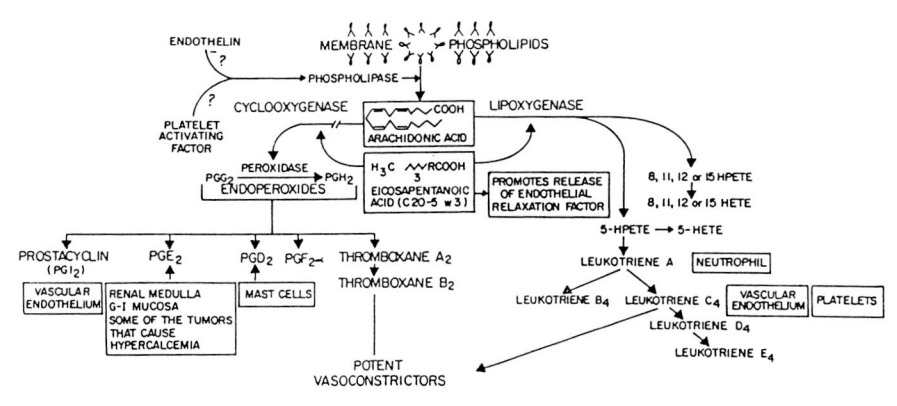

Figure 3-2. Diagram of potential inhibitory effect of EPA on endothelial hormones and autocoids, which may play a role in prolonging the life of hemodialysis vascular accesses.

aspirin thus prevents platelet aggregation and vasoconstriction while not interfering with the inhibition of clot propagation in vasodilators. Because the capacity of endothelial cells to generate prostacyclin decreases with age, diabetes, smoking, and atherosclerosis, its theoretical role in thrombosis and atherosclerosis was attractive. With the demonstration that the infusions of prostacyclin in vitro could inhibit mitogens (including platelet-derived growth factor) that produced vascular proliferation of the intima,[16] the cyclooxygenase theory of intimal hyperplasia and vascular thrombosis seemed confirmed. The only question that seemed to remain was that of which is the best mechanism of inhibition.

Eicosapentanoic Acid

Eicosapentanoic acid (EPA) has been shown to be a competitive inhibitor of cyclooxygenase in normal subjects[17] and was known to reduce platelet aggregation in hemodialysis patients (figure 3-2).[18] Additionally, EPA has been shown to reduce intimal hyperplasia in autogenous vein grafts used for arterial bypass in dogs.[19-21] More important, EPA was more effective than aspirin or dipyridamole in reducing intimal hyperplasia in a direct comparison in animals.[19]

In 1986, we devised a small pilot study to examine the beneficial effects of EPA on graft patency, outflow stenosis, and intimal hyperplasia.[22] We examined the effect of intradialytic EPA administration on outflow stenosis and angiopatency in chronic hemodialysis patients. Seven consecutive patients undergoing construction of a new PTFE access who had suffered more than three episodes of graft thrombosis within the preceding 12 months were selected. Three patients were randomized to receive placebo and four to receive 3 gm of EPA at each of thrice-weekly dialysis treatments for six consecutive months. No outflow stenosis developed in the EPA group, but it did appear in two of the three patients receiving placebo (figures 3-3 and 3-4). However, no significant difference in graft survival or any biochemical, hematologic, or coagulation parameters were noted at six months (table 3-1). Because of the small size of the study, no real conclusions could be drawn concerning any demonstrated or theoreti-

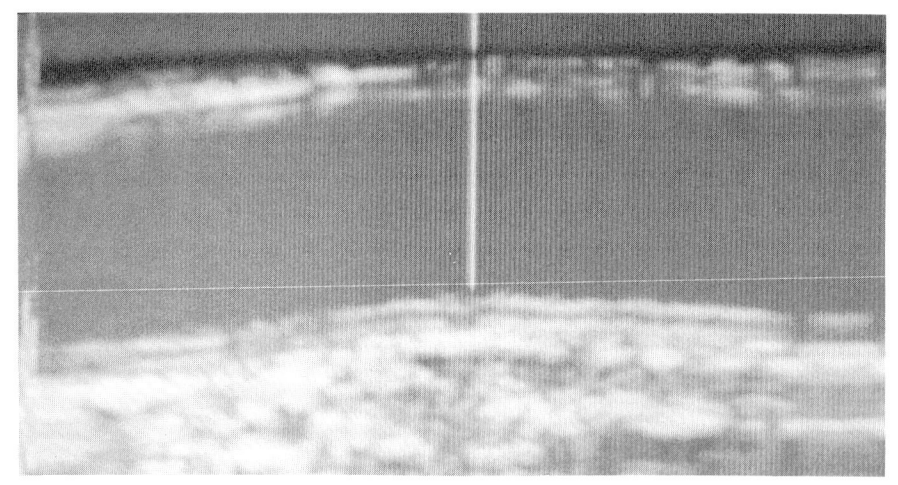

Figure 3-3. No intimal hyperplasia is seen at venous anastomosis (vertical line) in the fish oil group.

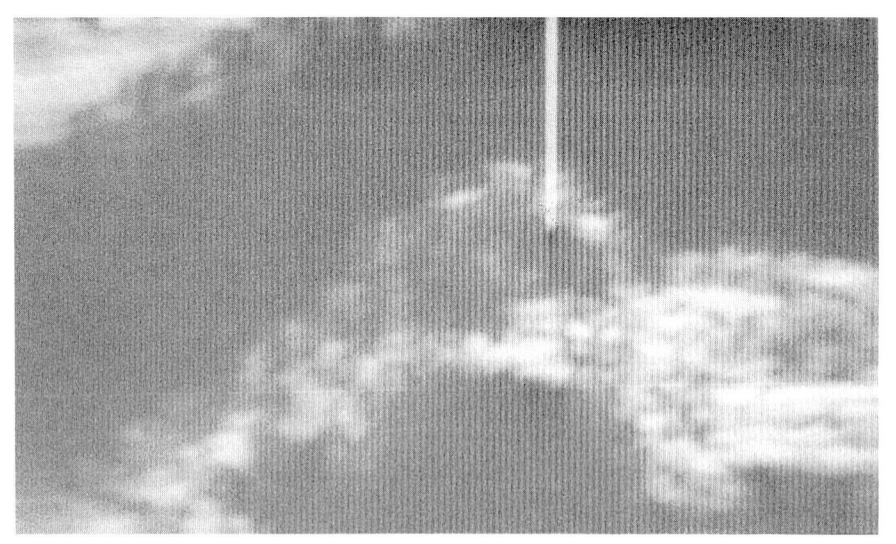

Figure 3-4. Intimal hyperplasia (vertical line) is seen at the venous anastomosis in the placebo group.

cal benefit. However, the absence of outflow stenosis in the treatment group gave promise and rationale for a large-scale study to determine the true benefits and risks of EPA supplementation of chronic maintenance hemodialysis for the possibility of a major therapeutic breakthrough in hemodialysis. Therefore, after gaining approval for a study, we applied for grant funding to set up a large prospective trial at Auburn University. The funding never came, and along the way, the cyclooxygenase theory was shattered.

Table 3-1. Metabolic, Hepatic, and Hemocytologic Parameters

	Ω-3 FA Before	Ω-3 FA After	Placebo Before	Placebo After
Metabolic mg/dl				
Glucose	107.7 ± 42.1	117.0 ± 45	134 ± 21	111.8 ± 44.4
Creatinine	13.9 ± 2.6	17.9 ± 2.9	19.2 ± 6.6	16.6 ± 5.2
BUN	58.9 ± 30.7	72.4 ± 12.9	53 ± 12.6	68.5 ± 17.1
Cholesterol	215 ± 58	187 ± 26	220 ± 60	206 ± 60
Hepatic				
SGOT, U/l	36 ± 14.1	35 ± 9.1	35.3 ± 11.4	26.3 ± 14.6
LDH, U/l	362 ± 150	313 ± 115	233 ± 57	174 ± 38
Albumin g/l	3.7 ± 0.4	3.8 ± 0.3	3.5 ± 0.2	3.8 ± 0.3
Hematologic				
Viscosity mm	1.5 ± 0.1	1.6 ± 0.0	1.7 ± 0.1	1.6 ± 0.1
BT, min	13.0 ± 5.7	7.2 ± 1.0	5.3 ± 1.5	7.2 ± 4.1
PT	13. ± 0.0	12.5 ± 0.4	13.3 ± 0.6	12.9 ± 0.5
PTT	22.5 ± 0.7	23 ± 0.5	24.3 ± 1.5	23.8 ± 0.8
WBC 1,000/μl	5.4 ± 2.3	8.5 ± 2.6	5.9 ± 0.9	6.2 ± 2.1
HGB, g/dl	24.8 ± 4.8	28.2 ± 6.1	32.5 ± 5.3	33.8 ± 3.9

End of the Cyclooxygenase Theory?

First came the reports of a lack of efficacy of aspirin and dipyridamole on intimal hyperplasia[23] and patency rates of hemodialysis accesses (personal communication from Lee Ann Mills, Boehringer-Ingelheim, 1989). Then, thromboxane synthetase inhibitors were shown to have even less effect than aspirin.[24] Meanwhile, prostacyclin production was demonstrated to be normal at the anastomotic site where intimal hyperplasia was produced. If thromboxane abolition and prostacyclin production were not the answer, then inhibition of cyclooxygenase could not be an effective pharmacologic intervention.

Present Status of EPA

If the cyclooxygenase inhibition theory was wrong, where does that leave EPA as a potential therapeutic inhibitor of intimal hyperplasia? We believe that

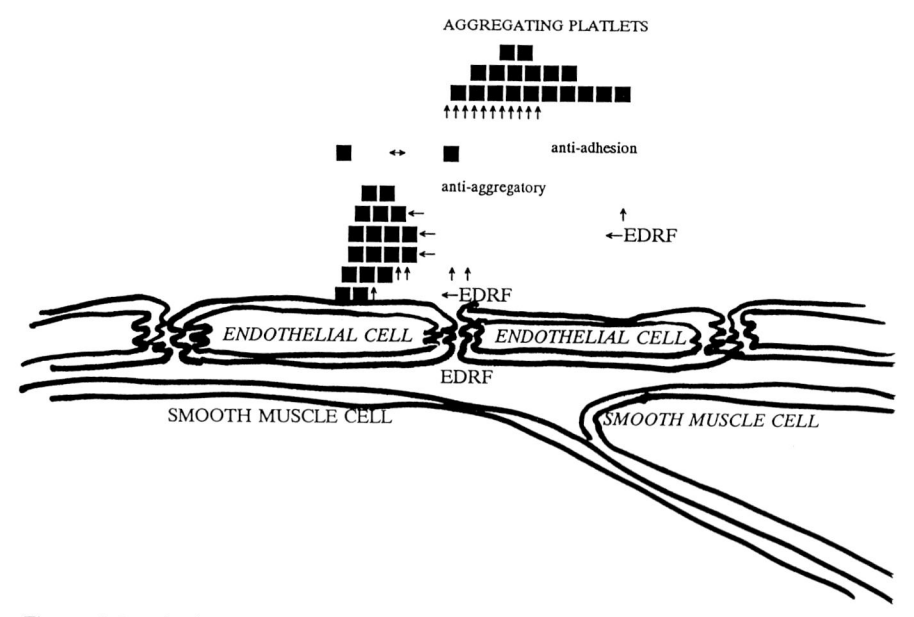

Figure 3-5. Antiaggregatory and antiadhesive effect of nitrate.

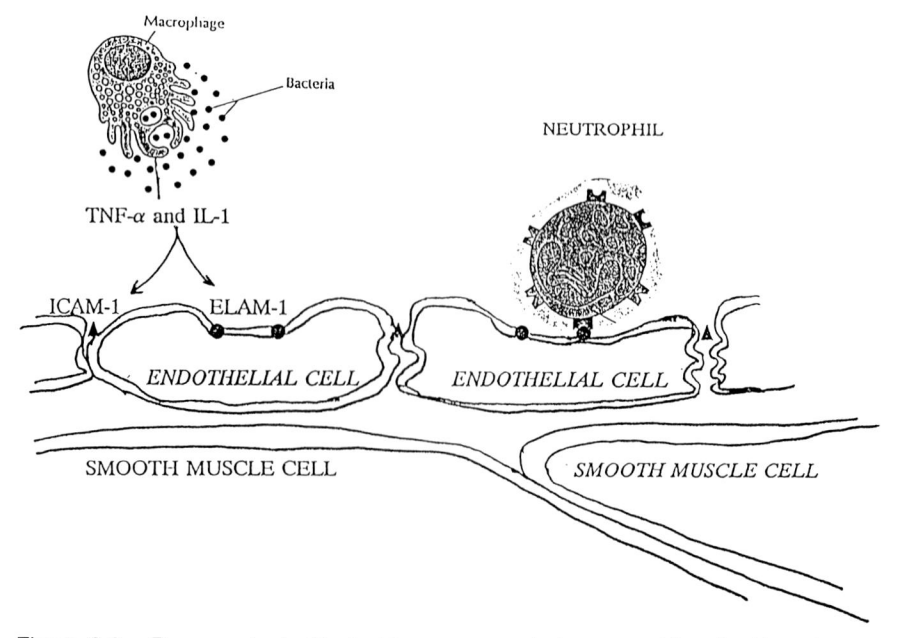

Figure 3-6. Procoagulant effect of tumor necrosis factor and interleukin-1: (1) decreased thrombomodulin; (2) increased TPA inhibitor. Exposure of ELAM results in less "rolling" and more "sticking" of monocytes as they circulate, which can result in the release of PDGF.

it is still a potentially potent drug. Indeed, our small pilot study proves very little.[25] In animals, it was more effective than aspirin in reducing intimal hyperplasia,[26] and more studies have shown a beneficial effect of aspirin[10-12,27,28] than those that have not.[29-31] However, EPA also promotes the release of endothelium-dependent relaxation factor (EDRF) (figure 3-2).[32,33] EDRF is nitric oxide that is produced by a healthy endothelium and, like prostacyclin, has an antiaggregating effect on platelets (figure 3-5).[34-36] More importantly, EDRF also has been shown to inhibit platelet adhesion to ECs,[37,38] something that PGI$_2$ cannot effect. With adherence thus inhibited, mediators such as TXA$_2$ and platelet-derived growth factor (PDGF) would not be released from platelets.

PDGF is a basic glycoprotein that acts as a mitogen and may be responsible for attracting smooth muscle cells (SMCs) from the media of the artery into the intima.[39] However, platelets are not the only source of PDGF; it can probably be produced also by injured smooth muscle, ECs, and activated macrophages.[39,40] Fortunately, EPA also inhibits PDGF,[41] decreases serum viscosity,[42] blunts endothelin, and inhibits lipoxygenase and inflammatory cytokines such as interleukin-1 (IL-1) and tumor necrosis factor.

Endothelin is the most potent vasoconstrictor known. Leukotriennes, the metabolic products of lipoxygenase, are inflammatory mediators that, together with IL-1 and human tumor necrosis factor (TNF), respond to tissue injury and promote coagulation and alter endothelial binding. IL-1 is a potent inducer of the biosynthesis and cell surface expression of procoagulant activity of human ECs (figure 3-6).[43] Together with TNF, IL-1 can decrease endothelial production of thrombomodulin and increase the synthesis of an inhibitor to plasminogen activator.[44] Furthermore, both cytokines stimulate the production of endothelial leukocyte adhesion molecules (ELAM-1) promoting neutrophil adherence to endothelial cells and inhibit the intercellular adhesion molecules (ICAM-1) that regulate EC integrity and adherence.[44]

Inhibition of these mediators would seem to make EPA a perfect drug to decrease platelet adherence, leukocyte adherence, vasoconstriction, and endothelial and smooth muscle proliferation and migration. However, history is replete with good theories that were wrong. Although we have been the only group to investigate EPA for the prevention of intimal hyperplasia and access thrombosis in hemodialysis patients, there have been several studies of the use of EPA to prevent intimal hyperplasia and stenosis after angioplasty that are divided between those claiming benefit[45,46] and those finding none.[47,48] Although this is disappointing, it is not unexpected, since EPA produces its effect through competitive inhibition (figure 3-7).[49] Only by overwhelming the amount of arachidonic acid substrate can the effect be achieved (table 3-2).[50] For that to happen, large doses of fish oil are necessary. To achieve the results of Dinarello, about 36 capsules of the most potent fish oil (500 mg) are necessary.[49] At one-sixth of that dose, we found that patients complained of fish odor breath, dysgeusia, and diarrhea. Because compliance was unreliable, we found it necessary to administer all doses ourselves. None of the studies failing to show any benefits for EPA had any provisions such as those to assure compliance. In the study failing to find benefit but claiming good compliance, the investigators felt that only 65% of the subjects took as much as 75% of their prescribed dose.[51] It is no wonder that they found no benefit. If EPA does work as we think that it should, it can only be successful if compliance is guaranteed.

48 PHARMACOLOGIC INTERVENTION TO PREVENT INTIMAL HYPERPLASIA

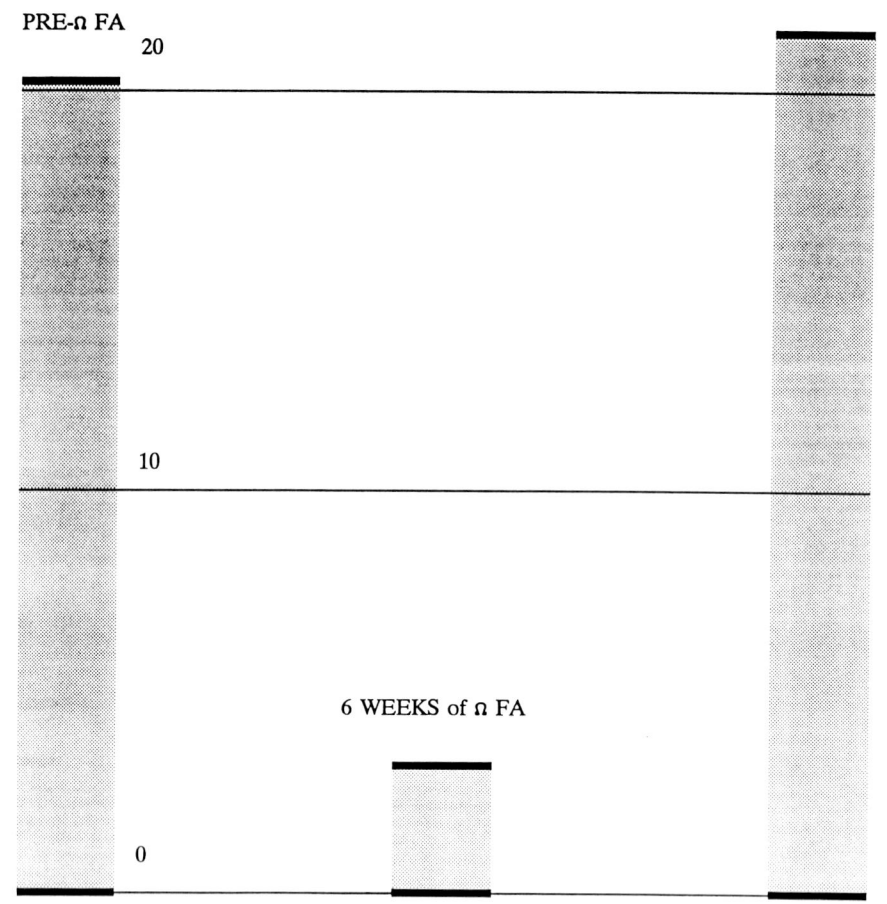

Figure 3-7. Effect of fish oil supplementation on fatty acid profile. (Data printed with permission of Dr. C. A. Dinarello, New England Medical Center.)

Other Possible Agents and Ongoing Studies

The goal of effective pharmacologic therapy would be to find a drug that: (1) intervenes only at the biologic mediators of intimal hyperplasia, but not in wound healing; (2) produces as few side effects as possible; (3) has as long a half-life as possible to minimize the effect of patient compliance; (4) has a good bioavailability in end-stage renal disease (ESRD) (many believe that drug levels in renal failure are as high or higher in renal failure patients as they are in normal people, but we have shown that this is not always the case, that the levels may indeed be very low for certain drugs in ESRD due to poor bioavailability);[52] and (5) has as few drug interactions as possible, since most ESRD patients take many medications. Although no ideal agent exists at present, five different

Table 3-2. Effect of Fish Oil Supplementation on Fatty Acid Composition in Blood Samples

Fatty acid	Before Ω-3 supplement	After Ω-3 supplement	10 weeks after end of Ω-3	20 weeks after end of Ω-3
AA (Ω-6)	13.8 ± 1.3	8.6 ± 0.7	9.5 ± 1.8	13.8 ± 2.6
EPA (Ω-3)	0.7 ± 0.1	3.8 ± 0.7	1.0 ± 0.3	0.6 ± 0.1
DHA (Ω-3)	2.3 ± 0.2	3.3 ± 0.4	2.4 ± 0.4	2.5 ± 0.7
AA/EPA	20.9 ± 2.2	2.4 ± 0.2	12.0 ± 2.1	23.9 ± 4.3

Source: N Engl J Med 1989;320:267 (reprinted with permission of Dr. C.A. Dinarello)

classes of agents are proposed, including antiplatelet, proendothelial, gylcocalyx regulating, antimigratory, and antiproliferative drugs. Unfortunately, all studies completed up to the present have been hampered by either small sample sizes or a lack of consideration of the pharmacokinetics of renal failure, often using doses of drugs that would be toxic in dialysis patients.

Antiplatelet Agents

The promise of these agents is based upon the documented role of platelets in the development of intimal hyperplasia. Even if cyclooxygenase inhibition is not as important as we had previously thought, experimental depletion of platelets will prevent the development of intimal hyperplasia in rabbits, as previously discussed. While there have been a number of agents studied in animal models and coronary artery bypass grafts that may prevent such a direct comparison of results,[53] all successes with normal platelets should be tested in renal failure before being accepted as therapy. EPA and aspirin have been the most successful agents of this group and (not coincidentally) the most studied. We previously discussed aspirin and EPA and we will present here a few of the less-well-studied agents.

SULFINPYRAZONE

Sulfinpyrazone was documented to prevent thrombosis of Scribner shunts even before aspirin.[54-56] Sulfinpyrazone is a congener of phenylbutazone (figure 3-8). Its antiproliferative and uricosuric properties are like that of phenylbutazone; it was developed because of the severe toxic side effects of the parent compound. Its main beneficial effect on platelets is through thromboxane inhibition and prevention of serotonin release from ECs. In hemodialysis patients, sulfinpyrazone has been documented to prevent a drop in antithrombin-III that occurs after dialysis. A chronic effect has been shown to decrease ADP-induced platelet aggregation and decreased quantities of platelet factor 4.[57] Indium 111 imaging of treated platelets has shown decreased deposition in bovine and Gore-Tex grafts at the venous anastomosis where intimal hyperplasia normally develops.[58]

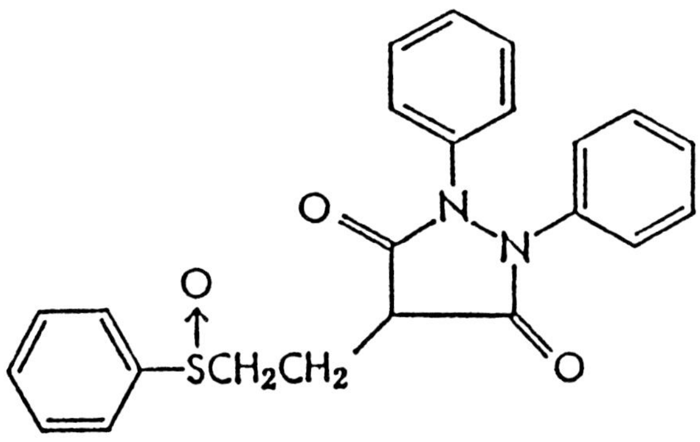

Sulfinpyrazone

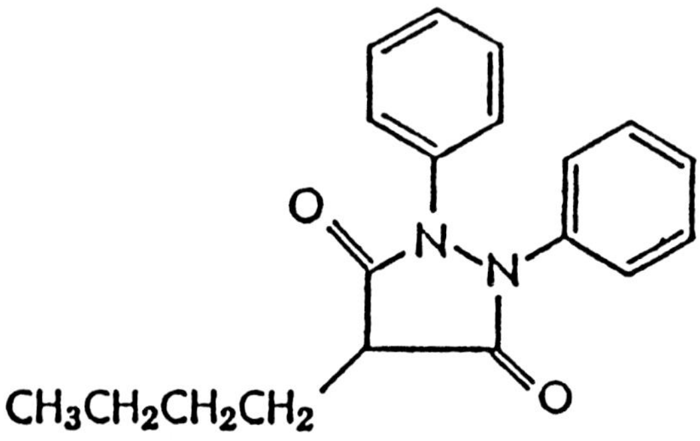

Phenylbutazone

Figure 3-8. Similarity of structure of sulfinpyrazone to phenylbutazone may explain some of its adverse side effects.

DIPYRIDAMOLE

Dipyridamole, a unique chemical with a pyrimidopyridine ring system, was originally marketed as a smooth muscle dilator. It has been subsequently thought to act as an antiplatelet agent through the inhibition of cyclic nucleotide phosphodiesterase activity with a promotion of prostacyclin production. It has been used in many studies in combination with the cyclooxygenase inhibitor aspirin. Independently, it has no effect of its own. A recent unpublished work sponsored by Boehringer in Boston found no benefit of dipyridamole in the prolongation of access patency. Although this drug should no longer be considered part of the antiplatelet pharmacologic armamentarium, the concept of antiplatelet activity through cyclic nucleotides may be useful when considering synergy with other drugs (see below).

IBUPROFEN

Ibuprofen, a propionic acid derivative, shares similar properties to other derivatives, including ketoprofen, indoprofen, flurbiprofen, fenoprofen, and naproxen. All are inhibitors of cyclooxygenase, with ibuprofen being roughly equivalent to aspirin in potency. In addition, ibuprofen may have the beneficial effect of decreasing TNF,[59] which can alter endothelial adhesion and, as noted above, has procoagulant activities. In a canine model, ibuprofen was more effective than aspirin, dipyridamole, verapamil and nifedipine in preventing platelet deposition acutely at the venous anastomosis;[59] unlike aspirin, the effect was dose-dependent up to 25 mg/kg/day. In addition, studies have found improved patency of PTFE microprostheses.[60-62] However, none of these studies were performed in renal failure, and no histologic proof was ever attempted to investigate the prevention of intimal hyperplasia.

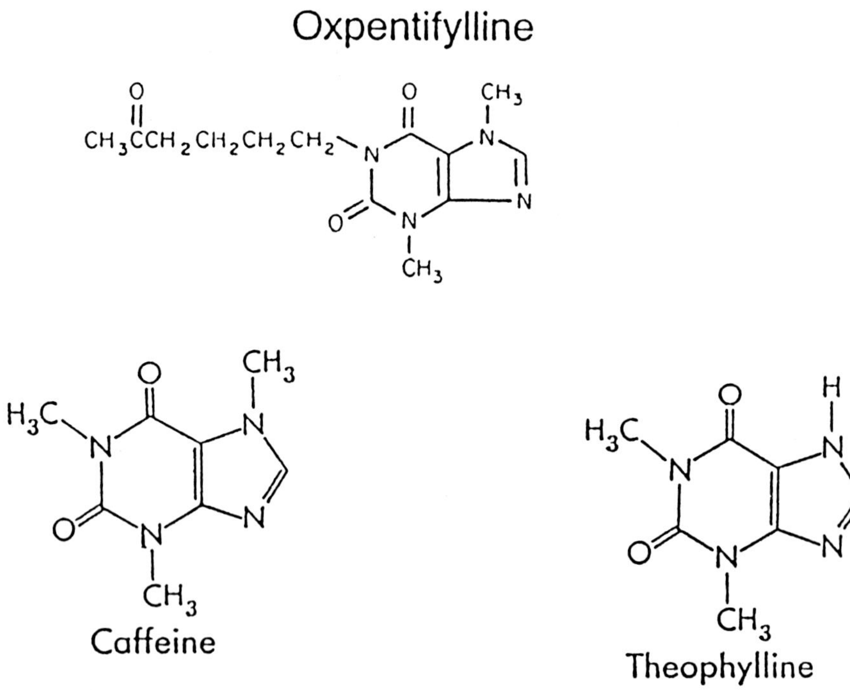

Figure 3-9. Pentoxifylline is a caffeine derivative. It shares pharmacokenetics and toxic symptoms of theophylline.

PENTOXIFLYLLINE

Pentoxiflylline is a methylxanthine with a structure similar to that of caffeine and theophylline (figure 3-9). Drugs of this class are primarily known for their effect on nucleotide phosphodiesterase resulting in CNS stimulation and smooth muscle relaxation. Pentoxifylline, however, improves the subnormal flexibility of erythrocytes in patients with claudication, thus improving blood flow to the ischemic limb. Unlike others of its class, it has no cardiotonic or smooth muscle effects. Although theophylline has been used for antiplatelet effects, presumably through phosphodiesterase inhibition of 5' CAMP,[63,64] pentoxifylline has been shown to be an even more potent inhibitor of ADP-induced platelet aggregation.[65] Indeed, in one direct comparison with aspirin, pentoxifylline was felt to be even more effective as an antiaggregate.[66,67] More interestingly, cyclooxygenase inhibition by aspirin and phosphodiesterase inhibition by pentoxifylline were synergistic.[68] Further, pentoxifylline decreases viscosity and leukocyte and platelet adhesion to EC walls[69] and promotes PGI2 release from ECs.[69,70] A group from Yugoslavia evaluated 51 ESRD patients who underwent a Scribner shunt as an acute access while waiting for development of a permanent access.[71] Twenty-six received pentoxifylline (400 mg t.i.d.) and 25 were given placebo. The mean numbers of thrombi per patient were 1.69 ± 1.29 with pentoxifylline and 3.28 ± 1.99 with controls (p < 0.005). No appreciable side effects were seen.

NITRATES AND NITRITES

Nitrates and nitrites have been used as vasodilators since 1847, when Constatine Herring found that a small quantity of oily nitroglycerine on the tongue could both relieve angina and produce very uncomfortable headaches. However, only in the past few years have we come to realize that the empiric use of organic nitrates for vasodilatation only mimicked the endothelium's natural production of EDRF, which is now known to be nitric oxide. All nitrogen-oxide-containing substances (including nitroprusside) can activate cyclic AMP and cyclic GMP in smooth muscle. However, it was shown more recently that by inhibition of nucleotide phosphodiesterase, nitric oxide induces an increase of cyclic GMP, which inhibits both platelet aggregation and significant adhesion to EC membranes.[37] Apparently, cyclic AMP controls platelet aggregation, but cyclic GMP controls both adhesion and aggregation.

Unfortunately, despite their great theoretical benefit, there has been no investigation of the use of nitrites in hemodialysis patients. Hypotension is a major side effect, but methemoglobin has been a problem of nitrites, including amyl nitrite.

TICLOPIDINE

Ticlopidine is a drug that alters the platelet membrane directly, independent of any effect on prostaglandins. A thienopyridine, it reduces platelet aggregation on surfaces, improves RBC deformity, reduces blood viscosity, and inhibits platelet-activating factor.[72] In one single-blind crossover study, ticlopidine significantly reduced platelet adhesion to the subendothelium,[73] and in a combined Canadian-American study, it effected a 30.2% reduction in stroke, myocardial infarction, or vascular death when compared to placebo.[74] Like pentoxyfylline, it has also been shown to reduce the incidence of intermittent claudication.[75-77]

Although ticlopidine was originally reported to reduce intimal hyperplasia,[78,79] more recent studies have not demonstrated any benefit.[80] No recent study has been conducted, but several studies were performed on ESRD patients

Table 3-3. Antiplatelet Agents

Cyclooxygenase inhibitors	Cyclic nucleotide promotors
1. Aspirin*	Dipyridamole
2. Fish oil (EPA)†	Pentoxifylline*†
3. Ibuprofen/NSAID	Sulfinpyrazone*
	Nitrates
	Ticlopidine
	Prostacyclin

* Clinical studies showing improved graft survival in hemodialysis patients
† Clinical studies showing reduction of intimal hyperplasia in hemodialysis patients

in the 1980s.[81,82] In 1985, 42 ESRD patients undergoing the construction of an A-V fistula were randomized to placebo or ticlopidine 250 mg b.i.d. for four weeks. Despite the short duration of the study, eight patients in the placebo group suffered thrombosis, compared to only two in the ticlopidine-treated group. The difference was statistically significant.[82]

We might divide the antiplatelet agents into two distinctive groups (table 3-3). In one group are the cyclooxygenase inhibitors, i.e., aspirin, EPA, sulfinpyrazone, and ibuprofen. In the other would be those agents affecting cyclonucleotides, including pentoxifylline, dipyridamole, and nitrates. Agents in both groups have been reported to inhibit platelet aggregation and prolong access patency. Only EPA and aspirin have been investigated for prevention of intimal hyperplasia in vascular accesses for hemodialysis. On the other hand, only agents affecting cylonucleotide levels have been shown to have an effect on platelet adherence to the endothelium that would prevent platelet deposition and release of platelet metabolic products such as thromboxane A_2 and PDGF. It is worth noting that the original combinations of aspirin and dipyridamole would have made use of these theoretical differences. We now know that dipyridamole has no independent effect. However, both pentoxifylline and nitrates are synergistic with aspirin in preventing platelet aggregation.[28,68] Are they synergistic in prolonging access patency and/or reducing intimal hyperplasia? What would be the best theoretical pharmacologic combination? These questions remain unanswered.

Proendothelial Agents

As with platelets, a central role for endothelium seems to exist from the empiric observation that the very presence of endothelium or platelets seems to determine the presence, absence, and degree of intimal hyperplasia. Endothelial seeded grafts had significantly less intimal hyperplasia than unseeded grafts,[24] and the degree of endothelial cell luminal coverage of the anastomotic site is inversely related to the amount of anastomotic intimal hyperplasia ($R = -0.6$, $P > 0.05$).[82]

PROSTACYCLIN

Under the cyclooxygenase theory, the main importance of the endothelium would be primarily its production of prostacyclin, which is a powerful vasodilator that inhibits platelet aggregation through the activation of adenylate cyclase, resulting in an intracellular increase in cyclic AMP (figure 3-1).[83] Mechanical or chemical deviation of cell membranes results in the formation of prostacyclin.[84] Pulsatile pressure, bradykinins, serotonin, PDGF, IL-I, and adenine nucleotides stimulate its production.[85] The capacity of ECs to generate PGI_2 decreases with age, smoking,[86] diabetes, and atherosclerosis. In addition, infusions of PGI_2 have been shown to prevent intimal thickening[16] and to directly inhibit the proliferation of cultured vascular SMCs.[87] Therefore, it is quite natural to apply a protective role for prostacyclin against both intimal hyperplasia and atherosclerosis. Prostacyclin production has been suggested to be normal at the vascular anastomotic site in animals developing intimal hyperplasia, thus limiting the potential for its efficacy in achieving long-term patency. However, the question of preventing acute graft thrombosis in patients with diabetes and severe atherosclerotic vascular disease who may have damaged endothelium and deficient prostacyclin production remains to be investigated.

DEFIBROTIDE

Defibrotide is a single-stranded polydeoxyribonucleotic sodium salt obtained from mammalian lungs that can stimulate PGI_2 from the vascular endothelium of various animal species.[88] Moreover, it may promote another endothelial function, that of fibrinolysis. Initially, it was shown to reduce intimal hyperplasia after thrombi were electrically induced in dogs.[89] In humans, it has reduced the incidence of intimal hyperplasia in renal transplant grafts,[90] prevented thrombosis of subclavian catheters used for total parenteral nutrition,[91] and reversed the acute renal failure associated with endothelial injury in hemolytic uremic syndrome and thrombotic thrombocytopenic purpura.[92] More recently, cyclosporin-treated rats have been found to have an increase in PGI2 produced by defibrotide that was thought to confer a protective effect against cyclosporin-produced glomerular injury.[93]

ANGIOTENSIN-CONVERTING ENZYME INHIBITORS

The major antihypertensive effect of angiotensin-converting enzyme (ACE) inhibitors is from the inhibition of angiotensin-converting enzyme and not from bradykinin production. However, bradykinins activate ECs to cause arachidonic acid mobilization and PGI_2 production.[94] Recent studies have found improved endothelial function and morphology in spontaneous hypertensive rats with a reduction of intimal hyperplasia when ACE inhibitors were used.[95] ACE inhibitors act on substrates other than bradykinin and angiotensin I, including autocoids and enkephalins. The potential role of this class of drug is more properly classed with the antiproliferative agents rather than the proendothelial, and a full discussion of its beneficial effects on the prevention of intimal hyperplasia will be deferred until a later section.

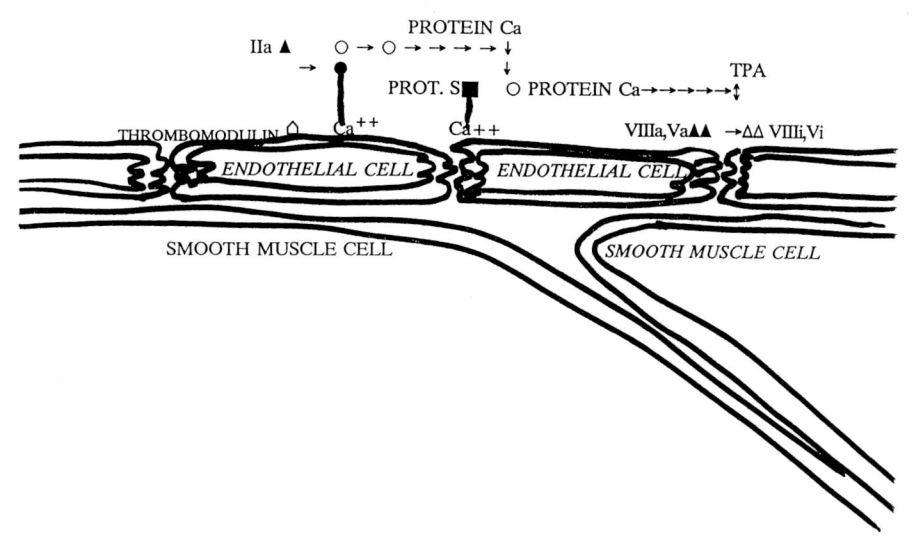

Figure 3-10. Anticoagulant effects of protein C: (1) proteolyzes any active Va or VIIIa; (2) destroys TPA inhibitor.

CALCIUM CHANNEL BLOCKERS

Calcium channel blockers are well known for inhibiting the entry of calcium into muscle cells and for blocking calcium mobilization from intracellular stores. Their effects upon the cardiac function and vascular smooth muscle is well known. However, interference with intracellular calcium stores by experimental calcium channel blockers was at one time thought to preserve the function of EDRF and PGI$_2$ in ECs damaged by atherosclerosis.[96,97] Indeed, verapamil has been shown to inhibit intimal hyperplasia in experimental vein grafts, but no effect was demonstrated on either the endothelium or platelets.[98] Like the ACE inhibitors, calcium channel blockers appear to play a role in preventing intimal hyperplasia, but that role involves more than the endothelium.

DANACRINE (DANZOL)

Danacrine is a weak androgen. Androgens have been shown to directly stimulate erythrocyte colony-forming units (CFU-e)[99] in bone marrow and have been employed for decades in the treatment of chronic renal failure.[100] Recently, there has been some suggestion that Danzol may stimulate the production of protein C.[101] Protein C is a zymogen serine protease that regulates blood coagulation by inactivating thrombin-activated blood coagulation factors V, VII.[102] Protein C, a vitamin-K–dependent protein normally synthesized by the liver, contains a gamma-carboxyglutamic acid residue like vitamin-K–dependent clotting factors. Found in circulating blood, it is bound to EC cell surface phospholipids by calcium bridges. Any thrombin that is diffused away from a vascular injury site and onto EC membranes is attached to thrombomodulin that cleaves and activates protein C molecules bound to the EC surface (figure 3-10). The activated enzyme protease derived from protein C (protein CA) then complexes with protein S and proteolyses any factor VIII: CA and VA that may have diffused away from the injury site. Protein CA also then destroys an inhibitor of TPA. The endothelium, which normally produces anticoagulants and vasodilator, can become procoagulant with the synthesis and activation of factors V and VII[103,104] and the vasoconstrictor endothelin. The hereditary absence of protein C results in life-threatening thrombosis.

HEPARIN

Although heparin is a documented stimulant to EC migration, its major therapeutic benefit appears to ensue from inhibition of SMC migration and proliferation. Therefore, discussion of this drug will be deferred until a later section.

NITRATES

In addition to their effect on platelets, nitrates can improve endothelial dysfunction caused by hypercholesterolemia. The normal EC maintains its own pool of L-arginine just to synthesize EDRF through its metabolism to citrulline.[103] Infusion of L-arginine into the atherosclerotic arteries of 15 patients undergoing cardiac catheterization restored normal endothelial function that had been lost.[104]

TISSUE PLASMINOGEN ACTIVATOR

Tissue plasminogen activator (rTPA) is an extrinsic activator of plasminogen preferentially bound to fibrin. It can be synthesized by ECs and it is certainly important in clot lysis. We have reported its benefit in both access and subclavian thrombolysis.[105] However, long-term patency of hemodialysis accesses preserved by thrombolysis and angioplasty is poor. In one study, only slightly over half were patent at six months,[106] and there is no known effect of rTPA on intimal hyperplasia while that of angioplasty greatly stimulates intimal hyperplasia.

In summary, although we realize that the endothelium appears to play a protective role against intimal hyperplasia, pharmacologic intervention to promote that role has been even less successful than antiplatelet therapy. However, prostacyclin, iliprost, and defibrotide have shown promise in early studies.

Gylocalyx Regulation

In order to understand the mechanisms under which the endothelium can be transformed from a surface preventing coagulation to that of a procoagulant, one must understand that the glycocalyx is a 100-angstrom-thick layer of fibronectin, proteoglycans, collagen, and elastin that acts as a filter and regulatory barrier between the blood and the endothelial membrane.[107] Through this barrier are many fingerlike projections that allow the endothelial membrane direct access to the blood (figure 3-11). They respond to injury by unmasking latent C3b Fc receptors that activate complement and subsequently the coagula-

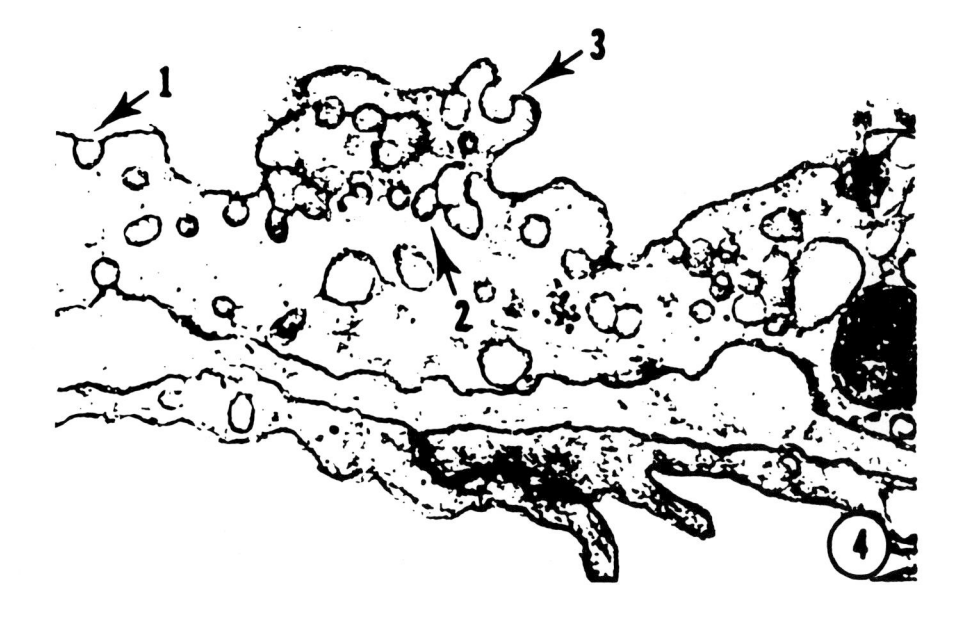

Figure 3-11. The glycocalyx. Arrow signifies a pit (calveola). (Reprinted with permission of Una S. Ryan, Ph.D., and the New York Academy of Science.)

tion cascade and neutrophil adhesion.[108] The degree of injury to invoke these changes is quite slight and undiscernible by most of our crude methods, something that oftentimes presents a problem for the investigation and the use of endothelial-seeded grafts. In addition to the projections are nests of enzymes on the endothelial surface membrane sitting in the pits (caveolae)[107] where only molecules of a particular size are allowed to enter and peculate. Here angiotensin and bradykinin come into contact with the converting enzyme.

Endothelial injury is followed by remodeling of the glycocalyx. Similarly, after the implantation of a new PTFE graft, this also becomes the first phase in construction of a new intima or pseudo-intima. Fibronectin and heparan sulfate, produced by ECs, are thought to be necessary for the growth of a new intima into PTFE grafts. Although canine new intima responds with complete new endothelialization, human intima is always incomplete, resulting in a pseudointima. Although proteoglycans constitute only 5% of the normal vessel dry weight, they become prominent in the extracellular matrix of intimal hyperplasia.[109] Proteoglycans are predominantly chondroitin sulfate, dermatan sulfate, and heparan sulfate. In contrast to ECs that produce heparan sulfate proteoglycan, SMCs produce chondroitin sulfate and dermatin sulfate, which promote cell migration and proliferation.[110,111] As intimal hyperplasia proceeds, the new glycocalyx grows from a normal 100-angstrom size to lumen occlusion, and the proteoglycans are replaced by Type I collagen and elastin from SMCs and fibroblasts.[109] Bringing control of the growth of the glycocalyx back under standard inhibitory factors could conceivably play a major role in preventing lumen occlusion.

COLCHICINE

Colchicine is an alkaloid of the autumn crocus, so named because it was known in ancient times to grow in Colchis in Asia Minor. Known as a poison as early as the sixth century, it was used in experimental biology to arrest spindle formation in metaphase by the beginning of the twentieth century. Its therapeutic effect in gout is by virtue of the inhibition of microtubular formation in leukocytes, preventing ingestion of uric acid crystals and glycoprotein synthesis by leukocytes. Therefore, it became logical to use colchicine to inhibit the glycoprotein overproduction by SMCs in intimal hyperplasia. A few favorable reports have been published on such inhibition in experimental models where vascular injury was induced in the laboratory.[112,113] No studies in dialysis patients have appeared.

HEPARIN

As discussed above, heparan sulfate (which is nearly identical to heparin sulfate in name and chemical structure; its biologic activity differs only in having less anticoagulant potential) constitutes one of the important proteoglycans in the glycocalyx, but there is also evidence that it can influence vascular wall structure and alter the accumulation and distribution of each of the major components of the glycocalyx.[114] Most probably, that effect is mostly mediated through its antiproliferative effect; we will reserve its discussion for that section.

DIMETHYL SULFOXIDE

Controversy has surrounded dimethyl sulfoxide (DMSO) for nearly 30 years since its clinical potential was announced to enhance the cutaneous absorption of topical steroids.[115] Recently, DMSO also has been shown to reduce the secretory organelles in SMCs.[116] It has been shown to decrease glycoprotein reduction in cultured SMCs that may be associated with smooth muscle migration into the intima.[117] In vitro, it appears to interfere with serum growth factors and reverses TPA inhibitors.[118] A possible mechanism for interference with PDGF may be to prevent a PDGF-mediated phosphorylation of nuclear pp64 through serine/threonine and tyrosine pathways.[119] If confirmed, such a mechanism will establish a true place for DMSO in the antiproliferative/antimigratory categories, but

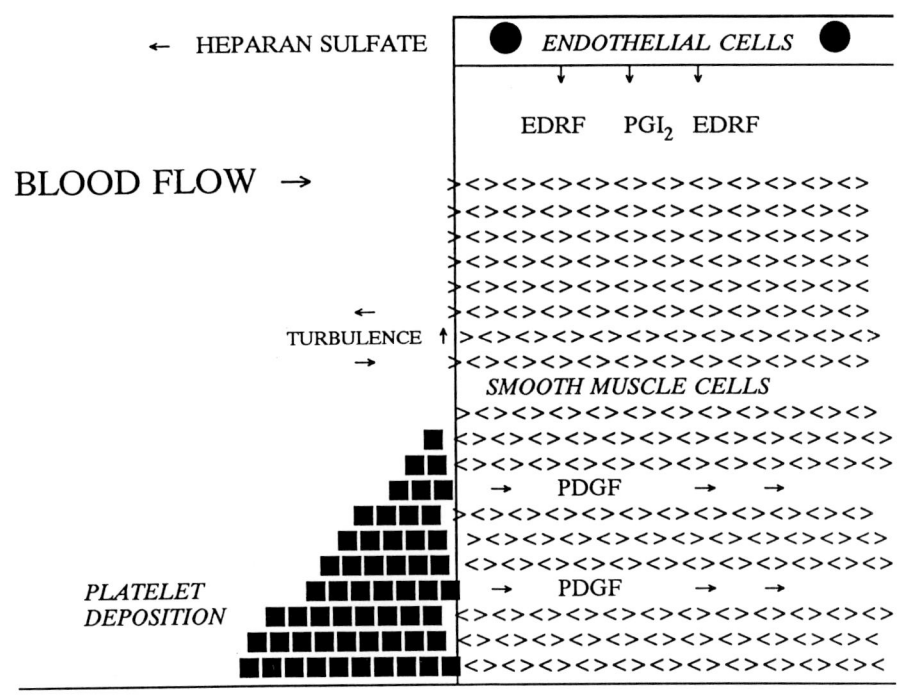

Figure 3-12. Wound healing with formation of pseudointima (deposition of protein, white cells, and monocytes) and neointima (granulation tissue, endothelial proliferation, smooth muscle proliferation, fibroblast proliferation).

at present any role or efficacy of DMSO remains true to the history of the drug—controversial.

FISH OIL

In addition to its many other mechanisms of potentially inhibiting intimal hyperplasia, fish oil may also inhibit proteoglycan synthesis. This, however, is not mediated through EPA, but through vitamin A and retinoids that are found in large quantities in fish oil. Retinoic acid has long been known to affect proteoglycan synthesis, has been used as treatment for keloid overproduction, and has recently been shown to be useful in the treatment of promyelocytic leukemia by inhibiting proteoglycan synthesis.[120] Now it is also being investigated for the overproduction of glycocalyx.[109]

Although several of the agents in this group have exciting theoretical potential, clinical studies of efficacy in hemodialysis patients are lacking. The potential role of any of the agents in this group is unknown.

Antimigratory Agents

After fibronectin has been elaborated onto the new PTFE access, endothelial SMC migration begins (figure 3-12). In dogs, re-endothelialization is complete,

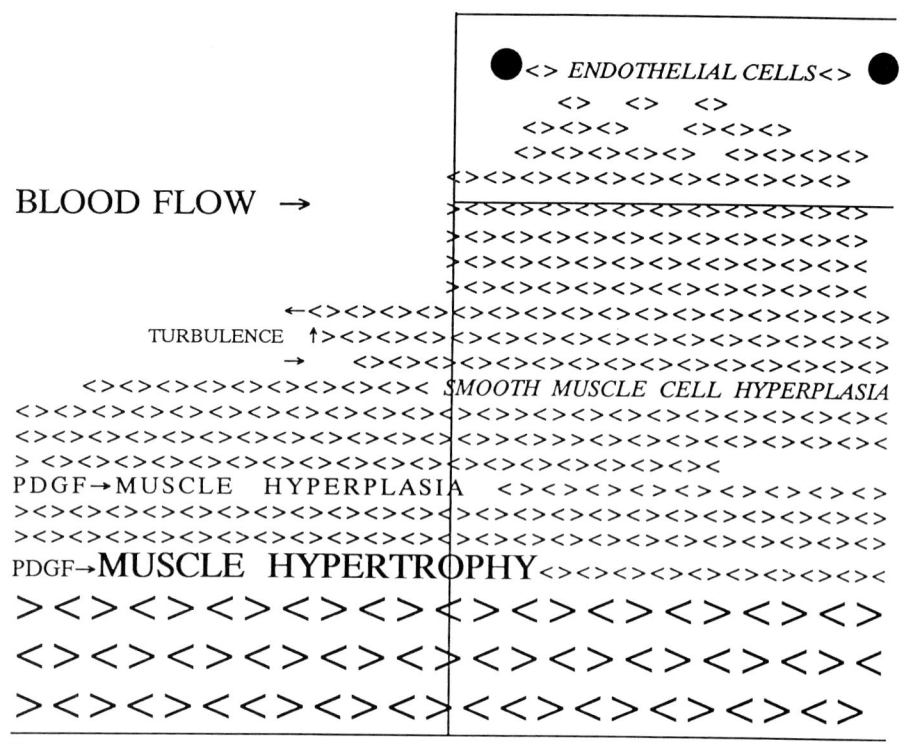

Figure 3-13. Intimal hyperplasia: (1) smooth muscle cell hypertrophy, hyperplasia, and migration; (2) glycocalyx expansion; (3) decreased lumen.

and a new intima is formed; in humans, endothelial migration stops and smooth muscle migration continues. It is the smooth muscle and fibroblasts that elaborate the chondroitin sulfate and dermatin sulfate. Similar events occur after endothelial injury such as angioplasty, which also leads to intimal hyperplasia. In both cases, once SMCs migrate into the neointima, they proliferate and elaborate the proteoglycans, resulting in a thickened intima (figure 3-13). Inhibition of that migration will be discussed in this section, with inhibition of proliferation referred for our final class of agents. However, because migration and proliferation appear to be stimulated by PDGF, a number of agents are common to both groups. Some exert a strong antimigratory effect other than just a generalized PDGF effect. The mechanism by which PDGF accomplishes chemoattraction of SMCs is through a lipoxygenase-derived product, 12-L-hydroxy-5,8,10,14, eicosatetraenoic acid (12HETE).[121] 12HETE is the most powerful chemoattractant known for SMCs. Nakuo was first to show that 12HETE, synthesized by platelets, macrophages, and granulocytes, was the major stimulant to smooth muscle migration after endothelial injury[122] and was responsible for the age-related smooth muscle migration that occurs in atherosclerosis.[122] Hyperglycemia has been shown to increase the effect of 12HETE and may contribute to the promotion of vascular disease in diabetics.[125] Pharmacologic efforts to prevent smooth muscle migration in endothelial injury have been primarily directed against the production of 12HETE by lipoxygenase inhibitors.

EPA

As noted earlier, EPA is a potent inhibitor of PDGF and is a competitive inhibitor of lipoxygenase. Both effects combine to provide antimigratory effects, benefits that have been discussed in prior sections. In addition, we will note only that although EPA inhibits smooth muscle migration, it enhances EC migration, which may be of great benefit for complete endothelialization of human PTFE grafts.[126]

CAFFEIC ACID

Studies of the medicinal effects of the Chinese plant *Artemisia rubrites naki* showed that it contains three specific inhibitors of lipoxygenase. Caffeic acid, the most potent, produced noncompetitive inhibition.[127] Later it was shown to selectively inhibit lipoxygenase but not cyclooxygenase.[128] Furthermore, it has been shown to prevent PDGF release of 12HETE and prevent smooth muscle migration.[129]

CALCIUM CHANNEL BLOCKERS

In addition to their effect on endothelial cells discussed in a previous section, calcium channel blockers have been shown to inhibit SMC migration.[130] In cell culture, SMC migration was initiated by the strong chemoattractant 12HETE and was stimulated by calcium ionophore A23187. Nicardipine inhibited smooth muscle migration. Trifluoperazine, a specific inhibitor of calmodulin, also inhibited 12HETE-induced smooth muscle migration.[130] The results suggest that smooth muscle migration is a highly calcium-dependent process and that the 12HETE might act at the initial stage of migration by enhancing calcium influx through SMC plasma membrane. This indeed may be the mechanism for documented reduction of intimal hyperplasia by verapamil in animal controls.

COLCHICINE

In addition to its effect on glycocalyx regulation, colchicine drastically inhibits 12HETE-induced smooth muscle migration, suggesting that actin-containing microfilaments and microtubules are involved in smooth muscle migration.[130]

GLYCYRRHETINIC ACID

Glycyrrhetinic acid (GRHA) is a licorice derivative known for the mineralocorticoid activity it produces as a result of inhibition of 11B hydroxysteroid dehydrogenase, which catalyzes the conversion of active cortisol to inactive cortisone as it is shuttled through the kidney.[131] Recently, topical GRHA has been used for this effect to prevent cutaneous breakdown of hydrocortisone in an effort to potentiate local inflammatory effect.[132] Similar work has shown that an injury response in the lung can be prevented by GRHA, but ECs may not have the ability to metabolize cortisol in any event, unlike epithelial cells.[133] More important, however, is that GRHA has lipoxygenase-inhibiting properties similar to caffeic acid.[134] This potential holds promise for the use of GRHA as an antimigratory drug, but its effect on cortisol concentration may produce prohibitive side effects.

Antiproliferative Drugs

Once SMCs migrate to the intima from the media, they proliferate and elaborate a thickened glycocalyx with chondroitin sulfate and dermatin sulfate (figure 3-13). This group of agents has been employed to stop smooth muscle proliferation. Again, PDGF is thought to be the major stimulus for the initiation of proliferation, and therefore most agents studied in this category are antimigratory agents as well.

EPA

EPA is a strong antagonist to the effects of PDGF, but it has been extensively discussed in preceding sections.[41,135]

TRIAZOLOPYRIDINE

Triazolopyridine is a pyridine compound similar to dipyridamole that was originally studied as a phosphodiesterase inhibitor and bronchodilator.[136] It was eventually marketed in Japan as a smooth muscle vasodilator and antianginal agent. Because its structure is similar to that of dipyridamole, initial studies focused on antiplatelet activity through PGI_2 and TXA_2, but other studies found that two hours after intravenous administration in rabbits, prostaglandin metabolites returned to normal.[137] Subsequently, it was found to inhibit PDGF-induced smooth muscle proliferation after endothelial injury in mice[138] and Sprague-Dawley rats.[139] Significantly, it reduces intimal hyperplasia in rabbits after angioplasty-induced endothelial injury.[140] One study found it even more successful than aspirin in the inhibition of intimal hyperplasia in a similar model.[141]

One particularly difficult side effect for the ESRD population is a high incidence of gastrointestinal intolerance and vomiting.[142]

ACE INHIBITORS

ACE inhibitors, in addition to their effects on bradykinin and prostacyclin production, also appear to prevent smooth muscle migration. Once angiotensin I (AI) has been converted to angiotensin II (AII) by endothelial-bound enzymes, AII can react with smooth muscle receptors, promoting the well-known vasoconstriction. However, AII also stimulates SMC hypertrophy.[143] The mechanism of AII-induced smooth muscle proliferation appears to occur in multiple steps, including promotion of synthesis of PDGF A chain, TGF-beta thrombospondin, and proto-oncogenes, L-myc and c-fos.[144] All of those effects were inhibited by cilazapril in rats.[144] Similarly, a significant reduction of smooth muscle mitotic activity was found in ramapril-treated rats after balloon angioplasty injury[145] and in captopril-treated New Zealand white rabbits.[146]

However, before we can embrace ACE inhibitors as a new member of our therapeutic armamentarium, a few words of caution are in order. First, in tissue culture, neither cilazapril nor its active metabolite cilazaprilate have had any effect on PDGF-induced smooth muscle proliferation.[147] Furthermore, despite in vivo success in rats and rabbits, recent studies have failed to show any beneficial effect in primates, prompting the investigators to suggest only species-specific benefit.[148]

HEPARIN

In 1916, a medical student investigating ether-soluble anticoagulants made the serendipitous discovery of phospholipid anticoagulant. Shortly thereafter, glycosaminglycan was discovered; it was named heparin because it was found in abundance in the liver. Since that time, heparin has been used for its effect on the clotting cascade and antithrombin III,[149] while effects have been noted on lipoprotein lipase, aldosterone, platelets, and the immune system. As described above, heparan sulfate is secreted by ECs and is an important proteoglycan in the glycocalyx. In fact, heparin appears to regulate the growth of both ECs and SMCs. The actions are diametrically opposed: while stimulating endothelial cell growth, heparin inhibits smooth muscle proliferation[150] and differentiation.[151] Vascular damage releases fibroblast growth factor that binds heparin, thus removing the inhibitor to smooth muscle proliferation while simultaneously eliminating the stimulation of EC growth.[151] As a consequence, the loss of heparin theoretically would both prevent the endothelialization of PTFE grafts while promoting smooth muscle migration into the pseudointima with resulting intimal hyperplasia.

In a number of recent studies, heparin has reduced intimal hyperplasia after vascular access implantation[152] and vascular injury.[153,154] In one human study of 212 infragenicular vein grafts, 16 subjects suffered thrombosis within one month after surgery. Direct infusion of heparin (10 U/min) and nitroglycerin for 52 hours after thrombectomy contributed to prolonged salvage of 80% of the thrombosed vein grafts.[155] In another study, subcutaneous administration of low-molecular-weight heparin also significantly reduced the incidence of intimal hyperplasia.[156] Because the antiproliferative effect appears to be disassociated from the anticoagulant effect, much promise appears in the study of heparin fragments with no anticoagulant hazards.

LOVASTATIN

Lovastatin is a competitive inhibitor of HMG-CoA reductase. This enzyme catalyzes the conversion of HMG-CoA to mevalonate, which is an early and rate-limiting step in the biosynthesis of cholesterol. It is currently marketed as the most successful inhibitor of cholesterol, but because cholesterol is an integral part of the cell membrane, lovastatin is now being investigated as an antiproliferative agent to reverse the effects of PGDF.[157] In tissue culture, it has been demonstrated to inhibit both smooth muscle and endothelial proliferation as well as PGI2 production, but the anti-EC activity occurs above therapeutic dosing.[158] In rabbits with endothelial injury induced by balloon angioplasty, significant reduction of intimal hyperplasia was seen after treatment with lovostatin.[157]

Because there are no clinical studies, we must conclude that the early laboratory investigations suggest promise, but much more work is needed before human studies may begin.

GLUCOCORTICOIDS

Corticoids are well known for their effects on inflammation and therefore have been suggested as a possible treatment for preventing an injury response after angioplasty.[159] In fact, some early tissue culture studies suggested an inhibitory effect of cortisol on smooth muscle proliferation.[160] More recent work, however, has been less sanguine, suggesting that glucocorticoids may promote such insalubrious factors leading to intimal hyperplasia as: (1) inhibition of endothelial production of prostacyclin;[161-163] (2) inhibition of endothelial production of endothelium-dependent relaxation factor;[164] (3) increased endothelin release[165] (which increases PDGF);[166] (4) increased calcium uptake by smooth muscles;[167] and, of course, (5) resultant smooth muscle proliferation.[168]

Although it is doubtful that steroids will play a significant role in preventing long-term thrombosis, we believe that they may indeed play a role in preventing acute thrombosis in patients with an exaggerated allergic response to PTFE material.

KETANSERIN

Ketanserin is a serotonin inhibitor that could just as appropriately been classed with the antiplatelet group, but we have chosen to list it with antiproliferative agents because the serotonin (5-HT) released from platelets (figure 3-1) is a mitogen for smooth muscle.[169,170] Although 5-HT is less potent than PDGF, both are released from the same platelet granule, and 97% of that granular release is accomplished within 40 minutes after attachment of the platelet to the EC. Therefore, as might be expected, ketanserin infusion appears to prevent early—but not late—thrombosis after angioplasty-induced injury.[170]

Although ketanserin has an obvious theoretical benefit, the clinical demonstration is much less apparent.

MISOPROSTOL

Misoprostol is a synthetic prostaglandin E_1 (PGE1) analogue that increases gastric bicarbonate and mucous production; it is used extensively for cytoprotection from ulceration induced by nonsteroidal anti-inflammatory agents. However, recent studies have evaluated vascular protection from cyclosporine-induced damage in the glomerular capillary bed.[171] Because many of its properties are similar to those of PGI2, we could have listed this drug also in the proendothelial section, but more important, PGE1 has been shown to inhibit DNA synthesis in arterial smooth cells stimulated by platelet growth factor[172] while not interfering with EC growth.[173] Therefore, misoprostol sustains the potential of an antiproliferative drug.

Implications for Future Therapy

As has been demonstrated, there is no perfect pharmacologic intervention. If we assume that inhibition of all five phases are equally important, fish oil

Table 3-4. Summary of Drugs Studied to Prevent Intimal Hyperplasia

Drugs	Platelet	Proendo-thelial	Gylcocalyx	Migratory	Proliferative
Fish oil*	✓		✓	✓	✓
Heparin		✓	✓	✓	✓
Nitrates	✓	✓			✓
ACE inhibitors		✓			✓
Calcium channel blockers		✓		✓	
Colchicine			✓	✓	
Pentoxyphylline*	✓				
Aspirin*	✓				
Sulfinpyrazone*	✓				
NSAID	✓				
Ticlopidine*	✓				
Iloprost		✓			
Misoprostel		✓			✓
Defibrotide		✓			
Danacrine		✓			
Caffeic acid				✓	
GHRA				✓	
Triazolopyradine					✓
Lovastatin					✓
Ketanserin					✓

* Only agents studied in hemodialysis vascular accesses

would theoretically be the most effective (table 3-4). However, patient compliance with such large drug doses is very difficult, considering the side effects. We are attempting to develop an intravenous fatty acid emulsion like intralipid or liposyn that is of a fish oil base rather than the respective soybean oil or safflower oil. Such a preparation could be given while the patients are on dialysis in high concentrations, thus eliminating the difficulties with compliance and at the same time providing a nonatherogenic fatty acid emulsion substitute for the intradialytic parenteral nutrition protocols.

Work needs to be continued on the effect of pharmacologic combinations such as topical nitrates applied during dialysis or heparin bound to PTFE, which may be able to promote endothelialization and inhibit myointimal hyperplasia without relying on patient compliance. As shown in the table, although a number of these agents have shown great promise in animal or angioplasty models, very little work has been done in hemodialysis patients. Indeed, only aspirin, sulfinpyrazone, fish oil, and pentoxifylline have been investigated and suggested to be of any benefit. We are only at the beginning of understanding how to design an effective pharmacologic intervention.

References

1. Boyd SJ, Dennis MB, Nogami RT, Cole JJ, Scribner BH. Prophylactic coumadin and AV cannula function. J Appl Physiol 1974; 37:6–7.
2. Wing AJ, Curtis, JR, DeWardener HE. Reduction of clotting of Scribner shunts by long-term anticoagulation. Br Med J 1967; 3:143–45.
3. Biggers JA, Remmers AR, Glassford DM. The risk of anticoagulation in hemodialysis patients. Nephron 1977; 18:109–13.
4. Leonard A, Shapiro FL. Subdural hematoma in regularly hemodialyzed patients. Ann Intern Med 1975; 82:650–58.
5. Brautbar N, Menz CL, Winston MA, Shinanberger JH. Retroperitoneal bleeding in hemodialyzed patients. A cause for morbidity and mortality. JAMA 1978; 239:1530–31.
6. Canadian Coopertive Study Group. A randomized trial of aspirin and sulfinpyrazone in threatened stroke. N Engl J Med 1978; 299:53–59.
7. Harter HR, Burch JW, Majerus PW. Prevention of thrombosis in patients on hemodialysis by low dose aspirin. N Engl J Med 1979; 301:577–79.
8. Glasham RW, Walker F. A histologic examination of Quinton/Scribner shunts. Br J Surg 1968; 55:189–92.
9. Jenkins AM, Buist TAS, Glover SD. Medium term follow-up of forty autogenous venin and forty polytetrafluoroethylene (GORE-TEX) grafts for vascular access. Surgery 1980; 88:667–72.
10. Green RM, Roederscheimer LR, DeWeese JA. Effect of aspirin and dipyridamole on expanded polytetrafluoroethylene graft patency. Surgery 1982; 92:1016–26.
11. McCann RL, Hagen P-O, Fuchs JC. Aspirin and dipyridamole decrease intimal hyperplasia in experimental vein grafts. Ann Surg 1980; 191:238–43.
12. Hagen P-O, Wang Z-G, Mikat EM. Antiplatelet therapy reduces aortic intimal hyperplasia distal to small diameter vascular prostheses (PTFE) in nonhuman primates. Ann Surg 1982; 195:328.
13. Friedman RJ, Stemerman MB, Wenz B, Moore S. The effects of thrombocytopenia on experimental arteriosclerotic lesion formation in rabbits. J Clin Invest 1977; 60:1191–1201.
14. Moncada S, Gryglewski R, Bunting S, Vane JR. An enzyme isolated from arteries transforms prostaglandin endoperoxides to an unstable substance that inhibits platelet aggregation. Nature 1976; 263:663–65.
15. Van der Ouderaa FJ, Buytenhek M, Nugteren DH, Vandorp DA. Acetylation of prostaglandin endoperoxide synthetase with acetylsalicylic acid. Eur J Biochem 1980; 109:1–8.
16. Willis AL, Smith DL, Vigo C, Kluge AF. Effects of prostacyclin and orally active stable mimetic agent RS-93472-007 on basic mechanisms of atherosclerosis. Lancet 1986; 2:682–83.
17. Dyerberg J, Bang HO, Stofferson E. Eicosapentaenoic acid and prevention of thrombosis. Lancet 1978; 2:117.
18. Rylance PB, Gordge MP, Saynor R, Parson V, Weston MJ. Fish oil modifies lipids and reduces platelet aggregability in hemodialysis patients. Nephron 1986; 43:196–202.
19. Landymore RW, Macaulay MA, Cooper JH. Effects of cod liver oil on intimal hyperplasia in vein grafts used for arterial bypass. Can J Surg 1986; 29:129–131.
20. Landymore RW, Kinley CE, Cooper JH. Cod liver oil for prevention of intimal hyperplasia of autogenous vein grafts used for arterial bypass. J Thorac Cardiovasc Surg 1985; 89:351–57.

21. Cahill PD, Sarris GE, Cooper AD. Inhibition of vein graft intimal thickening by eicosapentaenoic acid: Reduced thromboxane production without change in lipoprotein levels or low density lipoprotein density. J Vasc Surg 1988; 7:108-118.
22. Diskin CJ, Lock S, Tanja J. Intradialytic fish oil to decrease intimal hyperplasia (abst). Eur Dialysis & Transplant Assoc 1989; 160.
23. Graham LM, Brother TE, Vincent CK. The effect of duration of acetylsalicylic acid administration on patency and anastomotic hyperplasia of PTFE grafts (abst). Trans Am Soc Artif Intern Organs 1989; 35:83.
24. Endean ED, Boorstein JM, Hees PL, Cronenwett JL. Effect of thromboxane synthetase inhibition on canine autogenous vein grafts. J Surg Res 1986; 40:297-304.
25. Diskin CJ, Thomas CE, Zellner CP, Lock S, Tanja J. Fish oil to prevent intimal hyperplasia and access thrombosis. Nephron 1990; 55:445-47.
26. Boyle JM, Johnston B. Acute upper gastrointestinal hemorrhage in patients with chronic renal disease. Am J Med 1983; 75:409-12.
27. Hasegawa T, Hasegawa S, Fukushima K, Watanabe N, Yokoyama H. Prosthetic replacement of the superior vena cava treated with antiplatelet agents. Surgery 1987; 102:498-506.
28. Chesebro JH, Fuster V, Elveback LR. Effect of dipyridamole and aspirin on late vein-graft patency after coronary artery bypass operations. N Engl J Med 1984; 310:209-14.
29. Brothers TE, Vincent CK, Darvishan D. Effects of duration of acetylsalicylic administration on patency and anastomotic hyperplasia of ePTFE grafts. Trans Am Soc Artif Intern Organs 1989; 35:558-60.
30. Gershlick AH, Syndercombe-Court YD, Murday AJ, Lewis CT, Mills PG. Adverse effects of high dose aspirin on platelet adhesion to experimental autogenous vein grafts. Cardiovasc Res 1985; 19:770-76.
31. Gershlick AH, Syndercombe-Court YD, Murday AJ, Lewis CT, Mills PG. Activation of platelets by autogenous vein grafts is not prevented by acetylsalicylic acid and dipyridamole. Cardiovasc Res 1984; 18:391-396.
32. Shimokawa H, Lam JY, Chesebro JH. Effects of dietary supplementation with cod liver oil on endothelium dependent responses in porcine coronary arteries. Circulation 1987; 76:898-905.
33. Boulanger C, Schini VB, Hendrickson H, Vanhoutte PM. Chronic exposure of endothelial cells to eicosapentaenoic acid potentiates endothelium derived relaxation factor. Br J Pharmacol 1990; 99:176-81.
34. Furlong B, Henderson AH, Lewis MJ, Smith JA. Endothelium dependent relaxation factor inhibits in vitro platelet aggregation. Br J Pharmacol 1987; 90:687-92.
35. Radomski MW, Palmer RMJ, Moncada S. The anti-aggregating properties of vascular endothelium: Interactions between prostacyclin and nitric oxide. Br J Pharmacol 1987; 92:639-46.
36. Radomski MW, Palmer RMJ, Moncada S. Comparative pharmacology of endothelium dependent relaxation factor, nitric oxide and prostacyclin synthesis in platelets. Br J Pharmacol 1987; 92:181-87.
37. Radomski MW, Palmer RMJ, Moncada S. The role of nitric oxide and cGMP in platelet adhesion to vascular endothelium. Biochem Biophys Res Commun 1987; 148:1482-89.
38. Moncada S, Radomski MW, Palmer RMJ. Endothelium derived relaxation factor. Identification as nitric oxide and role in control of vascular tone and platelet function. Bio Pharmacol 1988; 37:2495-2501.
39. Libby P, Warner SJC, Salomon RN, Birniyi LK. Production of platelet derived growth factor-like mitogen by smooth muscle cells from human atheroma. N Engl J Med 1988; 318:1493-98.
40. Leibovich SJ, Ross R. A macrophage dependent factor that stimulates the proliferation of fibroblast in vitro. Am J Pathol 1976; 84:501-13.
41. Fox PL, Dicorleto PE. Fish oils inhibit endothelial production of platelet derived growth factor-like protein. Science 1988; 241:453-56.
42. Vanacker BAC, Bilo HJB, Popp-Snijders C. The effect of fish oil on lipid profile and viscosity of erythrocyte suspensions in CAPD patients. Nephrol Dial Transplant 1988; 2:557-61.
43. Bevilaqua MP, Pober JS, Majeau GR, Cotran RS, Gimbrone MA. Interleukin I induces biosynthesis

and cell surface expression of procoagulant activity in human vascular endothelial cells. J Exp Med 1984; 160:618–23.
44. Cotran RS, Pober JS. Cytokine-endothelial interaction in inflammation, immunity and vascular injury. J Am Soc Nephrol 1990; 1:225–35.
45. Dehmer GJ, Popma JJ, Vandenberg EK, Eichhorn EJ. Reduction in rate of early stenosis after coronary angioplasty by a diet supplemented with n-3 fatty acids. N Engl J Med 1988; 319:733–38.
46. Milner MR, Gallino RA, Leffingwell A, Pichard AD. Usefulness of fish oil supplements in preventing clinical evidence of restenosis after percutaneous transluminal coronary angioplasty. Am J Cardiol 1989; 64:294–99.
47. Reis GJ, Boucher TM, Sipperly ME, Silverman DI. Randomized trial of fish oil for prevention of restenosis after coronary angioplasty. Lancet 1989; 2:177–81.
48. Grigg LL, Kay TWH, Valentine PA. Determinants of restenosis and lack of effect of dietary supplementation with eicosapetaenoic acid on the incidence of coronary artery restenosis after angioplasty. J Am Coll Cardiol 1989; 13:665–72.
49. Dinarello CA. The endogenous pyrogens in host defense interactions. Hosp Prac 1989; 24:121–128.
50. Endres S, Ghorbani R, Kelley VE, Georgilis K. The effect of dietary supplementation with n-3 polyunsaturated acids on the synthesis of interleukin 1 and tumor necrosis factor by mononuclear cells. N Engl J Med 1989; 320:265–271.
51. Diskin CJ, Ravis W, Capagna KD, Clark CR. Pharmacokinetics of sulindac in ESRD. Nephron 1988; 50:397.
52. Remuzzi G, Marchesi D, Schiepeti A, Poletti E. Aspirin and thrombosis in patients undergoing hemodialysis. N Engl J Med 1980; 302:1420–21.
53. Kaegi A, Pineo GF, Shimizu A. Arteriovenous shunt thrombosis. N Engl J Med 1974; 290:304–06.
54. Kohler H. Prophylaxis of shunt thrombosis in terminal renal insufficiency. Klin Wochenschr 1977; 55:49–56.
55. Mitchie DD, Wombolt DG. Use of sulfinpyrazone to prevent shunt thrombosis in arteriovenous fistula and bovine grafts of patients on chronic hemodialysis. Curr Ther Res 1977; 22:196–204.
56. Dmoszynski-Gianopoulou A, Janika L, Sokowska B, Ksia zek A. The effect of sulfinpyrazone and alpha tocopherol on platelet activation and function in hemodialyzed patients. Int Urol Nephrol 1990; 22:561–66.
57. Ritchie JL, Lindner A, Hamilton GW, Harker LA. In 111-oxine platelet imaging in hemodialyzed patients; detection of platelet deposition at access site. Nephron 1982; 31:333–36.
58. Dewanjee MK, Pumphrey CW, Murphy KP, Rosemark JA. Evaluation of platelet inhibiter drugs in a canine bilateral femoral graft implant model. Trans Am Soc Artif Intern Organs 1982; 28:504–13.
59. Koepesky KR, Dewanjee MK, Lim MF. The effect of ibuprofen on platelet depostion in GORE-TEX and autogenous vein grafts. Am J Cardiol 1981; 47:455.
60. Claus PL, Gloviczki P, Hollier LH. Patency of polytetrafluoroethylene microarterial prostheses improved by ibuprofen. Am J Surg 1986; 144:180–85.
61. Gloviczki P, Hollier LH, Dewanjee MK, Trastek VK. Quantitative evaluation of ibuprofen treatment on the thrombogenicity of expanded polytetrafluoroethylene vascular grafts. Surgery 1984; 95:160–68.
62. Narayanan S. Inhibition of in vitro platelet inhibition and release and fibrinolysis. Clin Lab Sci 1989; 19:260–65.
63. Parker MT, Turrentine MA, Johnson GS. VonWillebrand factor in lysates of washed canine platelet. Am J Vet Res 1991; 52:119–25.
64. Huang ZS, Lee TK. Comparison of in vitro platelet aggregation and its inhibition by three antithrombotic drugs between human and guinea pig. Proc Natl Sci Counc Rep China 1991; 15:8–14.
65. Raithel D. Prevention of re-occulusion after prosthetic bypass operations in the femoro-popliteal region: A comparative study of pentoxifylline versus acetylsalicylic acid. Vasc Surg 1987; 208–14.
66. Lucas M. Prevention of post-operative thrombosis in peripheral arteriopathies. Pentoxifylline vs. conventional antiaggregants: A six-month randomized follow-up study. Angiology 1984; 35:443–50.
67. Weithman KU, Just M, Schlotte V, Seiffge D. Stimulatory effects of vascular prostaglandins on the

antiaggregatory activities of pentoxifylline-acetylsalicylic acid combinations in vitro. Vasa 1989; 18:273-76.
68. Schroer RH. Antithrombotic potential of pentoxifylline. A hemorrheologically active drug. Angiology 1985; 36:387-98.
69. Weithman KU. Reduced platelet aggregation by pentoxifylline stimulated prostacyclin release. Vasa 1981; 10:249-52.
70. Radmilovic A, Boric Z, Naumovic T, Stamenkovic M, Musikic P. Shunt thrombosis prevention in hemodialysis patients—double blind, randomized study: Pentoxifylline vs placebo. Angiology 1987; 38:499-506.
71. Saltiel E, Ward A. Ticlopidine: A review of its pharmacodynamic and pharmacokinetics properties, and therapeutic efficacy in platelet-dependent disease states. Drugs 1987; 34:222-62.
72. Orlando E, Cortelsazzo S, Nosari I. Inhibition of ticlopidine of platelet adhesion to human venous subendothelium in patients with diabetes. J Lab Clin Med 1988; 112:583-88.
73. Mirsen TR, Hachinskin VC. Transient ischemic attacks and stroke. Can Med Assoc J 1988; 138:1099-1105.
74. Palareti G, Poggi M, Torricelli P, Balesti V. Long-term effects of ticlopidine on fibrinogen and haemorheology in patients with peripheral vascular disease. Thromb Res 1988; 52:626-29.
75. Balsano F, Coccheri S, Librettit A. Ticlopidine in the treatment of intermittent claudication. J Lab Clin Med 1989; 114:84-91.
76. Janzon L, Bergqvist D, Boberys J. Ticlopidine an updated review of its pharmacology and therapeutic use. Drugs 1990; 40:238-59.
77. Hirosumi J, Nomoto A, Ohkubo Y, Sekiguchi C. Inflammatory responses in cuff induced atherosclerosis in rabbits. Artherosclerosis 1987; 645:243-54.
78. Courbier R. Basis for an international classification of cerebral arterial diseases. J Vasc Surg 1986; 4:179-83.
79. Itoh T, Shiba E, Kambayashi J, Watese M. The pathogenesis of thrombosis in venous prostheses. Eur J Vasc Surg 1990; 4:625-31.
80. Grontoft KC, Mulec H, Gutierrez A, Olander R. Thromboprophylactic effect of ticlopidine in arteriovenous fistulas for hemodialysis. Scand J Urol Nephrol 1985; 19:55-57.
81. Kobayashi K, Maeda K, Koshikawa S, Kawaguchi Y. Antithrombotic therapy with ticlopidine in chronic renal failure patients on chronic maintenance hemodialysis—a multicenter collaborative double blind study. Thromb Res 1980; 20:255-61.
82. Graham LM, Brothers TE, Vincent CK, Burkel WE, Stanley JC. The role of endothelial cell lining in limiting distal anastomotic intimal hyperplasia. J Biomed Mater Res 1991; 25:525-33.
83. Tateson JE, Moncada S, Vane JR. Effects of prostacylin on cyclic AMP concentrations in human platelets. Prostaglandins 1977; 13:389-97.
84. Piper P, Vane Jr. The release of prostaglandins from the lung and other tissues. Ann NY Acad Sci 1971; 180:363-85.
85. Forsberg EJ, Feurstein G, Shohami E, Pollard HB. Adenosine triphosphate stimulates inositol phospholipid metabolism and prostacyclin formation in adrenal medullary endothelial cells by means of P2 purinergic receptors. Proc Natl Acad Sci USA 1987; 84:5630-34.
86. Dadak CH, Leitner C, Sinzinger H, Silberbauer K. Diminished prostacylin formation from the endothelium of umbilical arteries in babies born to women who smoke. Lancet 1981; 1:94.
87. Sinzinger H, Fitscha P, Wagner O, Kaliman J. Prostaglandin E1 decreases activity of arterial smooth muscle cells. Lancet 1986; 2:186-87.
88. Niada R, Mantovani M, Prino G, Pescador R. Antithrombotic activity of a polydeoxyribonucleotidic substance extracted from mammalian organs: A possible link to prostacyclin. Thromb Res 1981; 23:233-46.
89. Ulutin ON, Tunali H, Ugur MS. Effect of defibrotide in electrically induced thrombosis in dogs. Haemostasis 1986; 16 (suppl) 1:9-12.
90. Bonomini V, Vangelista A, Stefoni S, Scolari MP. Use of defibrotide in renal transplantation in man. Haemostasis 1986; 16: (suppl) 1:48-50.

91. Grosso P, Martello L, Petrini PL, Massei R. Prevention of vena caval thrombosis in catheterization: Comparison of calciheparin and defibrotide. Minerva Anestesiol 1989; 55:273–276.
92. Bonomini V, Vagelista A, Frasca G. A new antithrombotic agent in the treatment of acute renal failure due to hemolytic-uremic syndrome and thrombotic thrombocytopenic purpura. Nephron 1984; 37:144.
93. Rigotti P, Amodio P, Sacerdoti D, Ferraresso D, Borsato M. Effects of defibrotide on renal function and urinary prostanoid excretion. Nephron 1991; 59:477–81.
94. Crutchley DJ, Ryan JW, Ryan US, Fisher GH. Bradykinin-induced release of prostacyclin from bovine pulmonary artery endothelial cells. Biochim Biophys Acta 1983; 753:99–107.
95. Clozel M, Kuhn H, Hefti F. Effects of angiotensin converting enzyme inhibitors and hydralazine on endothelial function in the spontaneous hypertensive rat. Hypertension 1990; 16:541–43.
96. Habib JB, Bossaller C, Wells S. Preservation of endothelium dependent relaxation factor in cholesterol fed rabbits by treating with calcium channel blocker PN 200110. Circ Res 1986; 58:305–09.
97. Long CJ, Stone TW. The release of endothelium relaxation factor is calcium dependent. Blood Vessels 1985; 22:205–08.
98. El-Sanadiki MN, Cross KS, Murray JJ, Schuman RW. Reduction of intimal hyperplasia and enhanced reactivity of experimental vein bypass grafts with verapamil treatment. Ann Surg 1990; 212:87–96.
99. McGonigle RJ, Wallin JD, Shadduck RK, Fisher JW. Erythropoietin deficiency and inhibition of erythropoiesis in renal insufficiency. Kidney Int 1984; 25:437–44.
100. Lindholm DD, Fisher JW, Viera JA, Dombeck DH. Clinical effects of oral methoxymesterone in patients with dialysis controlled uremia. Trans Am Soc Artif Intern Organs 1973; 19:475–83.
101. Gonzalez R, Alberca I, Sala N, Vincente V. Protein C deficiency-response to Danzol and DDAVP. Thromb Haemost 1985; 53:320–22.
102. Matsuda M, Sugo T, Sakata Y, Murayama H. A thrombotic state due to an abnormal protein C. N Engl Med 1988; 319:1265–68.
103. Cerveny J, Fass DN, Mann KG. Synthesis of coagulation factor by cultured aortic endothelium. Blood 1984; 63:1467-74.
104. Rogers GM, Schuman MA. Prothrombin is activated on vascular endothelial cells by factor Xa and calcium. Proc Natl Acad Sci USA 1983; 80:7001-05.
105. Moncada S, Palmer RMJ, Higgs EA. Biosynthesis of nitric oxide from L-arginine. Nature 1987; 327:425–26.
106. Drexler H, Zeiher AM, Meinzer K, Just H. Correction of endothelial dysfunction in microcirculation of hypercholesterolemic patients by L-arginine. Lancet 1991; 338:1546–50.
107. Diskin CJ, Thomas CE, Lock S, Campagna KD. Subclavian vein thrombosis treated with recombinant tissue plasminogen activator. Nephrol Dial Transplant 1990; 5:400–02.
108. Davis GB, Dowd CF, Bookstein JJ, Lang EV, Halasz N. Thrombosed dialysis grafts. AJR 1987; 149:177–81.
109. Ryan US, Ryan JW. The ultrastructural basis of endothelial surface functions. Biorheology 1984; 21:155–70.
110. Ryan US. Immunologic properties of endothelial cells. Trans Am Soc Artif Intern Organs 1985; 8:58–64.
111. Forrester JS, Fishbein M, Helfant R, Fagin J. A paradigm for restenosis based on cell biology: Clues for the development of new therapies. J Am Coll Cardiol 1991; 17:758–69.
112. Wight TN. Cell biology of arterial proteoglycans. Arteriosclerosis 1989; 9:1–20.
113. Bassols A, Massague J. Transforming growth factor beta regulates the expression and structure of extracellular matrix chondroitin/dermatan sulfate proteoglycans. J Biol Chem 1986; 263:3039–45.
114. Chaldakov GN. Antitubulins—a new therapeutic approach for atherosclerosis. Atherosclerosis 1982; 44:385–90.
115. Chaldakov GN, Vankov VN. Morphological aspects of secretion in the arterial smooth muscle cell, with special refernece to Golgi complex and microtubular cytoskeleton. Atherosclerosis 1986; 61:175–92.

116. Kuncl RW, Duncan G, Watson D, Anderson K. Colchicine myopathy and neuropathy. N Engl J Med 1987; 316:1562–68.
117. Stroughton RB, Fritsch W. Influence of dimethylsulfoxide on human percutaneous absorption. Arch Dermatol 1964; 90:512–14.
118. Katsuda S, Okada Y, Nakanishi I, Tanaka J. Inhibitory effect of dimethyl sulfoxide on the proliferation of cultured arterial smooth muscle cells. Exp Mol Pathol 1988; 48:48–58.
119. Okada Y, Katsuda S, Matsui Y, Minamoto T, Nakanishi I. Altered synthesis of collagen types in cultured arterial smooth muscle cells during phenotypic modulation by dimethyl sulfoxide. Acta Pathol Japn 1989; 39:15–22.
120. Nagashunmugan T, Srinivas S, Shanmugan G. Effect of DMSO on mouse embryo fibroblasts: Inhibition of plasminogen activator inhibitor deposition and interference with early events of serum stimulated growth factors. Biol Cell 1989; 66:307–15.
121. Shawver LK, Duel TF. Nuclear pp64 is phosphorylated in both serine/threonine and tryosine through complex pathways regulated by 12-0-tetradecanoylphorbol-13-acetate and platelet derived growth factor. Biochem Biophys Commun 1990; 167:918–26.
122. Warrell RP, Frankel SR, Miller WH, Scheinberg DA, Itri LM. Differentiation of acute promyelocytic leukemia with trentinoin (ALL transretinoic acid). N Engl J Med 1991; 324:1385–93.
123. Nakao J, Ito H, Chang WC, Koshihara Y, Murota S. Aortic smooth muscle migration caused by platelet derived growth factor is mediated by lipoxygenase products of arachidonic acid. Biochem Biophys Res Commun 1983; 112:866–71.
124. Nakao J, Ooyama T, Ito H, Chang WC, Murota S. Comparative effects of lipoxygenase products of arachidonic acid on rat smooth muscle cell migration. Atherosclerosis 1982; 44:339–42.
125. Nakao J, Ito H, Kanayasu T, Murota S. Stimulatory effect of insulin on aortic smooth muscle cell migration induced by 12-L-hydroxy-5,8,10,14, eicosatetraenoic acid and its modulation by elevated extracellular glucose levels. Diabetes 1985; 34:185.
126. Kanayasu T, Morita I, Nakao-Hayashi J, Ito H, Murota S. Enhancement of migration in bovine endothelial cells by eicosapentaenoic acid pretreatment. Atherosclerosis 1991; 87:57-64.
127. Koshihara Y, Neichi T, Murota S, Lao A. Selective inhibition of 5 lipoxygenase by natural compounds isolated from Chinese plants, Artemisia rubripes Nakai. FEBS Lett 1983; 158:41-44.
128. Koshihara Y, Neichi T, Murota S, Lao A. Caffeic acid is a selective inhibitor of leukotriene biosynthesis. Biochim Biophys Acta 1984; 792:92-97.
129. Nakao J, Koshihara Y, Ito H, Murota S, Chang WC. Enhancement of endogenous production of 12-L-hydroxy5,8,10,14-eicosatetranoic acid in aortic smooth muscle by platelet derived growth factor. Life Sci 1986; 37:1435-42.
130. Nakao J, Ito H, Ooyama Y, Chang WC, Murota S. Calcium dependency of aortic smooth muscle migration induced by 12-L-hydroxy-5,8,10,14, eicosatetraenoic acid. Effect of A23187, nicardipine, and trifluoperazine. Atherosclerosis 1983; 46:309-19.
131. Farese RV, Boglieri EG, Shacleton CHL, Irony I, Gomez-Fontes R. Licorice-induced hypermineralocorticoidism. N Engl J Med 1991; 325:1223-27.
132. Teelucksingh S, Mackie ADR, Burt D, Mcintyre MA. The potentiation of hydrocortisone activity in the skin by glycyrrhetinic acid. Lancet 1990; 33:1060-63.
133. Schleimer RP. Potential regulation of inflammation in the lung by local metabolism of hydrocortisone. Am J Respir Cell Mol Biol 1991; 4:166-173.
134. Inoue H, Saito H, Koshihara Y, Murota S. Inhibitory effect of glycyrrhetinic acid derivatives on lipoxygenase and prostaglandin synthesis. Chem Pharm Bull 1986; 34:897-901.
135. Painter TA. Myointimal hyperplasia: pathogenesis and implications. Artif Organs 1991; 15:42-55.
136. Davies GE. Antibronchoconstricter activity of two new phosphodiesterase inhibitors, a triazolopyazine (ICI 58 301) and trizolopyrimidine (ICI 63 197). J Pharm Pharmacol 1973; 25:681-89.
137. Block HU, Hoffman-Henroth I, Taube C, Neibisch M, Mest HJ. Inhibition of thromboxane B2 formation of blood platelets by trapidil. Prostaglandins Leukot Med 1987; 30:77-86.
138. Ohnishi H, Yamaguchi K, Shimada S, Suzuki Y, Kamagai A. A new approach to atherosclerosis and trapidil as an antagonist to platelet derived growth factor. Life Sci 1981; 28:1641-46.

139. Tiel M, Sussman II, Gordon PB, Saunders RN. Suppression of fibroblast proliferation in vitro and myointimal hyperplasia in vivo by triazolopyrimidine. Artery 1983: 12:33-50.
140. Liu MW, Roubin GS, Robinson KA, Black AJR. Trapidil in preventing restenosis after balloon angioplasty in the atherosclerotic rabbit. Circulation 1990; 81:1089-93.
141. Liu MW, Roubin GS, Robinson KA, and Black AJR. Trapidil: A platelet-derived growth factor antagonist in preventing re-stenosis after balloon angioplasty in the atherosclerotic rabbit. Circulation 1988; 78 (suppl II):290.
142. Akahori F, Ichimura T, Masaoka T, Arai S. Emetic effect of triazolopyrimidine, a pyrimidine compound, in dogs. Vet Hum Toxicol 1985; 27:381-85.
143. Geisterfer AA, Peach MJ, Owens GK. Angiotensin produces hypertrophy, not hyperplasia of aortic smooth muscle cells. Circ Res 1988; 62:749-56.
144. Powell JS, Rouge M, Muller RK, Baumgartener HR. Cilazapril suppresses myointimal hyperplasia after vascular injury: Effects on growth factor induction in vascular smooth muscle cells. Basic Res Cardiol 1991; 86 (suppl 1):65-77.
145. Capron L, Heudes D, Chajara A, Bruneval P. Effect of Rampril, a converting enzyme inhibitor, on the response of rat thoracic aorta to injury with a balloon catheter. J Cardiovasc Pharmacol 1991; 18:207-11.
146. O'Donohoe MK, Schwartz LB, Radic ZS, Mikat EM. Chronic ACE inhibition reduces intimal hyperplasia in experimental vein grafts. Ann Surg 1991; 214:727-32.
147. Powell JS, Muller RK, Kuhn H. The proliferative response to vascular injury is suppressed by angiotensin-converting enzyme inhibition. J Cardiovasc Pharmacol 1990; 16 (suppl 4):S42-S49.
148. Hanson SR, Powell JS, Dodson T, Lumsden A, Kelly AB. Effect of angiotensin-converting enzyme inhibition with cilazapril on intimal hyperplasia in injured arteries and vascular grafts in the baboon. Hypertension 1991; 18 (suppl II):70-76.
149. Diskin CJ, Weitberg A. Minidose heparin therapy. Arch Intern Med 1980; 140:263-66.
150. Hammele H, Betz E, Herr D. Human endothelial cells are stimulated and smooth muscle cells are inhibited in their proliferation and migration by heparins. Vasa 1991; 20:207-15.
151. Bjornsson TD, Dryjski M, Tluczek J, Mennie R. Acidic fibroblast growth factor promotes vascular repair. Proc Nat Acad Sci USA 1991; 88:8651-55.
152. Hirsch GM, Karnovsky MJ. Inhibition of vein graft intimal hyperplasia lesions in the rat by heparin. Am J Pathol 1991; 139:581-87.
153. Seuter F, Bayer AG. Pharmacologic inhibition of experimental atherosclerosis. Z Kardiol 1989; 78 (suppl 6):117-19.
154. Norman PE, House AK. Heparin reduces intimal hyperplasia seen in microvascular vein grafts. Aust NZ J Surg 1991; 61:942-48.
155. Walsh DB, Zwolak RM, McDaniel MD, Scheinder JR, Cronenwett JL. Intragraft drug infusion as adjunct to balloon catheter for salvage of thrombosed infragenicular vein graft. J Vasc Surg 1990; 11:753-59.
156. Wilson NV, Salisbury JR, Kakkar VV. Effect of low molecular heparin on intimal hyperplasia. Br J Surg 1991; 78:1381-83
157. Gellman J, Ezekowitz MD, Sarembock AA, Azrin MA. Effect of lovastatin on intimal hyperplasia after balloon angioplasty: A study in hypercholesterolemic rabbit. J Am Coll Cardiol 1991; 17:251-59.
158. Falke P, Mattiasson I, Stavenow L, Hood B. Effects of competitive inhibiter of 3-hydroxy-3 methylglutaryl coenzyme A reductase on human and bovine endothelial cells, fibroblasts, and smooth muscle cells in vitro. Pharmacol Toxicol 1989; 64:173-76.
159. Liu MW, Roubin GS, King SB. Restenosis after coronary angioplasty. Potential biologic determinants and role of intimal hyperplasia. Circulation 1989; 79:1374-87.
160. Jarvelinen H, Halme T, Rnnemaa T. Effect of cortisol on proliferation and smooth muscle synthesis of human aortic smooth muscle cells in culture. Acta Med Scand 1982: 660:114-22.
161. Baily JM. Glucocorticoids inhibit prostacyclin synthesis in endothelial cells. Biofactors 1991; 3:97-102.

162. Medow MS, Intrieri L, Moatter T, Gerritsen ME. Dexamethasone effects on microvascular endothelial cell lipid composition. Am J Physiol 1989; 257:512-19.
163. Fujimoto M, Sakata T, Tsruta Y, Iwagami S, Teraoka H. Glucocorticoid treatment reduces prostacyclin synthesis in response to limited stimuli. Thromb Res 1991; 61:11-21.
164. Radomski MW, Palmer RM, Moncada S. Glucocorticoids inhibit the expression of an inducible but not the constitutive nitric oxide synthesis in vascular endothelial cells. Proc Nat Acad Sci USA 1990; 87:10043-47.
165. Kanse SM, Takahashi K, Warren JB, Ghatei M, Bloom SR. Glucocorticoids induce endothelin release from vascular smooth muscle but not endothelial cells. Eur J Pharmacol 1992; 199:99-101.
166. Jaffer FA, Knauss TC, Poptic E, Abbound HA. Endothelin stimulates PDGF in cultured human mesangial cells. Kidney Int 1990; 38:1193-98.
167. Hayashi T, Nakai T, Miyabo S. Glucocorticoids increase CA2+ uptake and [3H] dihydropyridine binding in A7r5 vascular smooth muscle cells. Am J Physiol 1990; 261:C106-C114.
168. Yashunari K, Kohno M, Balmforth A, Murakawa K. Glucocorticoids and dopamine 1 receptors on vascular smooth muscle cells. Hypertension 1990; 13:575-81.
169. Clowes AW, Reidy MA, Clowes MM. Mechanism of stenosis after arterial injury. Lab Invest 1983; 49:208-15.
170. Nemecek GM, Coughlin SR. Stimulation of smooth muscle mitogenesiss by serotonin. Proc Nat Acad Sci USA 1990; 83:674-78.
171. Moran M, Mozes MF, Maddux MS, Veremis S. Prevention of acute graft rejection by the prostaglandin E1 analogue misoprostol in renal transplant recipients treated with cyclosporine and prednisone. N Engl J Med 1990; 322:1183-88.
172. Nilsson J, Olsson AG. Prostaglandin E1 inhibits DNA synthesis in arterial smooth muscle cells stimulated by platelet-derived growth factor. Atherosclerosis 1984; 53:77-82.
173. Patrice T, Harb J, Foultier MT, Berrada A. Endothelial growth regulation by PE1 analogue misoprostol and indomethacin. Dig Dis Sci 1989; 34: 1681-85.

PANEL DISCUSSION

Moderator:
  Mitchell L. Henry, M.D.
Panelists:
  Charles J. Diskin, M.D.
  Mark F. Fillinger, M.D.
  J. Michael Lazarus, M.D.

Discussant: Dr. Lazarus, I heard from you that we are having problems with increasing graft failures. You spent a great deal of time defending EPO and telling us this is not causing the graft failures, but you really didn't give us a clue as to what you really think is causing the graft failures. I feel that you probably have to have some idea, having looked at the data this long. The second item I would like for you to address is the concept of the increasing pressures of high-flux dialysis that are being used in your units. We have heard today that intimal hyperplasia is the major cause of graft failure. Increased flows result in hemodynamic abnormalities that cause tissue injury. What do you think about the increasing flows that are being used in dialysis units, and do you think this is one of the reasons we are seeing increasing problems with the grafts?

Dr. Lazarus: As I said at the beginning of my talk, it is not clear to me why we are seeing this sudden burst of increased hospitalization for accesses since 1989. I listed those things that I think might contribute. It is the same as mortality in dialysis programs. Most of us are inclined to say we take sicker people, that they are older, they are diabetic, that they have bad vascular disease, and that is clearly the problem. Why it should occur since 1989 is not clear. It's also the time period, as I suggested, when high-flux, high-flow dialysis occurs. Our concern was that it was EPO, and the data just do not support that concern. It is still intriguing to me, and I think possibly we could break down this data for different types of accesses, to examine their blood pressure prior to access failure. I don't have the answer, and I left that intentionally vague. I am concerned about flow, and I would be interested to see what some of the surgeons say about blood flows of 400 to 500 (cc/min), which is standard in dialysis units now.

Moderator: Any time you are changing the characteristics of your dialysis pattern, i.e., high-flux dialysis, then you are altering blood flow within those grafts even more than they were with "regular" flows. We clearly know from the introductory remarks, as well as Dr. Fillinger's discussion, if you interrupt "normalized abnormal" blood flow, you may contribute significantly to increasing problems.

Discussant: I think you can go even further. The one thing that is emerging as a paradigm is increasing access problems. We have presented a model of complex biologic phenomenon of intimal hyperplasia and thrombosis of these grafts, but that model is really one of wound healing and repair. Those are the normal mechanisms. It's going to be complex, and they are going to be biologically relevant. I don't think we can block all of the wound healing to prevent intimal hyperplasia. We have intermittent changes in local hemodynamics with repeated vessel injury and repair. It might well be that it's the local, abrupt changes in hemodynamics, stimulating vessel injury, followed by repair. They then get dialyzed again, setting up the environment to produce these hemodynamic changes all over again.

Dr. Lazarus has suggested that the platelet is a central player here. One striking piece of information was how the platelet dysfunction in uremic patients improves to normal when you give them EPO. How significant do you think it is that you have returned platelet function to normal in these individuals, as a contributing factor to graft failure?

Dr. Lazarus: That was clearly a concern in the initial studies when we were in phase 2. Everyone was concerned that we were going to return platelet function to normal. I had never seen a pulmonary embolus in a dialysis patient until we used EPO. Now we have concern that platelet function is going to be so good that you may even see those routinely. But if you talk to the people who manufacture EPO, they say there is no evidence for that happening.

Dr. Ferguson: I think the local environment must mediate repeated injury. It sets up a local environment of repair, which is proliferative in nature in terms of wound healing. You then change the hemodynamics. All those things that Dr. Henry talked about—Reynolds numbers, turbulence, and flows—are changing frequently. You're setting up a local environment that is very conducive to proliferation, especially if you have better "wound healing" properties mediated by platelets. It seems to me that a good prospective study would be one that would take an in-depth look at platelet function in dialysis patients to test out the hypothesis. You're doing a great deal with color flow Doppler; but this could be combined with, perhaps, platelet aggregometry or adhesion assays. It might be one thing that we should be monitoring and targeting to address this perceived increase in vascular access failure.

Discussant: I am concerned that you haven't stratified the data. You are seeing a tremendous increase in admissions. It may not be that the surgeries are worse than they were; the surgeries may in fact be improving. With prolonging the graft much longer, we are having many more secondary interventions. My question is, have you stratified the data in terms of primary grafts, secondary patency in terms of autogenous versus graft material and in terms of duration?

Dr. Lazarus: No, we did not look at graft survival. That was clearly only hospital admissions. It may be that now we have techniques to go back and repair PTFEs over and over again, and these data may reflect that. Why it should occur temporally in the first quarter of 1989 is not clear to me. I know of nothing that happened in 1989 that abruptly changed practice habits.

Discussant: In fact, your numbers have increased. You started off with about 14,000, and now you're up to 30,000. There may be a tremendous bias just secondary to the numbers, and unless you stratify it, you are not going to see any of that.

Discussant: Do you have any evidence whether different PTFE graft locations or configurations affect outcome? Specifically, is it the size of the vein used for outflow that affects survival rates? For example, if you place a graft directly into the femoral vein in a leg graft, is survival longer than when one is sewn in a lower arm graft?

Moderator: Certainly the configuration is important. The problem with a lot of the studies addressing your question specifically is that there haven't been randomized prospective studies looking at placement. Much of the information we have is from one institution that uses upper arm grafts solely, compared to another institution that uses lower arm grafts. It's not done in a scientific manner. For example, femoral grafts are rarely put in as a primary procedure, in contrast to a forearm loop in a prospective trial. That's not done routinely because we know there is greater morbidity with leg grafts. There are data to show that a straight graft in the forearm has outcome inferior to a loop graft configuration in the forearm. The comparative data are not very good.

Dr. Fillinger: It is my impression in using PTFE that upper grafts are very poor in terms of the survival because the angle of inflow is usually very perpendicular. I think there is an enormous amount of turbulence in that area. I have recently been using grafts from the brachial artery at the elbow crossing the shoulder joint and sewing it into the axillary vein, taking off a piece of the pectoralis minor muscle for exposure. I have been impressed that the patency rate is longer, and I've wondered whether or not it is just because I am putting it into a vein that is about 10 to 12 mm in diameter. The angle of inflow, the diameter of the vein, and the rate of flow through the graft all make a big difference in the amount of turbulence that is produced, the amount of vibration, and the amount of kinetic energy that is lost at the anastomosis. What you are seeing may be simply that when you put it into a larger diameter vein, it takes a lot longer for that vein to become thick enough to cause a hemodynamically critical stenosis. From the work that I've done in the lab, it's unlikely that the basic process of hyperplasia is going to be substantially altered by a simple change in graft geometry or where the graft is placed. Hyperplasia probably continues to occur. It just takes a lot longer for it to become critical in the larger vein.

Moderator: If you throw all the publications on vascular access into a big pot and look for the best procedure to accomplish long-term survival, it is the forearm loop graft.

Discussant: Dr. Lazarus, we have seen an increase in numbers of patients in our dialysis units, and the demand on our nursing personnel has increased. We have found some poor techniques insofar as how nurses are achieving hemostasis after removing their needles—sending patients home with rather tight bandages, for example. I wonder if that might be contributing to some of these failures.

Dr. Lazarus: This is a large population of 14,000 to 26,000 patients. It is hard for me to believe that either surgical technique or nursing technique over a patient population that large would surface in this study as an answer to this problem. It certainly can be a factor, though.

Discussant: Dr. Fillinger, you have done outstanding work in relating the geometry of grafts and intimal hyperplasia, and you have found that by limiting inflow you can limit intimal hyperplasia, particularly by using tapered grafts 4 mm to 7 mm. Is there any way to limit inflow in order to minimize intimal hyperplasia?

Dr. Fillinger: From the data in the animal model we found that tapered grafts reduced the amount of perivascular, perianastomotic kinetic energy loss. The amount of turbulence at the anastomosis may have been related specifically to the size of the vessels in question and the amount of flow that we had through the grafts. That may be the clinical situation Dr. Henry was discussing. When you use an inflow of the radial artery, the flow within the graft may be such that the tapered geometry is not important. But when you get into the high-flow rates in our model, say a liter per minute, then it becomes more important. We have some as yet unpublished data demonstrating that there is clearly a change as the flow within a graft is increased. At a certain point, the flow reaches a critical level at which the pressure drop across that venous anastomosis begins to generate vibration. Unfortunately, that critical point is around 300–500 cc per minute, which brings up some of the questions about high-flux dialysis. If you are going to do high-flux dialysis, you need grafts that are flowing higher to begin with. It's not just the flux that is occurring while the patients are on dialysis, but the bigger grafts carry more flow when the patient is off dialysis as well. With high-flux dialysis, it is going to be increasingly difficult to try to limit that perivascular vibration and energy loss.

Discussant: Dr. Lazarus, I was wondering at what point you looked at that data and determined how many of those patients had some sort of acute dialysis prior to starting chronic dialysis. I am impressed that I never place an access anymore in someone who doesn't have a central venous dialysis catheter. I wonder what role the proximal strictures are playing in readmitting patients for multiple revisions?

Dr. Lazarus: I can't break out those data. This is too big a data base from too many units to do that, but time relation is certainly a possibility. I don't know if anyone else has a comment about IJ catheters and subclavians.

Moderator: I think that if you look at the incidence of catheters in Dow's study in Detroit, it was very high in those patients who didn't have the access created ahead of time. From a temporal standpoint, I suppose that is a very reasonable hypothesis.

Dr. Lazarus: What also happens with increased flow is that we pick up venous stenosis a lot quicker and a lot better. I used to ignore problems with venous stenosis, but with a blood flow of 400 cc per minute, I can no longer do that. The surgeon gets a call from me a lot more often now, simply related to minor defects that in the past we might have ignored.

SECTION II

4

COLOR FLOW DOPPLER PHYSICS AND CLINICAL APPROACHES

Samuel P. Martin, M.D., and Kathleen S. Bubb, R.V.T.

DIALYSIS-ACCESS-RELATED MORBIDITY is the single most pressing issue facing the nephrologist and access surgeon today. Despite attempts to modify the problems by manipulating biologic factors, we still are far from any semblance of success. While these efforts are ongoing, we must face and try to modify the actual course of events. If the clinician could identify sources of potential failure prior to their clinical appearance, perhaps this morbidity could be avoided. Our emphasis thus is currently on diagnosing the problem prior to thrombosis of the access.

Color flow imaging is a high-technology, noninvasive diagnostic tool that has the potential for wide application in hemoaccess. Traditionally, angiography has been our chief diagnostic tool because of its reproducibility. Unfortunately, angiography cannot demonstrate intimal integrity, it gives limited hemodynamic information, and it is not practical as a surveillance procedure. Even with the advent of duplex imaging, angiography was still the modality of choice because ultrasound and conventional Doppler technology combined did not yield sufficient information regarding the graft-blood interface.[1] Color flow imaging now provides a means of obtaining that missing information, but because of a lack of understanding of this "black box," many clinicians fail to realize its potential. Despite the combination of complex physical principles and sophisticated computer software, information produced by color flow ultrasound is as easily interpreted as an angiogram. Our purpose here is to explain the basics of this technology, to place them in context in light of their shortcomings, and to demonstrate their use in access evaluation.

The authors would like to thank Clinical Diagnostic Systems for providing us with the photographic material for this presentation. Special thanks go to sonographers Lori Knowles, Janet Nelson, and Lori Huffman for their diligence in obtaining the pathological case studies.

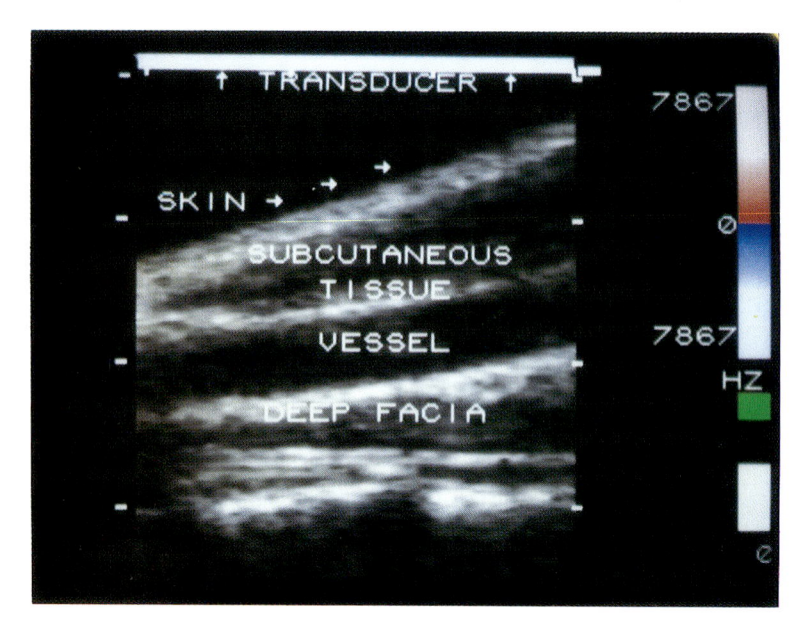

Figure 4-1. Sound waves emitted from the transducer pass through the body. The various tissues and structures send a reflection back to the transducer, indicating location and strength.

Principles

Ultrasound refers to sound waves having a frequency exceeding the limit of human hearing, which is 20,000 Hz. In vascular imaging, typical frequencies range from 5 MHz to 10 MHz. Ultrasound images are made from reflections from sound waves transmitted into the body from a transducer.[2] These sound waves pass through the internal structures and send a reflection or "echo" back to the transducer (figure 4-1). The returning echoes are processed to create a gray-scale or B-mode image that displays location by the depth and lateral position of the reflecting structure and displays brightness by the amplitude or strength of the returning echo. The changes in amplitude of these acoustic reflections occur as a result of differences in tissue densities. For example, an acute thrombus will not reflect as brightly as a chronic thrombus or a calcified plaque.

Transducers

B-mode scanning produces images that are two-dimensional. In order to obtain "real time" information, the ultrasound transducer must produce a num-

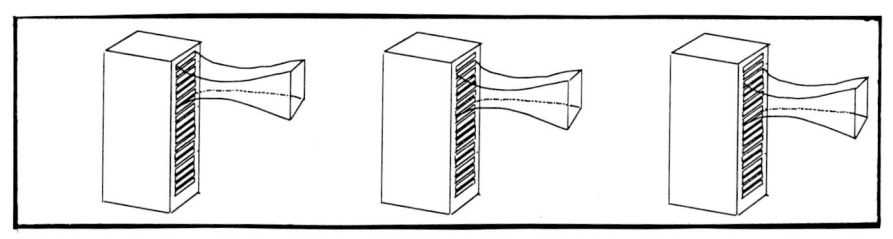

Figure 4-2. Linear array transducers have multiple elements in a line that are sequentially fired to form the image.

ber of images per second.[3] Most commonly used in vascular imaging are the mechanical linear array transducers (figure 4-2), which have multiple elements arranged in a line.[5] These elements are fired in sequence to provide a two-dimensional moving picture. The frequency of the transducer will determine the depth of penetration as well as the quality of the image. The higher frequency transducers (7.5 MHz and 10.0 MHz) offer superior resolution but very little depth of penetration. The lower frequencies (3.5 MHz and 5.0 MHz) provide greater imaging depth but sacrifice image quality. A simple rule is that as frequency increases, imaging depth decreases but lateral resolution increases.

Doppler Ultrasound

Doppler ultrasound detects the movement of blood cells. This movement can be laminar, turbulent, accelerated, diminished, or, in the extreme case, nonexistent. The Doppler effect or Doppler shift is a change in the frequency of sound as a result of motion between the transducer and the blood cells. A positive shift occurs when the transmitted sound and the blood cells are approaching each other. A negative shift occurs when the transmitted sound and the blood cells are moving away from each other.[4]

Two types of Doppler instruments are routinely used to evaluate blood flow (figure 4-3).[6] A continuous-wave Doppler has two crystals, one constantly transmitting a signal and the other constantly receiving a signal. Continuous-wave Doppler has the advantage of being able to measure very high velocities. However, the information is generated from the entire length of the sound beam, so there is no depth resolution. In pulsed-wave Dopplers, one crystal alternately sends and receives signals. This type of instrument makes it possible to select the area to be investigated, but it is limited in its ability to accurately measure very high velocities.

Spectral analysis is the processing of the many varied Doppler-shifted frequencies. The Doppler spectrum demonstrates the direction of flow, the maximum and minimum velocities, and the amount of turbulence (figure 4-4).

Systems that incorporate imaging with Doppler are known as duplex scanners. A fairly recent development in this area is the ability to calculate blood flow volume. Using the gray-scale image, the vessel walls are outlined. The system (QAD-PV Siemens Quantum, 1040 12th Ave. NW, Issaquah, WA 98027) tracks the changes in diameter throughout the cardiac cycle and uses these data

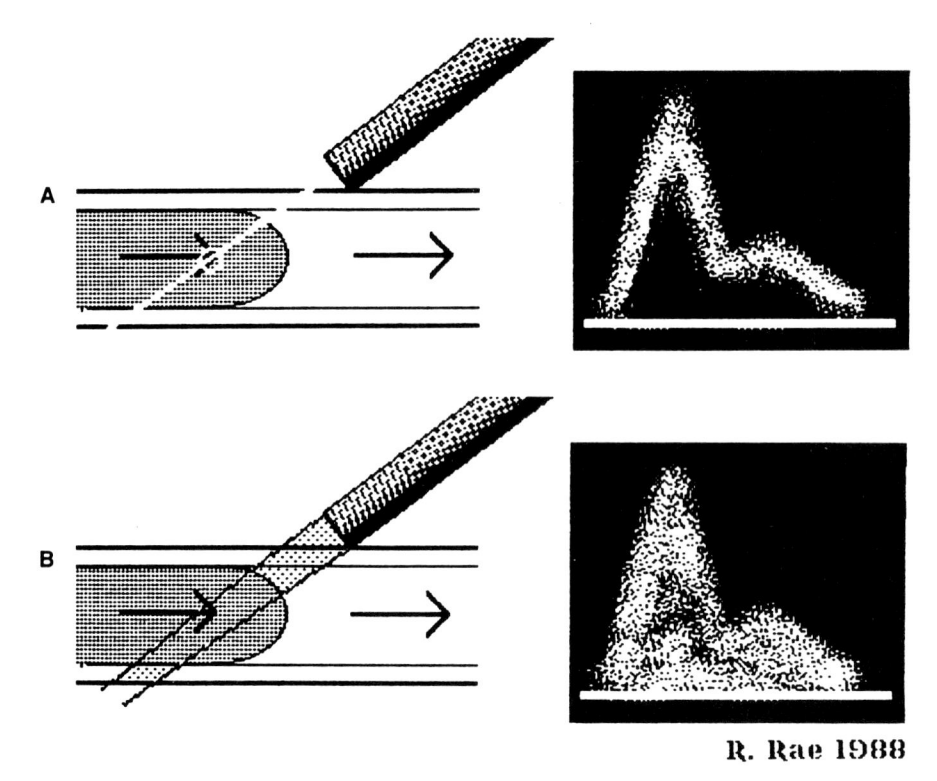

84 COLOR FLOW DOPPLER PHYSICS AND CLINICAL APPROACHES

Figure 4-3. (*Left*) Pulsed versus continuous-wave Doppler. The pulsed Doppler (A) allows discrete sampling of a particular flow stream from the center or edges of the vessel. The continuous-wave Doppler (B) samples the entire range of flow across the vessel.

Figure 4-4. (*Right*) The corresponding Doppler spectral displays demonstrate the individual velocities that make up the Doppler signal.

to calculate the vessel's cross-sectional area in real-time. Simultaneously, the Doppler produces a velocity profile from within the delineated vessel, then calculates the time average flow velocity (figure 4-5).[7] This method of calculation makes certain assumptions regarding vessel shape and flow characteristics; therefore, extreme care should be taken when making calculations and should be performed only under optimal circumstances.

Color Flow

Color Doppler is a pulsed ultrasound technique that codes Doppler information into color according to direction—either toward or away from the transducer (red or blue, respectively) (figure 4-6). Color hues represent the velocities of flow in either direction, the darker hues indicating lower velocities, and the lighter hues indicating higher velocities (figure 4-7). Color flow has the same limitations as pulsed-wave Doppler in relation to high-velocity flow.[10]

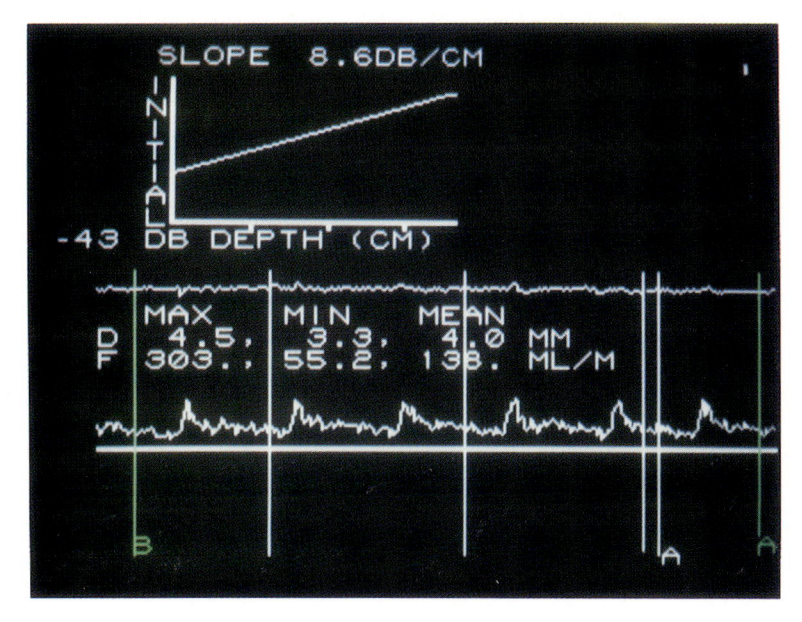

Figure 4-5. Volume flow wave form represents the mean of all velocities within the specific area of the vessel.

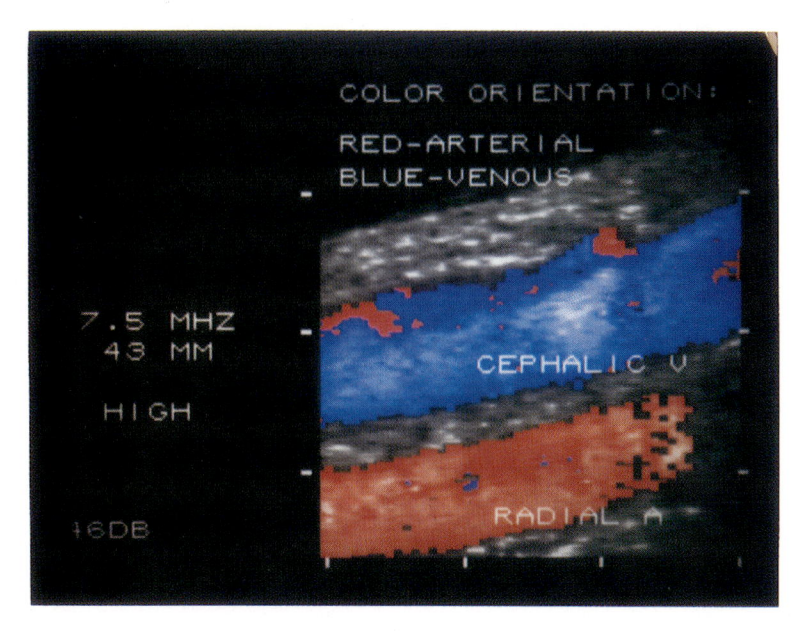

Figure 4-6. Color indicates flow toward the transducer (red) or away from the transducer (blue).

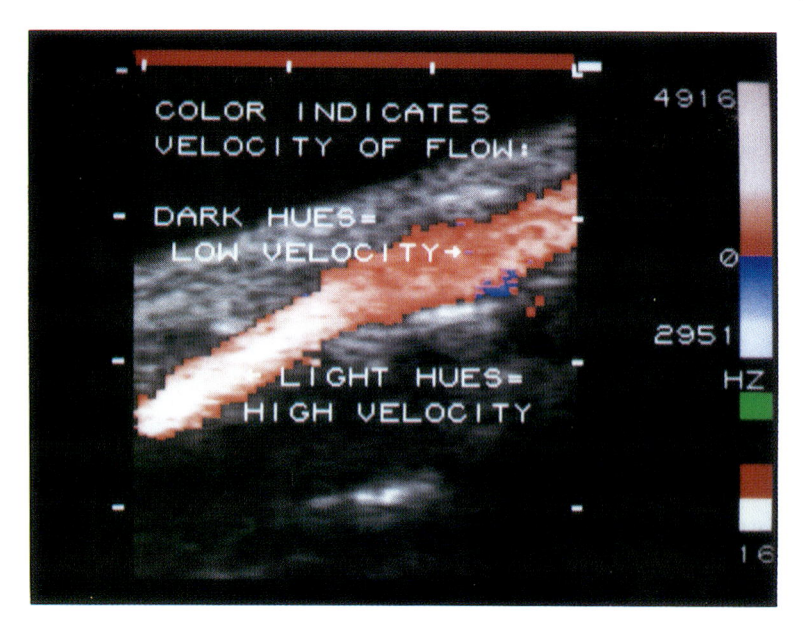

Figure 4-7. Color also indicates flow velocity. The darker hues are lower velocities, the lighter hues higher velocities.

Synchronous color imaging systems display gray-scale and color Doppler in real time.[10] Typically, they use a wedge attachment on the transducer; this creates a constant angle of incidence for acquisition of Doppler/color flow information but does not affect the gray-scale information.

Pitfalls and Artifacts

In ultrasound imaging, an artifact is anything not properly indicative of the structures imaged. One can see from the previous sections that each of the combined modalities that make up a color flow system has its limitations.

The most significant artifact is the obstacle of attenuation. The effect of attenuation is the loss of information or "shadowing" caused by strongly reflecting structures that are very dense or stiff. For example, as sound waves encounter bone, most of the energy is reflected back to the transducer. When this occurs, little or no information can be received from the structures that lie behind the bone (figure 4-8). This phenomenon occurs in color flow as well as gray-scale.

Enhancement can also give a distorted picture; this occurs when a structure appears to be abnormally bright. This is the result of the sound traveling through a medium with a lower attenuation than that of the surrounding structures (figure 4-9), such as fluid-filled cysts or seromas. Enhancement artifacts will affect the gray-scale image only.

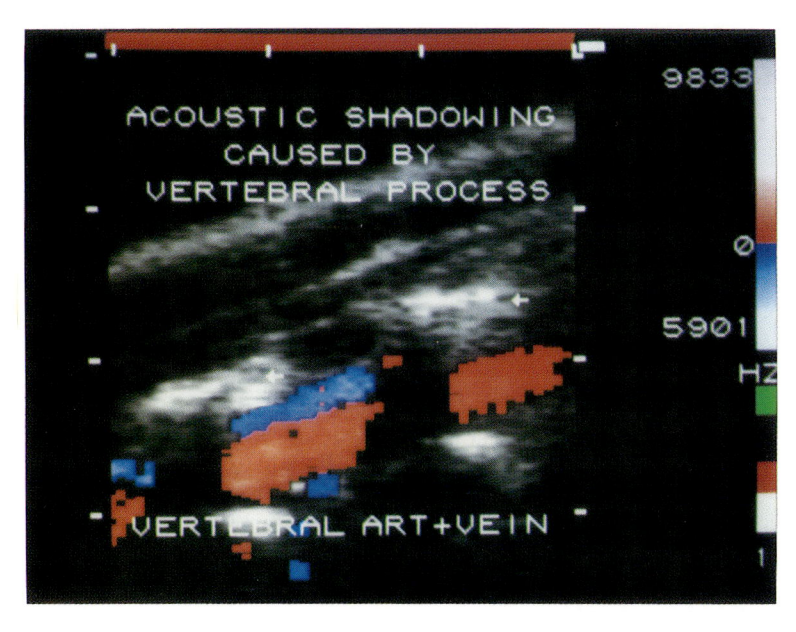

Figure 4-8. Loss of color and gray-scale information due to shadowing caused by bone.

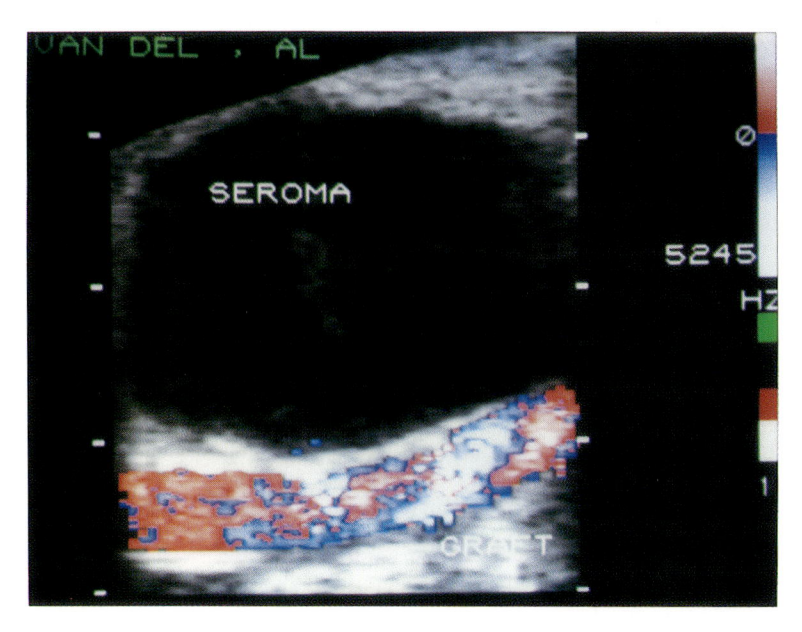

Figure 4-9. Sound traveling through a large seroma loses very little energy, causing enhancement of the graft and tissues directly below it.

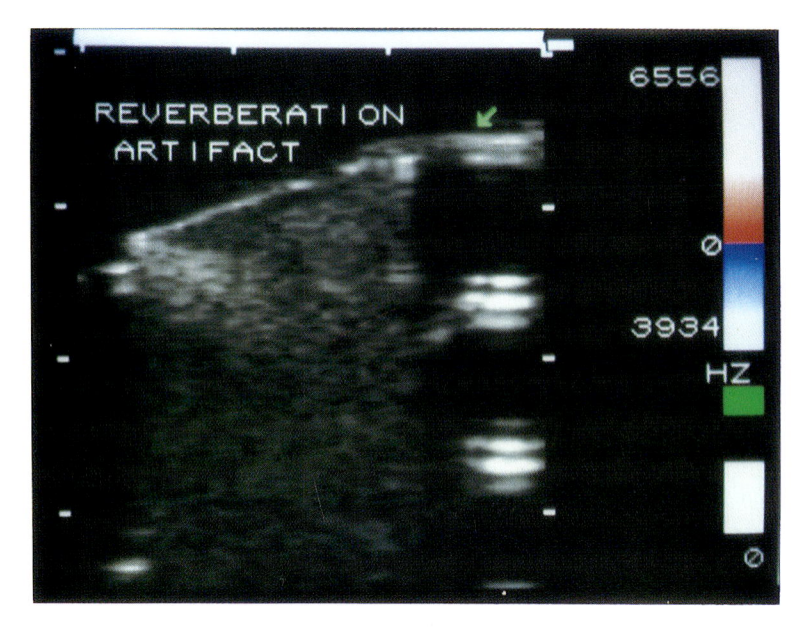

88 COLOR FLOW DOPPLER PHYSICS AND CLINICAL APPROACHES

Figure 4-10. Reverberation is caused by a strong reflector encountered in the near field.

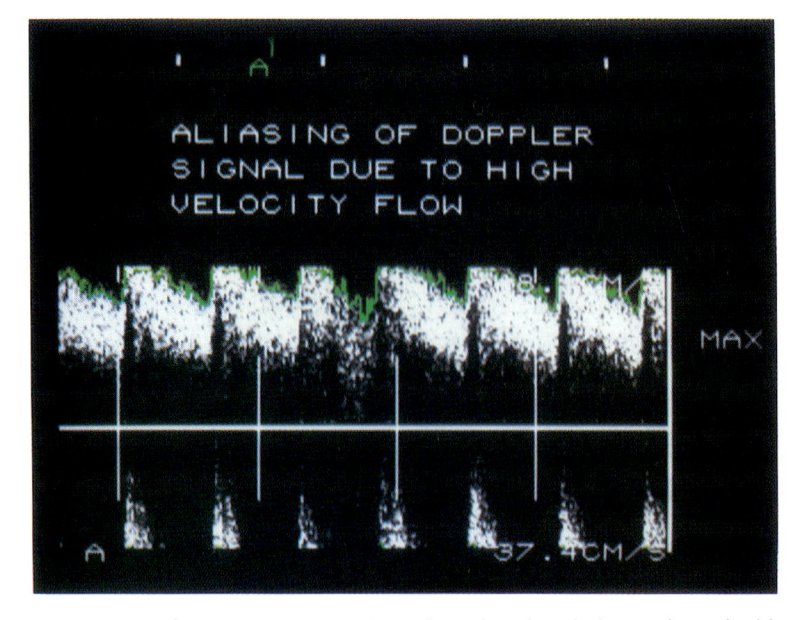

Figure 4-11. Spectral analysis of the Doppler signal shows the velocities that exceed the Nyquist limit as negative; they appear at the bottom of the display.

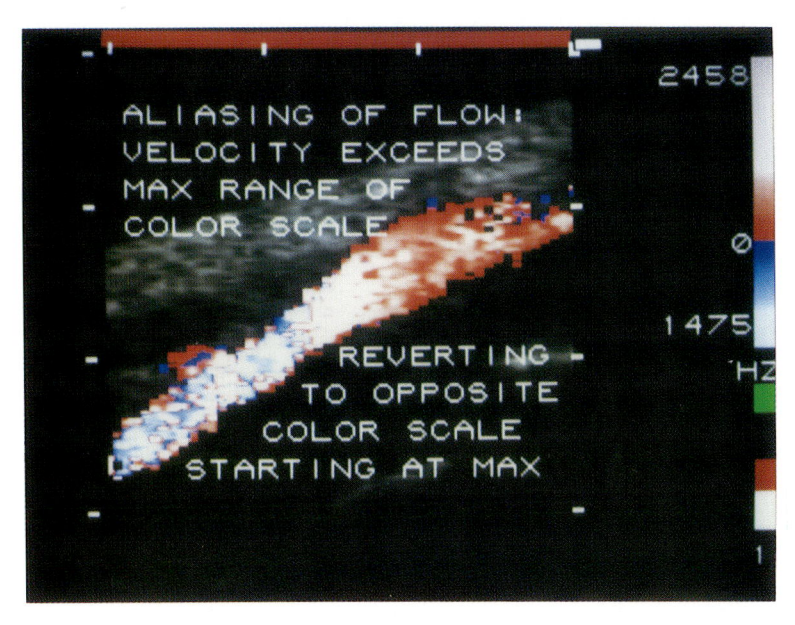

COLOR FLOW DOPPLER PHYSICS AND CLINICAL APPROACHES   89

Figure 4-12. Aliasing in color appears as a change from one color to the opposite color.

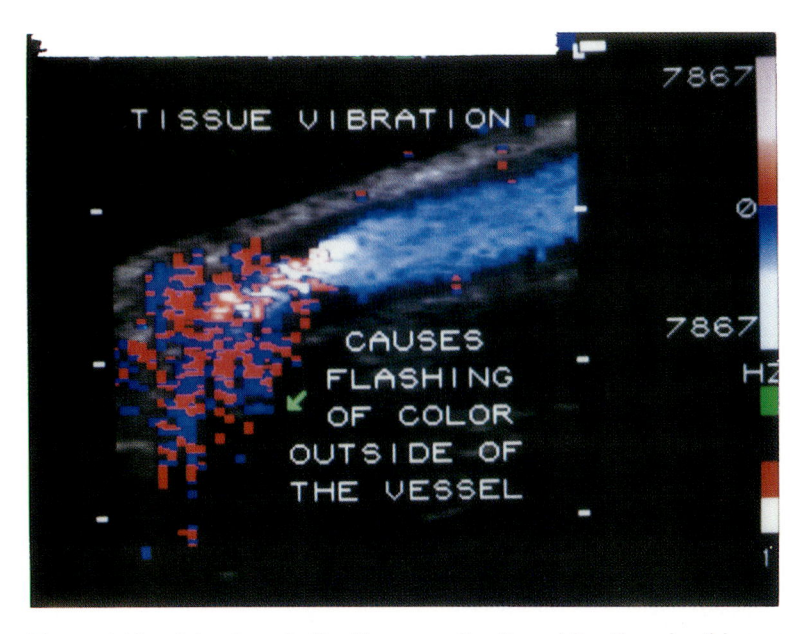

Figure 4-13. A bruit or thrill will cause vibration of the tissues; this appears as a flashing of color outside the vessel.

Reverberation artifact, easily detected, appears as multiple equally spaced reflections on the gray-scale image (figure 4-10). This occurs when two or more strong reflectors lie in the path of the sound wave and cause the reflections to "ping-pong" back and forth between the structures. Identification is easily made, since they are equally spaced on the display.

With pulsed-wave Doppler, there is a limit to the Doppler-shifted frequency that can be detected by the instrument. When that limit is exceeded, aliasing occurs, and velocities that exceed the Nyquist limit appear as negative (figure 4-11) (The Nyquist limit is the Doppler frequency at which aliasing occurs). In color flow, this will cause a shift from the lightest hues of one color spectrum to the lightest hues of the opposite color spectrum (figure 4-12). Lower-frequency transducers are less likely to produce aliasing.

Another form of color artifact is caused by tissue vibration, typically seen at stenotic areas or anastomotic sites and caused by blood flow turbulence. This vibration, detected by the machine, is displayed as a "flashing" of color outside of the vessel (figure 4-13). Because this flashing obscures the underlying gray-scale information, the color should be removed to allow for thorough evaluation.

Clinical Application

Vascular access pathology is unique in the field of vascular ultrasonography. The arterial system has its unique characteristics (predominantly related to flow) interfacing directly with the venous system and its special properties (predominantly related to wall compliance) frequently in contact with a synthetic graft. Stenoses and obstruction often have unique characteristics and locations.

Intimal hyperplasia is by far the greatest problem faced. This is seen in grafts and in outflow veins whose walls have dilated and subsequently hypertrophied with arterial pressure. The most critical site for this is the graft/vein interface (figure 4-14). One does not see hyperplasia nearly to the same extent with an autogenous arteriovenous (A-V) interface. Occasionally, hyperplasia is seen remotely in the outflow vein at a site of turbulence (figure 4-15). This can lead to occlusion without clinical symptoms if collaterals are present. Critical hyperplasia is rare within the graft, but is seen ostensibly secondary to the trauma of cannulation (figure 4-16). Angiography cannot differentiate clot versus hyperplasia, whereas duplex scanning can.

Color flow can easily differentiate pseudoaneurysms from seromas and hematomas (figure 4-17). We also are able to appreciate endograft changes secondary to the turbulent flow caused by pseudoaneurysms. Orifice diameter of pseudoaneurysms can easily be measured to determine if the graft can be salvaged and to plan a repair, be it suture, patch, or segmental graft replacement (figure 4-18).

Determination of the access volume flow can be useful as a predictor of access function and survival. An access that has a moderate stenosis in the pres-

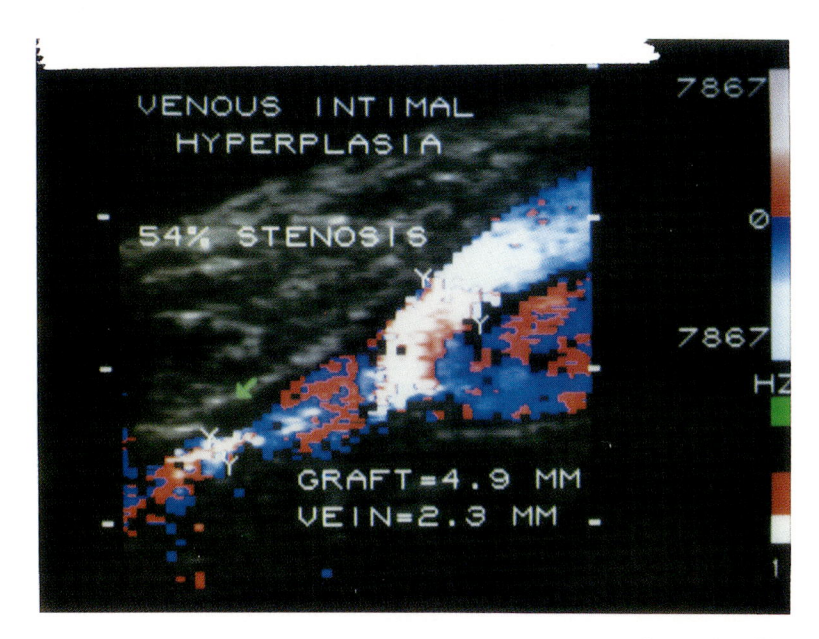

Figure 4-14. Formation of intimal hyperplasia in the outflow vein with a significantly reduced lumen.

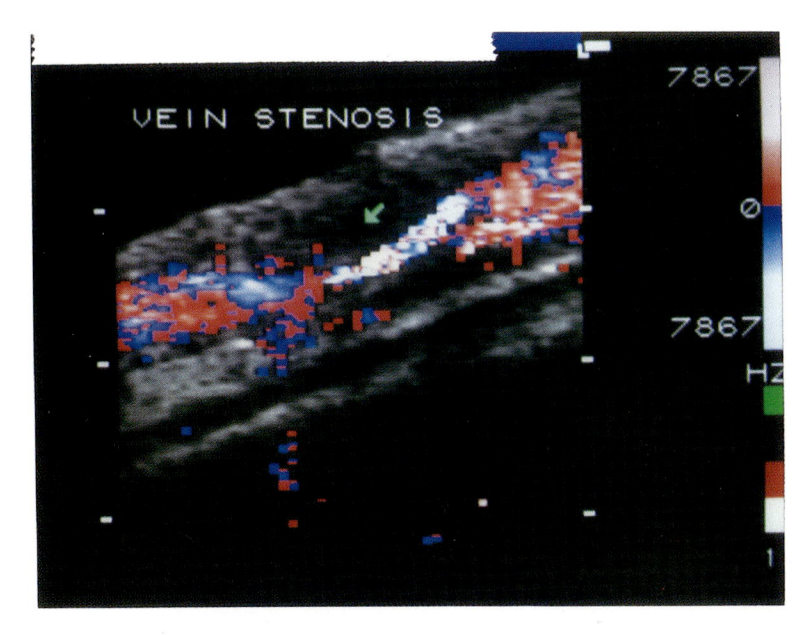

Figure 4-15. Stenotic segment of vein.

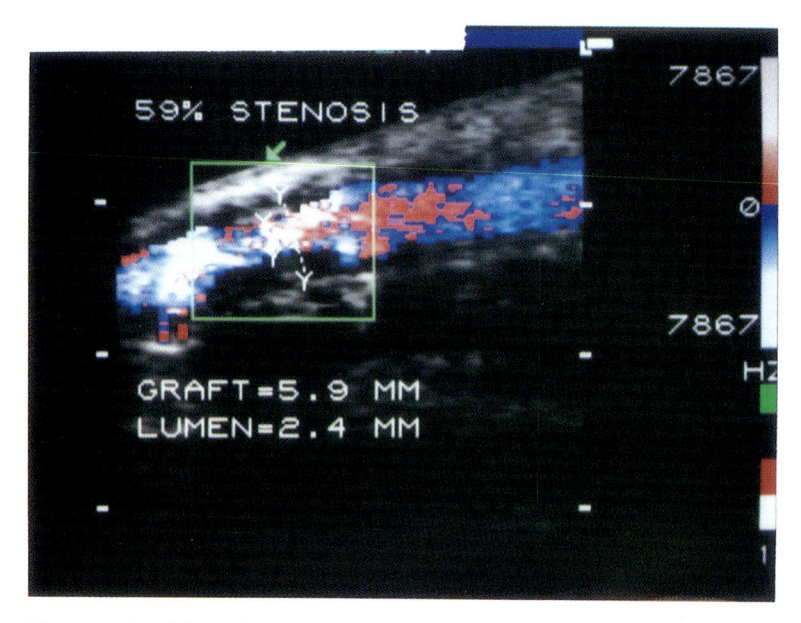

92 COLOR FLOW DOPPLER PHYSICS AND CLINICAL APPROACHES

Figure 4-16. Midgraft stenosis caused by repeated puncturing.

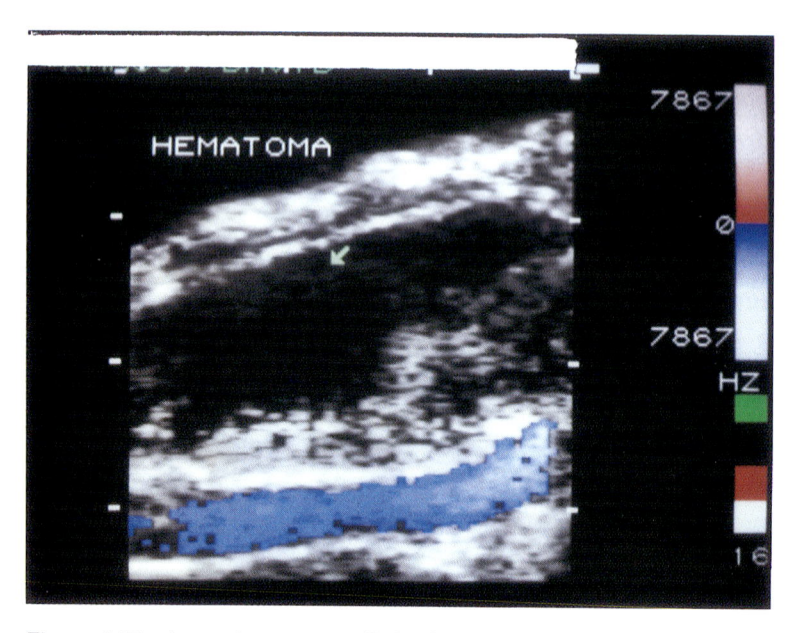

Figure 4-17. Large hematoma. Color flow confirms that this is not a pseudoaneurysm.

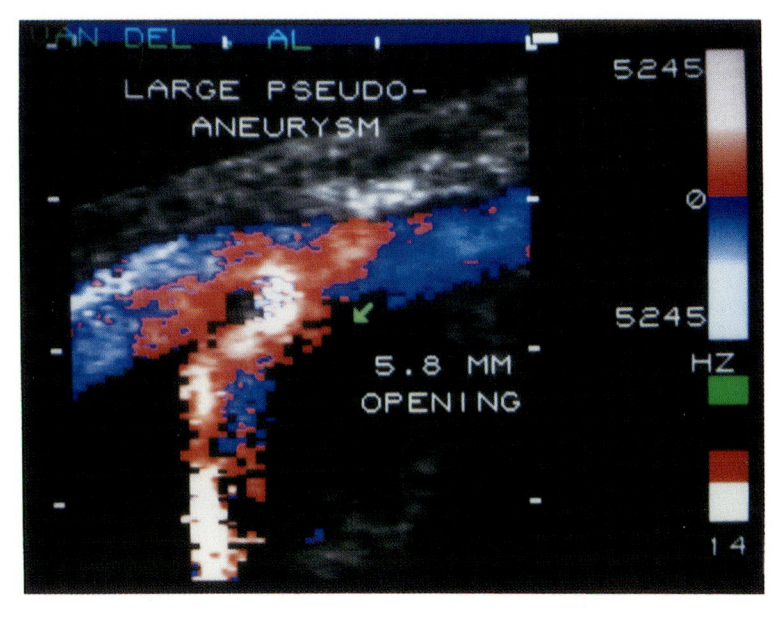

Figure 4-18. Large pseudoaneurysm lies deep to the graft with a 5.8 mm opening.

ence of decreased volume flow could be potentially at risk of failure. Data presented at the first vascular access symposium have helped us to establish values for volume flow in A-V fistulas and grafts.[11] We know that the total flow through the access should exceed the flow through the artificial kidney by at least 50%.[12] The use of ultrasound technology to determine access volume flow has, in our experience, produced reasonable, reproducible information and allows blood flow rates during dialysis to be adjusted accordingly.

Summary

Despite the complexities of the technology, color flow duplex scanning provides a cost-effective, sensitive, and specific diagnostic tool to study the dialysis access. Pathology is well demonstrated in a noninvasive manner while providing additional flow characteristics. We now have a tool useful in routine graft surveillance that may have an impact on access morbidity.

Definitions

duplex systems that combine gray-scale imaging and Doppler
hertz (Hz) unit of frequency; one hertz is one cycle per second or one com-

plete variation per second; one megahertz (MHz) is one million Hz[3]

B-mode returning echoes appear as spots on the line of travel of the emitted US pulse; the stronger the returning echo, the brighter the spot[4]

amplitude relates to the strength of the sound signal or wave; amplitude changes as sound propagates through the body[3]

real time a series of frames or pictures displayed in a rapid fashion so as to give the impression of constant motion[4]

transducer turns electrical into acoustic energy during transmission and turns returning acoustic into electrical energy during reception[4]

Doppler shift MHz = reflected frequency (MHz)-incident freq. MHz = ± 2 × reflector speed (m/s) × incident freq. (MHz) propagation speed (m/s)

volume flow equation[8] Q = 60 × TAV × Area

Q = Volume flow (ml/min)
TAV = time average velocity (m/sec)
Area = cross-sectional area (mm2)
60 = multiplier to express flow over one minute

volume flow criteria[9] (1) the flow is not turbulent, (2) flow is symmetrical (or nearly so), (3) all contributing flow is fast enough to be detected, (4) all the contributors to the volume flow are located between the delimiter limits, (5) vessel should be no smaller than 4 mm

References

1. Villemarette PA, et al. Use of color flow Doppler to evaluate vascular access graft function. Vasc Tech 1989; 13:164.
2. Case TD, Marick KW. Introduction to duplex ultrasound, principles and techniques. Milpitas, CA: Diasonics, 1985; V: 3.
3. Kremkau FW. Diagnostic ultrasound principles, instrumentation and exercises. 3d ed. Philadelphia: WB Saunders, 1989; 6,18,48.
4. Edleman SK. Understanding ultrasound physics, fundamentals and exam review. Houston: ESP Publishers, 1990; 47,69,72,85.
5. Zwiebel WJ. Introduction to vascular ultrasonography. 2d ed. Philadelphia: WB Saunders, 1986; 2:27.
6. Hagen-Ansert, SL. Textbook of diagnostic ultrasonography. St. Louis: Mosby, 1989; 37, 884.
7. QAD-PV operators manual. Issaquah, WA: Quantum Medical Systems, 1988; 45-46.
8. Hayes A. Measurement of volume blood flow in peripheral vessels using ultrasound. Dec. 4, 1989, personal correspondence from Acuson to Acuson users.
9. Powis RL. Volume flow calculations using the QAD-1. Oct. 11, 1991, personal correspondence from Quantum Medical Systems to Kathy Sargent.
10. Powis RL. Color flow imaging: understanding its science and technology. Diagnostic Med Sonography, 1988; 236–45.
11. Anderson CB, et al. Physiology and hemodynamics of vascular access. In: Sommer BG, Henry ML, eds. Vascular access for hemodialysis. Chicago: Pluribus Press, 1989; 19.
12. Kootstra G, Jorning PJG. Access surgery. Ridgewood: Bogden & Sons, 1983: 45.

5

CORRELATION OF COLOR FLOW DOPPLER AND ANGIOGRAPHY

William H. Bay, M.D.

A FREQUENT CAUSE FOR HOSPITALIZATION of many hemodialysis patients is failure of their dialysis vascular access. According to data from the National Medical Care clinical data base, 16.2% of all hospitalizations for hemodialysis patients are related to vascular access complications (E.G. Lowrie, personal communication). In the future, significant patient benefits will be derived from therapies that reduce the incidence of vascular access stenosis and thrombosis. Patients will also prefer a noninvasive technique for evaluation of the hemodialysis vascular access inasmuch as the current gold standard is contrast fistulography, performed as either standard angiography or digital subtraction angiography (DSA). Both the physician's and patient's expectation is that early diagnosis of a vascular access stenosis will permit either angioplasty or surgical repair to diminish the risk of future graft failure (figure 5-1). This report reviews the experience with one noninvasive technique, color flow Doppler ultrasound (CFD), applied in a large hemodialysis population. The CFD findings in regard to stenoses are correlated with the angiographic results.

Methods and Results

Chronic hemodialysis patients in a freestanding dialysis center were studied. These patients had rejected home dialysis, and many were not transplant candidates because of age or other medical conditions. The average age of the patients was 57 years. There were 51 males and 49 females, and 40% of the patients were diabetic. Sixty-nine percent of the patients had polytetrafluoroethylene (PTFE) grafts and 31% had Brescia-Cimino fistulas. During the year prior

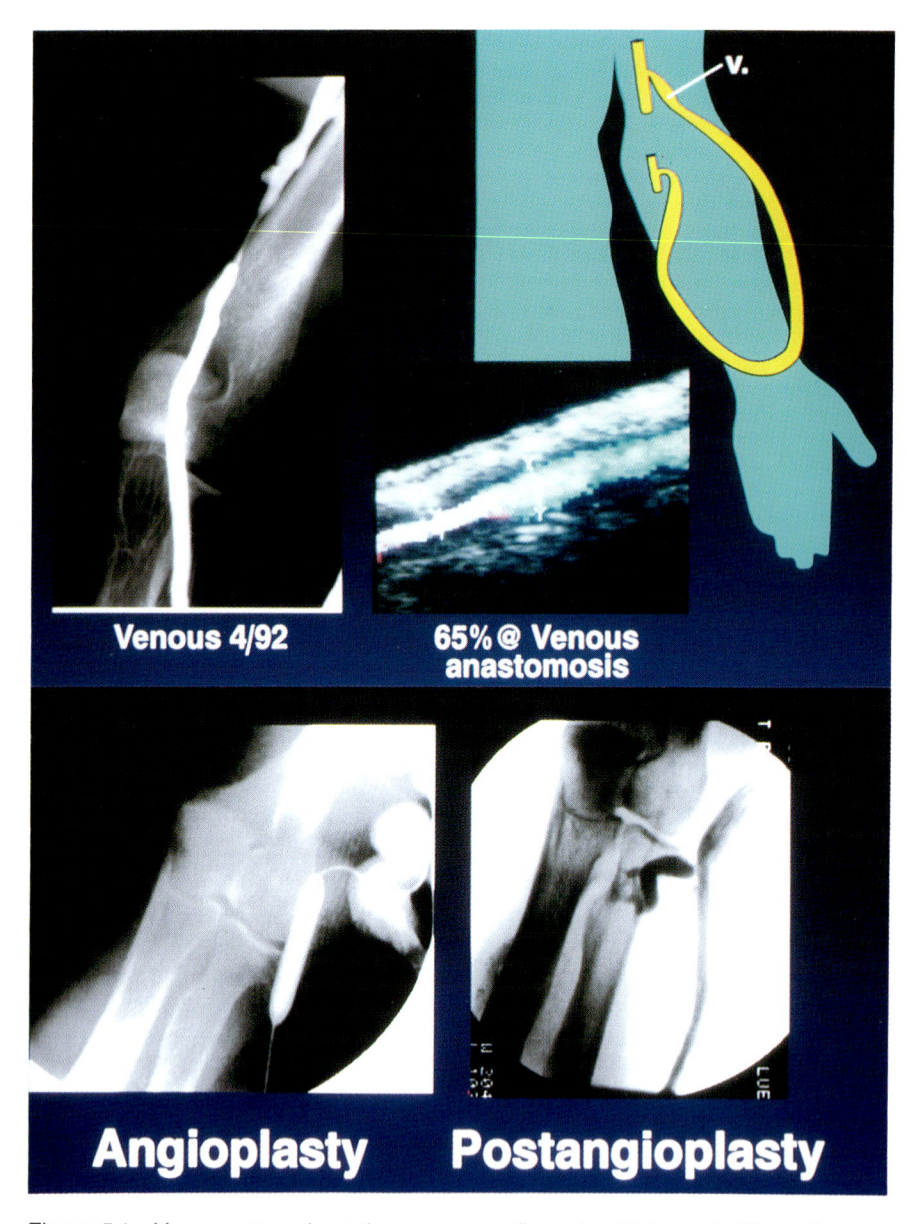

Figure 5-1. Venous stenosis at the venous outflow of a PTFE graft. *(Top left panel)* Fistulagram. *(Top right panel)* Simultaneous Doppler study and schematic presentation of the lesion area. *(Bottom left panel)* Angioplasty of the stenotic lesion. *(Bottom right panel)* Postangiographic fistulogram.

to this report, 18% of the patients had been admitted to Ohio State University Hospitals because of vascular access complications.

CFD was performed with a 7.4 MHz linear array transducer that provided high quality gray-scale images at relatively shallow depths. A wedge apparatus was applied to the transducer to create the angle of incidence necessary to perform CFD interrogation of blood flow. From 90 to 100 patients had CFD testing during October 1990, May 1991, October 1991, and April 1992. A fistulogram was recommended for all patients who had a vascular access stenosis of 50% or greater by CFD analysis. The clinical intention was to evaluate the stenosis and determine if a correctable lesion, either by angioplasty or surgery, was present. Not all patients with a CFD stenosis of >50% were evaluated, as some patients refused an angiogram; for others, the study was not completed. Patients with a vascular access stenosis of <50% by CFD were not evaluated by angiography. For this reason, the false-negative CFD stenosis rate cannot be determined. This report addresses only whether a stenosis of ≥50% by CFD can be confirmed by angiography.

All consenting patients underwent either an intra-arterial digital subtraction or a standard fistulogram. The angiographic technique was chosen by the radiologist. The angiogram as reported by the radiologist was compared to the CFD report as analyzed by the author.

The results of the October 1991 and April 1992 CFD surveys demonstrated that 7% of the patients had vascular access stenoses of ≥50%. Twenty patients were evaluated by angiography within four weeks of their CFD test. The confirmation rate of a CFD-documented stenosis by angiography was 96%—28 of 29 stenoses. In the nonconfirmed stenosis, there was a 54% narrowing at the distal end of the graft according to the CFD analysis that was not supported by angiography. There also was a separate stenosis noted by angiography that was not appreciated by CFD. In this case, one stenosis was detected by CFD, but two stenoses were found by angiography. The second stenosis documented by angiography was just proximal to the CFD-localized stenosis; however, both stenoses were believed to be significant and to require angioplasty.

Three patients with Brescia-Cimino fistulas had a ≥50% stenosis demonstrated by CFD. In two of these patients, the stenosis was confirmed by DSA, an accuracy rate of 67%.

Discussion

CFD ultrasound is a noninvasive technology that should provide a high degree of accuracy for the analysis of hemodialysis vascular accesses. Dousset et al. studied 22 patients with PTFE grafts who had CFD-demonstrated stenoses of ≥50% and who also had DSA. There was an 86% (16 of 19 patients) correlation between the CFD-detected stenoses and the DSA findings.[1] The three false-negative CFD studies eventrated because additional stenoses were discovered in the subclavian vein by DSA. One patient had a stenosis described by CFD that was not corroborated by DSA but was confirmed in surgery. An additional CFD-detected stenosis was not verified by angiography.

Middleton et al. surveyed 17 patients with PTFE grafts. Sixteen grafts had stenoses of >50% by CFD, but 17 stenoses were observed by DSA. The CFD false-negative occurrence was a subclavian vein stenosis. The accuracy rate for PTFE grafts was 94%.[2] Middleton also studied six patients with Brescia-Cimino fistulas. Four stenoses were detected by CFD, but six stenoses were found by DSA. The accuracy rate for Brescia-Cimino fistulas in this study was 67%.

Table 5-1. Brescia-Cimino Fistulas and Doppler Sensitivity

Authors	Sensitivity (%)
Ohio State	67
Middleton	67
Nonnast-Daniel	100
Tordoir	81

In a report from Nonnast-Daniel et al., 51 patients were investigated, of whom 28 had CFD and angiography evaluation.[3] In all patients, there was angiographic verification of the CFD-demonstrated stenoses. In addition, five patients with CFD-established stenoses did not receive angiography, but their stenoses were confirmed in surgery. Nonnast-Daniel's findings suggested a 100% stenoses correlation between angiography and CFD for both fistulas and grafts.

In a larger analysis, Tordoir et al. evaluated 36 patients with arteriovenous (A-V) fistulas and 28 patients with PTFE grafts.[4] They found 83 stenoses in the 64 patients. The correlation between CFD documented stenoses and angiography for Brescia-Cimino fistulas was 81%, with a sensitivity of 79% and a specificity of 84%. In PTFE grafts, the correlation of CFD stenoses and angiography increased to 91%, with a sensitivity of 75% and a specificity of 96%. When efferent venous stenoses were examined from either a fistula or graft, Tordoir found an accuracy of 96%, with a sensitivity of 95% and a specificity of 97%. Glickman et al. also reported that they were successful using CFD to diagnose significant stenoses in 25 PTFE grafts; these were substantiated by angiography.[5]

When the results of this study are combined with the three other published results, CFD appears to be an unsatisfactory test for evaluation of the Brescia-Cimino fistula.[2-4] As shown in table 5-1, the correlation between the CFD findings and angiogram results ranges from 67% to 100%. The perfect correlation reported in Nonnast-Daniel's study of Brescia-Cimino fistulas probably is inappropriately elevated when the data are compared to the three other studies. If Nonnast-Daniel's data for Brescia-Cimino fistulas are excluded, the CFD correlation with angiography may be in the 66–75% range.[3] The more complicated vascular anatomy of fistulas with intricate venous run-off and varying arterial anastomoses may explain the decrease in accuracy.

When the Ohio State and the literature data[1-5] are consolidated for PTFE grafts (table 5-2), the range of correlation between CFD and angiography is 91%–100%. However, when evaluation of the subclavian area is eliminated from the data and the efferent vein accuracy value of Tordoir is employed, the correlation between CFD analysis and angiography results for PTFE grafts appears to be at least 95% (table 5-2). This superb agreement between CFD and angiography may be explained by the simple vascular anatomy of PTFE grafts. CFD easily evaluates the afferent artery, the arterial anastomosis, the PTFE graft, the venous anastomosis, and the vein of the upper arm excluding the area of the subclavian vein. Disregarding this last limitation, CFD results have a high degree of accuracy, equal to the findings observed with angiography.

Table 5-2. PTFE Grafts and Doppler Sensitivity

Authors	Overall (%)	Without subcl vein (%)
Ohio State	96	96
Dousset	86	100
Middleton	94	100
Nonnast-Daniel	100	100
Tordoir	91	96
Glickman	100	100

It is not surprising that CFD does not adequately evaluate the subclavian vein because of the superimposed clavicle. However, the most common PTFE graft complications are stenoses at the vascular anastomoses. CFD investigation is an excellent noninvasive test for these areas of the PTFE graft. If clinical signs such as elevated venous pressure, severe arm swelling, or recurrent graft insufficiency continue despite a normal CFD evaluation, then angiographic investigation of the subclavian vein anatomy is required. The mobility of CFD units can be beneficial because vascular graft assessment can occur in the dialysis facility and reduce the patient's time commitment for another medical appointment. For patients with PTFE grafts, the ease of obtaining a CFD without invasive risks may make this diagnostic approach preferable to an angiogram.

Whether CFD screening will be beneficial for determining which PTFE grafts may fail has yet to be decided. The corroboration of CFD with angiography anatomical results is excellent, but whether CFD-observed stenoses will foretell future graft insufficiency is unknown. Intuitively, periodic CFD surveys of hemodialysis accesses should detect progressive stenoses and permit corrective intervention. Figure 5-2 illustrates the increase in both an arterial and venous stenosis during a six-month period. However, if the cost of CFD is unreasonable for general screening of the dialysis population, clinical indicators of access dysfunction might dictate when CFD can be applied. Questions concerning the significance of elevated venous pressure, increased difficulty with dialysis needle placement, acute swelling of the access arm, and an increased recirculation rate as predictors of graft stenosis must be answered.

The predictive value of merging the anatomical findings of CFD with Doppler ultrasound measurement of access blood flow may better forecast graft failure, but pertinent studies to answer this question are not available. Finally, if CFD is used to detect vascular access lesions, does early intervention with angioplasty or surgical correction enhance graft survival?

Even with these prevailing unanswered questions, new issues are arising. Will the prescription of erythropoietin to raise hematocrits for hemodialysis patients influence their vascular access survival? Hematocrits elevated to the middle 30 range may amplify the thrombogenic tendencies in hemodialysis access grafts and accelerate graft thrombosis. To extend the longevity of PTFE grafts with higher hematocrit values, anticoagulation therapies such as aspirin,

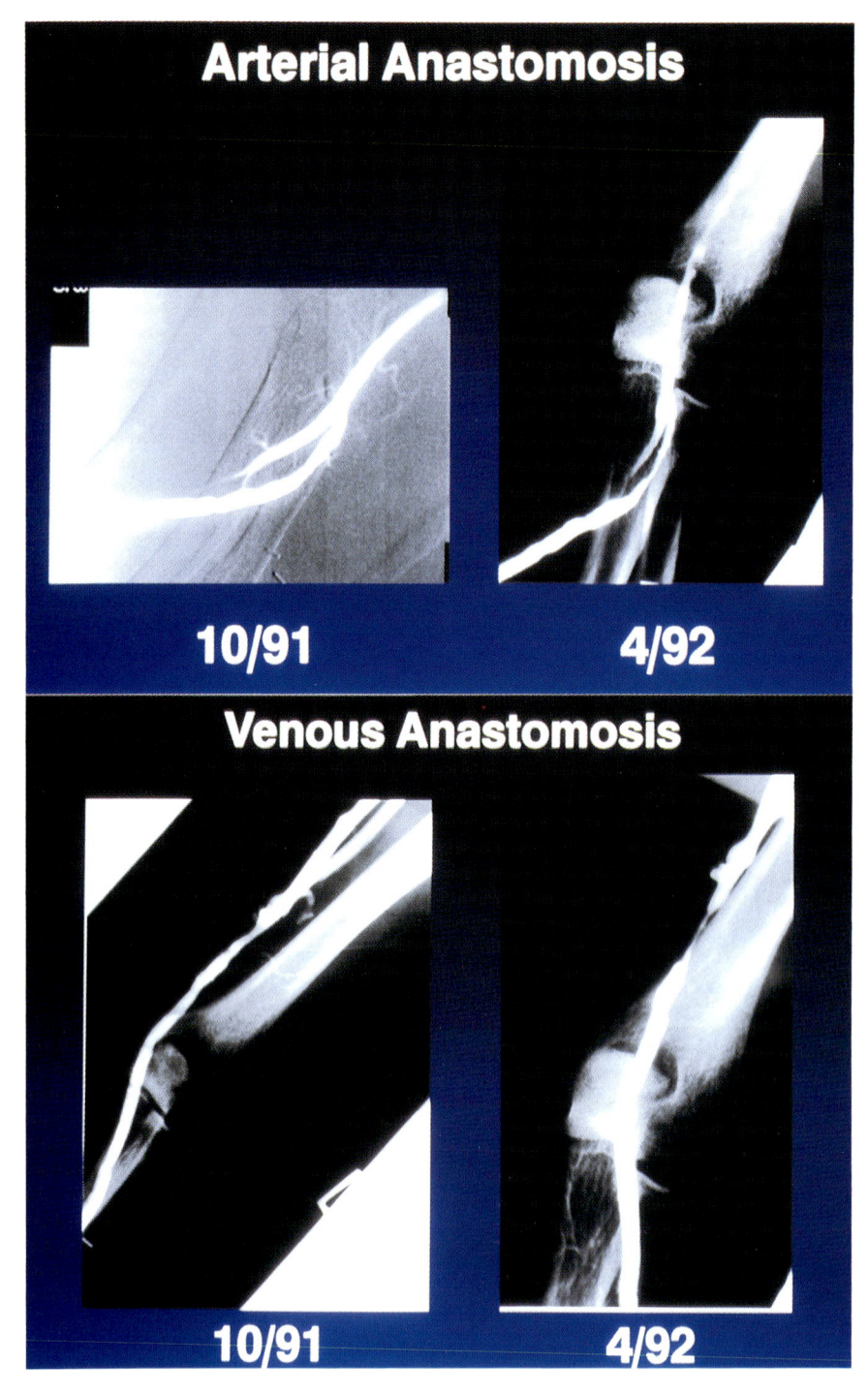

Figure 5-2. Progression of arterial and venous stenosis during a six-month period. *(Top left panel)* Arterial anastomosis 10/91. *(Top right panel)* Arterial anastomosis 4/92. *(Bottom left panel)* Venous anastomosis 10/91. *(Bottom right panel)* Venous anastomosis 4/92.

dipyridamole, or warfarin may have to be implemented. Further investigations are needed to clarify these concerns.

Many factors challenge the successful functioning of the dialysis vascular access, and vascular access failure for hemodialysis patients persists as the most frequent complication in these patients. New approaches for diagnosing access abnormalities such as CFD may reduce the morbidity of access failure. The use of CFD may allow early interventional therapy prior to graft failure. However, to fully comprehend the complicated intricacies of hemodialysis access failure, many additional clinical studies will be required.

References

1. Dousset V, Grenier H, Douws C, Senuita P, Sassouste G, Ada L, Potaux L. Hemodialysis grafts: color Doppler flow imaging correlated with digital subtraction angiography and function status. Radiology 1991; 181:89–94.
2. Middleton W, Picus D, Marx MV, Melson GL. Color Doppler sonography of hemodialysis vascular access: Comparison with angiography. AJR 1989; 152:633–39.
3. Nonnast-Daniel B, Martin RP, Lindert O, et al. Colour Doppler ultrasound assessment of arteriovenous haemodialysis fistulas. Lancet 1992; 339:143–45.
4. Tordoir JHM, de Bruin HG, Hoeneveld H, Eikelboom BC, Kitslaar PJEHM. Duplex ultrasound scanning in the assessment of arteriovenous fistulas created for hemodialysis access: Comparison with digital subtraction angiography. J Vasc Surg 1989; 10:122–28.
5. Glickman MH, Clark S, Goodrich V. Determination of outflow stenosis of arteriovenous fistulas for hemodialysis. Bruit 1985; 9:16–19.

6

CLINICAL USE OF COLOR FLOW DOPPLER

Barry S. Strauch, M.D., Robert S. O'Connell, M.D., Kenneth L. Geoly, M.D., Marietta Grundlehner, M.D., Y. Nabil Yakub, M.D., and David P. Tietjen, M.D.

FAILURE OF VASCULAR ACCESS FISTULAS AND GRAFTS is a leading cause of hospitalizations among hemodialysis patients.[1] This creates logistical problems for dialysis providers, vascular access radiologists, surgeons, and hospitals, as well as an extra burden for patients on dialysis therapy. For these reasons, we have evaluated various parameters in predicting failure of vascular access grafts and fistulas. The initial findings of this study have been previously reported.[2]

Color flow Doppler imaging (CFD) of vascular access grafts and fistulas has proven effective in evaluating anatomic vascular features as well as blood flow vascular parameters.[3] Comparison of CFD sonography with angiography has revealed a critical correlation with angiographic techniques.[4-6] Few studies, however, have attempted to test the predictive value of CFD for future thrombosis. In one study, a lower blood flow was found to have predictive value.[7] In a second study, multiple stenosis (>50% diameter reduction) correlated with vascular complications but did not predict thrombosis.[8]

In this study, we investigated the predictive value of CFD imaging of vascular access (polytetrafluoroethylene [PTFE] grafts and radial-cephalic fistulas) in a consecutive series of chronic hemodialysis patients. The maximum degree of vascular access narrowing was assessed as to its predictive value in forecasting access failure.

Recirculation of dialyzer blood has been associated with vascular access stenosis and thrombosis.[9] The value of the extent of recirculation in predicting clotting has not been studied, and the degree of recirculation that should necessitate further study is controversial. Earlier studies considered 20% recirculation as significant,[10] while a more recent study suggested 10%.[9] We investigated the role of abnormal recirculation as a predictor of vascular access thrombosis. We continue to use 20% as the lower limit for significance of percent recirculation because the more recent study had no patient above 10% in the screened group to study for correlation with clinical findings.

We investigated venous pressure in the dialysis circuit to predict vascular access clotting. Access volume flow, assessed by CFD, was also studied as a predictor. Last, we examined the change in grade of stenosis to explore the etiology of clotting in patients without positive predictive factors.

Methods

Seventy-three patients with grafts and 25 patients with fistulas at one outpatient dialysis center were screened with CFD. All current hemodialysis patients with PTFE grafts and radial-cephalic fistulas who were available were studied over a one-week period. Examinations were performed on a commercially available vascular ultrasound unit with CFD capability (QAD PV, Quantum Medical Systems, Issaquah, WA). The grafts and fistulas were examined with a 7.5 MHz transducer in the longitudinal plane (and transverse plane when needed) with and without color, from the arterial anastomosis, through the entire access, and into the draining veins as far as they could be imaged. Each examination was interpreted by one of the authors (R.S.O., a radiologist experienced in vascular ultrasound diagnosis). The degree of stenosis, measured in the longitudinal plane at the narrowest portion of the color stream, was recorded both directly in terms of millimeters of residual lumen and as a percent stenosis by comparing the minimal lumen to the diameter of a nearby normal segment of the graft or fistula.

Access volume flow was calculated using the time of velocity integral of a midstream spectrum obtained in a normal portion of the venous segment of the graft. The diameter of the graft was measured at the point of the spectral tracing. Care was taken to ensure that there were no wall irregularities at the area of measurement, that the graft had a constant diameter, that no turbulent flow was present, and that the Doppler angle was acceptable. Five cycles were averaged, with calculations performed by software built into the ultrasound unit.

Patients with grafts were classified into three groups: 1—a lesion of >50% diameter narrowing; 2—a lesion of 30–50% diameter narrowing; and 3—a normal study or a lesion of <30% diameter narrowing.

The percent recirculation was calculated by the method of Gotch[9,11] with the following formula:

$$\% \text{ recirculation} = 100 \times \frac{(S-I)}{(S-O)}$$

where S is concentration of blood urea nitrogen (BUN) in systemic blood flow as sampled in opposite limb, I is the BUN at the dialyzer blood inlet, and O is the BUN at the dialyzer blood outlet. Blood samples were obtained within the

Table 6-1. Classification of Cases and Basis for Incomplete Studies

	Cases	Completed study	Transplant	Moved or expired	Angioplasty
Group 1	21	14	2	3	2
Group 2	23	21		2	
Group 3	29	23	2	4	

Reason for not completing study (columns: Transplant, Moved or expired, Angioplasty)

Table 6-2. Patients Followed for Complete Six Months or Until Clotting Episode

	No. Patients	No. Clotted	Clotted (%)
Group 1*	14	8	57.1
Group 2	21	2	9.5
Group 3	23	3	13.0
Group 2 plus 3	44	5	11.4

*$p < 0.006$ for group 1 vs. 2
*$p < 0.008$ for group 1 vs. 3
*$p < 0.001$ for group 1 vs. 2 plus 3 combined

first 15 minutes of initiation of dialysis. BUN was determined by a commercial laboratory.

Venous pressure in the dialysis circuit was recorded within 15 minutes of initiation of dialysis at a blood flow rate of either 250 or 300 ml/min as ordered by the patient's physician. All subsequent venous pressure determinations were made at the same blood flow rate initially used for that patient.

The study was planned to end at six months to provide information for clinical decision making. All patients in the initial cohort were followed for the full six months unless they left the program, suffered a vascular access thrombotic episode, or underwent an elective angioplasty procedure.

After six months, we performed a repeat CFD study on all available patients in groups 2 and 3 who completed the initial six-month phase without a vascular access thrombosis.

To evaluate relationships between variables, the Fisher exact test was used for categorical variables, while both paired and unpaired *t*-tests were used for continuous variables.[12]

Results

Table 6-1 illustrates the division of cases with grafts into the three groups and gives the reasons for incomplete follow-up.

Table 6-3. Relationship of Access Volume Flow to Clotting (Grafts Only)

AVF (ml/min)	<200	<300	<400	<500	≥500
No. clotted	3	3	1	2	4
No. not clotted	2	0	2	5	35

As shown in table 6-2, of patients that completed follow-up, 57% of those in group 1 had clotting episodes within the six-month follow-up period. Only 9–13% of patients in groups 2 and 3 experienced clotting. The findings in group 1 as compared to the findings in group 2, group 3, and groups 2 and 3 combined were highly significant (p <0.006, <0.008, and <.001, respectively).

Recirculation of <20% was considered insignificant. In the group with clotting episodes (13 patients), recirculation as measured in 11 patients was <17% in all (<10% in seven patients). Recirculation in group 1 patients who completed the study was measured in 13 of 14 patients. None of the 13 had >16% recirculation.

Two patients in the original group 1 were above 20% (25% and 55%); the one who had a result of 55% underwent elective angioplasty. The patient with a result of 25% transferred from the program and was removed from the study. (It is known that he had a clotting episode one week after transfer to another facility.)

A third patient had a recirculation test at five months into the study. This revealed a dramatic rise from 7% to 80%. The patient underwent angioplasty and was removed from the study.

Patients with grafts without thrombotic episodes had an access volume flow (AVF) of 638.5 ml/min (± 46.2 S.E.) versus 357.0 ml/min (± 47.2 S.E.) in those with episodes of thrombosis (p < 0.001 by unpaired t-test). As shown in table 6-3, seven of the 13 patients with episodes of clotting had an AVF of <400 ml/min versus only four of 44 in those who did not clot. Two of the three patients in group 3 who clotted had AVF of <300 ml/min.

Eight patients with stenosis of >50% (group 1) also had AVF of < 400 ml/min. Five of these eight patients (62%) had an episode of clotting. The risk of clotting for patients in group 1 (57%) versus patients in group 1 with AVF of <400 ml/min (62%) was not statistically significant (p = 0.8).

In all patients who had episodes of thrombosis, a comparison was made of the average venous pressure over the two weeks prior to the performance of the CFD study with an average of two weeks prior to the episode of clotting and with the treatment just prior to the clotting episode. As shown in table 6-4, no significant difference was apparent. The average venous pressure at the time of the CFD study in the group that subsequently thrombosed (160.8 mm Hg ± 12.8 S.E.) did not differ significantly from that of those who did not thrombose (137.8 mm Hg ± 4.4 S.E.), (p > 0.1).

As shown in table 6-5, the fraction of loop grafts and that of straight grafts that thrombosed was quite similar to the division of straight and loop grafts in the study group.

The record of each patient with an episode of clotting was reviewed for the two weeks prior to clotting for difficulty with needle insertion. Of 78 treatments, only one was noted as difficult.

Table 6-4. Changes in Venous Pressure (mm Hg ± S.E.) in Patients with Thrombotic Episodes

(A) at time of Doppler	(B) > 2 weeks prethrombosis	(C) treatment prethrombosis	(B–A)*	(C–A)*
129.6 ± 2.9	133.3 ± 2.6	123.8 ± 3.6	3.7 ± 6.7	1.2 ± 7.5

*p = 0.59 for (A) vs. (B) and p = 0.88 for (C) vs. (A) as assessed by paired *t*-test

Table 6-5. Nature of Graft

	Loop* No. (%)	Straight* No. (%)
Thrombosed	9 (69.2)	4 (30.8)
Not thrombosed	35 (77.8)	10 (22.2)
Total	44 (75.9)	14 (24.1)

*p = 0.71 for loop versus straight grafts.

In patients in group 1 (>50% stenotic area), areas of stenosis in loop grafts were apparent in the venous limb in all but one patient; they tended to be most apparent from the midvenous limb to the venous anastomosis. Two patients had a stenotic access just distal to the venous anastomosis in the native vein segment. In patients in group 1 with straight grafts, areas of stenosis were most apparent in areas near the venous anastomosis.

Of 19 patients in group 2 who finished the six-month study period without thrombosis, 16 were available for a repeat CFD study. As shown in table 6-6, five patients progressed to group 1, and one patient fell into group 3.

Of 20 patients in group 3 who completed the six-month study period without thrombosis, 19 were available for a repeat CFD study. As shown in table 6-7, 10 progressed to group 2 and three went to group 1.

Of 25 patients with radial-cephalic fistulas, three were transplanted and 22 completed the study period. None of the 25 patients had a stenosis of ≥30% and none had an episode of thrombosis. These patients were not further assessed.

Discussion and Conclusion

We were unable to find any differences in simple clinical parameters (venous pressure or difficult needle insertion) that allowed for prediction of clotting in patients with grafts. The results do not allow us to evaluate prediction values for significantly abnormal recirculation. Only two patients in group 1 had initial recirculation above 20%. One of these patients moved from the facility

Table 6-6. Classification of Group 2—Cases with Repeat Studies

	Initial study	Repeat study
Group 1	—	5
Group 2	16	10
Group 3	—	1

Table 6-7. Classification of Group 3—Cases with Repeat Studies

	Initial study	Repeat study
Group 1	—	3
Group 2	—	10
Group 3	19	6

prior to the completion of the study, and the other underwent elective angioplasty. Of the patients who had a clotting episode, none of those measured had a recirculation above 16%.

Our study has revealed that stenosis of >50% in a graft as demonstrated by CFD is highly valuable in predicting a clotting episode within six months. Performance of CFD at six- to 12-month intervals would identify patients at high risk for thrombosis. These patients could then be treated for lesions before acute thrombosis of their grafts occurred. Whether such prophylactic measures will prove helpful remains to be tested.

Decreased access volume flow in grafts correlated with episodes of thrombosis as has previously been shown.[7] All but one patient who clotted had either AVF of <300 ml/min or stenosis of at least 30%. The ability to predict thrombosis was not significantly enhanced by combining stenosis of >50% with AVF of <400 ml/min.

The follow-up CFD studies suggest a rapid progression of stenotic lesions. Over half of patients in group 3 and nearly one third of patients in group 2 progressed at least one grade within six months. This rapid rate of change may explain why patients who did not fit into group 1 when first classified underwent thrombosis during the six-month study period.

Because no patients with fistulas had significant stenosis or clotted, we were unable to demonstrate the value of CFD in predicting thrombosis in these patients. Our study does not support routine performance of CFD on patients with fistulas. The data reconfirm that fistulas provide superior vascular access and should be chosen whenever possible.

In conclusion, CFD has proven to be a valuable tool in predicting hemodialysis access failure. Routine graft surveillance with this technology can identify graft problems prior to failure. The next step is to identify the long-term outcome following correction of the new-found underlying abnormality.

References

1. Eggers PW, Connerton R, McMullan M. The Medicare experience with end-stage renal disease: Trends in incidence, prevalence and survival. Health Care Manage Rev 1984;5:69-88.
2. Strauch BS, O'Connell RS, Geoly KL, Grundlehner M, Yakub YN, Tietjen DP. Forecasting thrombosis of vascular access with Doppler color flow imaging. Am J Kidney Dis 1992;19:554-57.
3. Tordoir JHM, de Bruin HG, Hoeneveld H, Eikelboom BC, Kitslaar PJEHM. Duplex ultrasound scanning in the assessment of arteriovenous fistulas created for hemodialysis access: Comparison with digital subtraction angiography. J Vasc Surg 1989;10:122-28.
4. Grant G, Tessler FN, Perrella RR. Clinical Doppler imaging. AJR 1989;152:707-11.
5. Evans RG. Doppler sonographic imaging of the vascular system. JAMA 1991;265:2382-87.
6. Middleton WD, Picus DD, Marx MV, Meison GL. Color Doppler sonography of hemodialysis vascular access: Comparison with angiography. AJR 1989;152:634-39.
7. Shackleton CR, Taylor DC, Buckley AR, Rowley A, Cooperberg PL, Fry PD. Predicting failure in polytetrafluoroethylene vascular access grafts for hemodialysis: a pilot study. Can J Surg 1987;30:442-44.
8. Tordoir JHM, Hoeneveld H, Eikelboom BC, Kitslaar PJEHM. The correlation between clinical and Doppler ultrasound parameters and the development of complications in arterio-venous fistulae for hemodialysis. Eur J Vasc Surg 1990;4:179-84.
9. Nordi L, Bosch J. Recirculation: Review, techniques for measurement and ability to predict hemoaccess stenosis before and after angioplasty. Blood Purif 1988;6:85-89.
10. Seidman MS, Lundis AP, Brown CD. Extent of blood recirculation during two-needle hemodialysis. Abstr Am Soc Artif Intern Organs 1979;8:56.
11. Gotch FA. The kidney. Philadelphia: WB Saunders, 1976.
12. Rumin AA, Hartz AJ, Kolbflesch, Anderson AJ, Hoffman RG. Basic biostatistics in medicine. New York: Appleton-Century-Crofts, 1980.

PANEL DISCUSSION

Moderator:
  Ronald M. Ferguson, M.D., Ph.D.
Panelists:
  Samuel Martin, M.D.
  William H. Bay, M.D.
  Barry S. Strauch, M.D.

Discussant: Low-flow grafts tend to have less perivascular vibration but appear to be more likely to thrombose. Did any of the presenters find grafts that did not have a significant amount of perivascular tissue vibration, and if you did, did you find any problem with clotting in that group of grafts?

Dr. Martin: No, all of them have some vibration. It is going to take some time to correlate the degree of tissue vibration with the eventual outcome of those grafts. That is, are the patients who have more perivascular vibration going on to have a graft with a shorter life span? We haven't had a chance to correlate that.

Discussant: Dr. Strauch, is there a way to select a subgroup of patients who need to be studied, or should all outpatients be studied regularly?

Dr. Strauch: A patient with a fistula is not going to get a lot of benefit by being screened on a six-month basis. It would appear that patients with PTFE grafts will benefit, as best we can tell at this point, from being screened on a regular basis at six months because of the rate of progression of lesions in this group. I have to emphasize that we haven't proven that intervening in a patient two to three months before they thrombose is going to help. However, if it does, it will serve to prevent the actual thrombosis and make an urgent situation into one that is relatively elective.

Dr. Martin: Our usual clinical criteria give us no information as to the predictability of graft thrombosis. As one of these grafts thromboses, the economic as well as morbidity issues increase significantly. The patient may have to be admitted and have a temporary access line placed, with those attendant costs and risks. Routine color flow surveillance may avoid this.

Discussant: Dr. Strauch, I have a question regarding your percent recirculation statistics. Would you please tell us at what blood flows these were drawn and was a systemic blood sample drawn? It seems to me that these percent recirculations were very low, at least compared to what we see in Philadelphia.

Dr. Strauch: Your observation of recirculation changing with blood flow is correct and is reported in an elegant paper in the literature. These measurements were done at 15 minutes into dialysis, and the patients had a blood flow rate of either 250 or 300 cc per minute. We were not a high-flux unit at that point, by the way. The technique was a peripheral draw of a BUN 15 minutes into dialysis and then one draw from the arterial and venous limbs of the dialyzer.

Discussant: When you define stenosis, are we talking about percent diameter reduction or area reduction? Are these studies being done postdialysis, especially when there is more hypotension?

Dr. Martin: We are talking about decreased vessel diameter. Certainly a more accurate measurement is the cross-sectional area reduction. It is important that we deal with the cross-sectional diameter, because when we are comparing it to the angiogram we must compare it to diameter. Historically, this has been a very important point that we saw when looking at carotid angiograms. We have to report it in terms of percentage diameter reduction as opposed to cross-sectional area, because otherwise we are talking apples and oranges. Later, when everybody feels more secure with the technology and we are operating on the basis of a color flow image solely, without an angiogram, we then can speak in terms of cross-sectional areas.

Discussant: When was the study completed?

Dr. Bay: In my report, a mobile color flow Doppler was used and was done during dialysis so the patients weren't inconvenienced by another appointment.

Discussant: What studies are being done preoperatively to evaluate a patient's arm or leg, to make sure that there are no abnormalities in either the venous outflow or arterial inflow that may cause a problem with the graft? At what percent stenosis do you recommend repairing?

Dr. Martin: In dealing with preoperative studies, we have not routinely done CFD or duplex imaging of the outflow veins unless the patient has a history of several access failures or we are concerned about an access being placed in an area where there has been a previous access. We occasionally have used it in an obese patient in whom we want to place an autogenous fistula to the outflow vein.

Dr. Bay: I think your second question regarding at what degree of stenosis do you repair the access is excellent. We are trying to do this by putting together a multicenter data base to answer these questions, one of the most pertinent of which is whether we can prevent thrombosis by intervening before thrombosis. The whole issue of reimbursement is a growing problem because it may mean that routine surveys are required to identify existing abnormalities that are not accepted by Medicare. A larger data base may allow us to find clinical signs of impending graft failure and thus avoid the need for the routine CFD.

Discussant: Do you feel comfortable enough with CFD to do intervention or a revision based solely on the CFD findings?

Dr. Martin: Yes, I think we have refined things to the point that now we are able to do this. I certainly would feel a little less comfortable in the autogenous fistula, but in the prosthetic grafts the results correlate well. I think it is another opportunity to save the patient and the system money, and we are ready to progress to that point now.

Moderator: If we were to use this to monitor all PTFE accesses, how much would it cost, especially if it was in the dialysis unit and they could just do it right there?

Dr. Martin: This varies from state to state, but the charge is about $200 to $250 to do the test.

SECTION III—
ABSTRACT PRESENTATIONS

7

INCIDENCE OF VASCULAR ACCESS THROMBOSIS IN PATIENTS TREATED WITH RECOMBINANT HUMAN ERYTHROPOIETIN

George Carty, M.D., and Daniel Hoheim, M.D.

SEVERE ANEMIA ASSOCIATED WITH end-stage renal disease (ESRD) is a major impediment to effective medical rehabilitation of dialysis patients. Until recently, treatment alternatives were blood transfusion and administration of androgens. Transfusions, while generally effective, carry considerable risks. Androgen therapy, with its own adverse effects, is effective only in a minority of patients. Recombinant human erythropoietin (EPO) has been found to be effective in correcting the anemia of hemodialysis patients.[1-4]

Concerns related to the use of EPO include a reported increase in vascular access clotting[1-5] resulting from transient increase in platelet counts[2,6] and normalization of bleeding times after reversal of anemia.[7,8] Maintenance of a patent vascular access in the hemodialysis patient population has always been vital and challenging. Having previously reviewed the experience with our own hemodialysis patients,[9] we decided to undertake a prospective study to determine the incidence of vascular access thrombosis in EPO-treated patients.

Materials and Methods

From September 1989 through August 1990, at varying starting dates 59 patients were placed on EPO (Epogen, Amgen, Inc., Thousand Oaks, CA), following standard accepted guidelines.[6] To secure a homogeneous patient population in terms of type of vascular access, only patients with polytetrafluorethylene (PTFE) grafts were included. Patients with Brescia-Cimino arteri-

Total Dialysis Patient Population

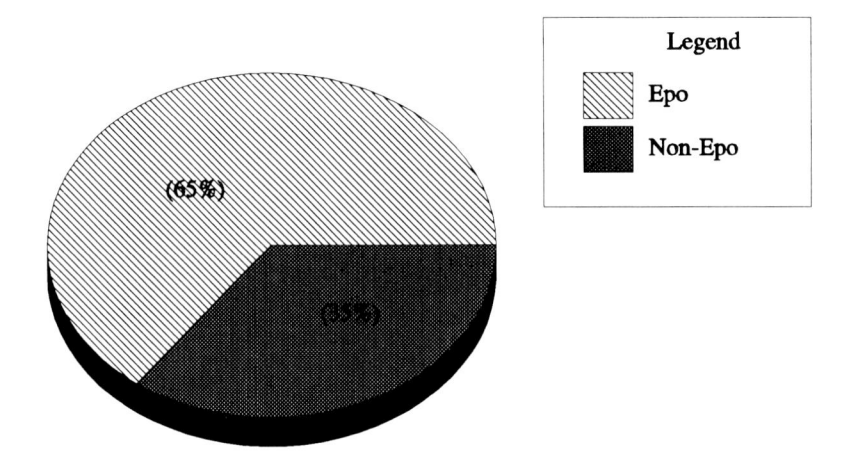

Figure 7-1. Total of patients on hemodialysis for the duration of the study period was 91. Of these, 59—64.8% of the entire dialysis patient population—were on erythropoietin therapy.

ovenous (A-V) fistulas were not entered in the study. Patient-months in this study totaled 231. The initial and final hemoglobin and hematocrit values were recorded and averaged. The number of vascular access graft thrombotic episodes was recorded. A-V conduits that thrombosed before the patient was on EPO for at least two weeks were not included.

Records of all outpatients treated at the hemodialysis unit of Saginaw (Michigan) General Hospitals from September 1983 to May 1992 were available for review. The incidence of thrombosis was tabulated as the total number of events per 100 graft-months. The incidence of thrombosis was also evaluated as it related to the total number of months at risk, for all accesses. The period September 1988 to August 1989 was chosen as the historical control, corresponding to a 12-month interval before the introduction of EPO therapy.

Statistical comparisons using unpaired student's t-test and chi-square test were carried out. A p value of $<.05$ was considered significant.

Results

A total of 59 patients were entered in the EPO group during the study period. The average duration at risk for thrombosis of these accesses was 15.75 months. Patients in hemodialysis during this period totaled 91, of whom 32 were in the non-EPO category (figure 7-1).

Table 7-1. Hemoglobin and Hematocrit at Beginning of Study

	Hemoglobin (gm %)	Hematocrit (%)
Patients on EPO	7.94 ± 0.2	23.58 ± 0.5
Patients not on EPO	9.26 ± 0.4	27.95 ± 0.5

Table 7-2. Hemoglobin and Hematocrit at End of Study

	Hemoglobin (gm %)	Hemaocrit (%)
Patients on EPO	8.72 ± 0.2*	26.04 ± 0.5*
Patients not on EPO	9.51 ± 0.4	28.32 ± 0.5

*$p < .01$ when compared to starting values in table 7-1

The average hemoglobin value of patients on EPO at the beginning of the study period was 7.94 gm% with an average hematocrit value of 23.58%, while the average hemoglobin value of the patients not on EPO was 9.26 gm% with a hematocrit value of 27.95% (table 7-1). The average final hemoglobin value in the 59 patients entered in the EPO group was 8.72 gm% and the average hematocrit value was 26.04%, with an increase of 10% and 12%, respectively, over the course of the study period (table 7-2). The difference between hemoglobin and hematocrit starting and ending values was statistically significant ($p < .004$ and $< .002$, respectively) for the EPO-treated group. As anticipated, the EPO group did not show a significant interval change in hemoglobin or hematocrit values (9.51 gm% and 28.32%).

There were 73 vascular access thrombotic episodes during the study period, for an overall thrombosis rate of 6.68 per 100 graft-months. Thirty-six of these thromboses occurred in 16 of 59 EPO-treated patients, and 37 episodes occurred in 19 of 32 non-EPO–treated patients (figure 7-2). The statistically significant difference ($p < .005$) suggested a higher rate of graft thrombosis in the nontreated patients (59% vs. 27%).

Figure 7-3 shows the yearly incidence of vascular access thrombosis over a three-year period in relation to the total number of grafts, as well as patients, at risk. EPO therapy was introduced in September 1989. The proportion of patients at risk who eventually required thrombectomy has not significantly changed over the past three years; however, the total number of thrombotic events has increased. When these data are expressed as the rate of thrombosis per patient, they reflect a statistically significant increase from 1.5 per patient per year in 1988 to 1.8 per patient per year in 1989 and to 2.1 per patient per year in 1990 ($p < .001$).

The annualized risk of vascular access thrombosis as presented in figure 7-4 for the past three years is grouped by "recurrent clotter" (more than one event per year) and "average patient" (single event per year). During the year of introduction of EPO, the annualized thrombosis risk per access was 80.2%. Twelve percent of the dialysis patient population accounted for 59% of all

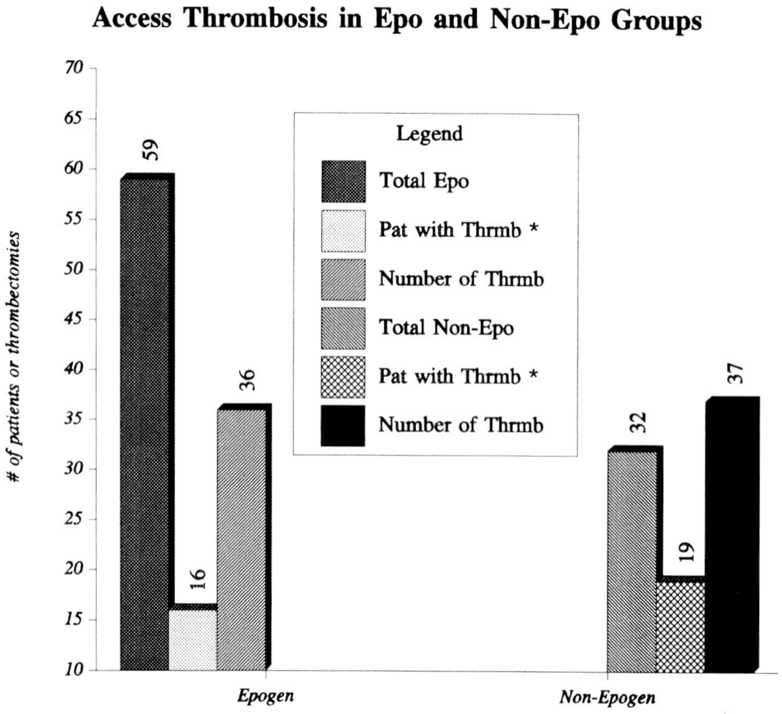

Access Thrombosis in Epo and Non-Epo Groups

Figure 7-2. Number of vascular access thrombosis patients, subgrouped by EPO and non-EPO–treated patients (*p < .01 when comparing both groups).

thrombotic events. Seven percent of the dialysis population accounted for 39% of the thrombotic events. If "recurrent clotters" are defined as those having three or more episodes of graft thrombosis during the study period and are excluded, the probability of clotting decreased to 38.3% per year. When "recurrent clotters" are defined as those patients with two or more thrombotic events during one calendar year and are excluded, the annualized risk of thrombosis fell to 18.6%. A significant difference was seen in the number of "recurrent clotters" present in the EPO-treated group (7 of 59) and in the non-EPO–treated group (11 of 32) during the length of the study. All thrombotic episodes in our series were considered to be a different event, even when they occurred within one week of each other and even if angiography demonstrated an uncorrected anatomic abnormality predisposing to thrombosis.

Discussion

At first glance, patients with ESRD should have few thrombotic problems. These patients have a low hematocrit and therefore a low blood viscosity, and there is a well-known bleeding tendency in uremia that is related to a qualitative platelet defect.[10] Still, grafts and fistulas often thrombose. The reduction in

**Annualized Risk of Vascular Access Thrombosis
Jan 1988-Dec 1990**

Figure 7-3. Total number of vascular access patients at risk, plotted against the total number of patients with thrombotic episodes and the total number of events.

**Annual Access Thrombosis
Jan 1988-Dec 1990**

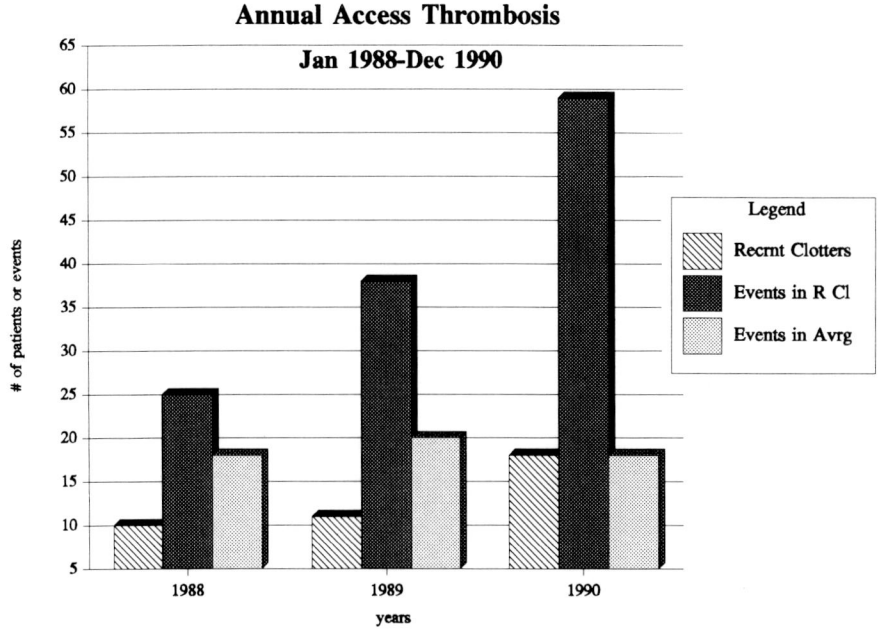

Figure 7-4. Yearly incidence of vascular access thrombosis grouped by "recurrent clotters" (two or more events per year) and "average patients."

failure rate through use of sulfinpyrazone suggests that platelets may be implicated.[11] Whole blood viscosity, or hematocrit, has also been found to be of importance in both arterial[12] and venous[13] thrombosis.

Although there has been no definitive evidence so far that the use of EPO does increase vascular access thrombosis, more frequent clotting was initially reported by Winerals et al.,[3] Casati et al.,[7] and Paganini et al.[14] in small groups of patients with autogenous fistulas as well as prosthetic grafts. It has been postulated that correction of the anemia with EPO may shorten bleeding time in uremic patients as blood viscosity increases.[15] A rise in platelet count, even though it remains within normal range, has also been reported, and it is suggested as a factor in vascular access thrombosis.[2]

Although a change in vascular access thrombosis rates has been observed over the past three years, our results show that the increase has occurred in the non-EPO–treated patients. The fraction of thrombotic episodes in patients labeled "recurrent clotters" has also increased throughout this period, whereas the total number of thrombotic events is equally distributed among the EPO and the non-EPO groups.

The findings of the current study suggest that there is a significant difference between the frequency of occurrence of vascular access thrombosis in EPO and non-EPO hemodialysis patients. However, this difference was expressed as a lower incidence of access thrombosis in the EPO-treated patients. Although higher hemoglobin and hematocrit values were obtained in all EPO-treated patients, their average hemoglobin and hematocrit values remained fractionally lower than those of the non-EPO patients.

The realities of patient care appear to have redefined the ideal parameters initially set forth, resulting in lower than expected hemoglobin and hematocrit values—and possibly lower platelet levels as well—in the treated group. It is conceivable that this circumstance alone may have been the determining factor in shifting the balance toward the nontreated group. Therefore, the 10% hemoglobin and 12% hematocrit increases among the EPO-treated patients were not clinically expressed as increased rate of access thrombosis.

For any given time interval, a lower total number of events appears to correlate well with the absence of many "recurrent clotters." It has been our experience that this subset of patients, with repeated episodes of access clotting without an anatomical graft abnormality, will significantly alter all data and is responsible for periodical changes in the annualized risk of access thrombosis. Whereas a similar percentage of the total dialysis patient population continue to have access thrombotic episodes, the total number of events has increased. The relative number of "recurrent clotters" has not changed, although the rate of thrombosis for this group significantly increased between 1988 and 1990, from 2.5 to 3.3 ($p < .001$) per patient per year. This can explain the overall rise in the number of thrombotic events per year for the entire dialysis population.

The expanding number of patients on maintenance hemodialysis makes it imperative to maintain vascular access patency and prevent complications, particularly in older individuals. Although new variables such as drugs or dialysate composition changes will be introduced from time to time and will require evaluation in terms of their potential influence in vascular access thrombosis rates, an essential factor appears to be the presence and random distribution of "recurrent clotters." It would seem appropriate that future efforts be directed to this rather small but extremely important subset of patients.

Summary

The results of this study show that patients currently on EPO do not have an increased incidence of vascular access graft thrombosis. Because all hemodialysis patients could potentially be placed on EPO therapy, a perfectly matched control group will not be available for a prospective, randomized study. Therefore, comparisons will need to be made with the previously generated historical controls.

Whereas increases in hematocrit and blood viscosity, as well as the relative number of platelets, are thought to predispose to vascular access clotting, the incidence of thrombosis appears to be lower in the EPO-treated patients. Long-term follow-up will be needed to ascertain if the distribution observed in the thrombosis rates continues to be statistically valid in the future.

References

1. Watson A. Adverse effects of therapy for the correction of anemia in hemodialysis patients. Semin Nephrol 1989; 9:30-34.
2. Bommer J, Alexiou C, Muller-Buhl U, Eifert J, Ritz E. Recombinant human erythropoietin therapy in hemodialysis patients—dose determination and clinical experience. Nephrol Dial Transplant 1987; 2:238-42.
3. Winearls C, Oliver D, Pippard M, Reid C, Cotes P, Downing M. Effect of human erythropoietin derived from recombinant DNA on the anaemia of patients maintained by chronic hemodialysis. Lancet 1986; 2:1175-78.
4. Raine AE. Hypertension, blood viscosity, and cardiovascular morbidity in renal failure: Implications of erythropoietin therapy. Lancet 1988; 1:97-99.
5. Ahmad R, Hand M. Recombinant erythropoietin for the anemia of chronic renal failure (letter). N Engl J Med 1987; 317:169.
6. Eschbach JW, Adamson JW. Guidelines for recombinant human erythropoietin therapy. Am J Kidney Dis 1989; 14:2-8.
7. Casati S, Passerini P, Moia M, Graziani G, Mannucci PM, Ponticelli C. Correction of clotting disturbances in chronic hemodialysis patients treated with human recombinant erythropoietin (rHuEPO). Kidney Int 1988; 33:662A.
8. Gordge MP, Leaker B, Patel A, Oviasu E, Cameron JS, Neild GH. Recombinant human erythropoietin shortens the uraemic bleeding time without causing intravascular hemostatic activation. Thromb Res 1990; 57:171-82.
9. Carty GA, Davis VH. Mid-graft stenosis in expanded polytetrafluorethylene hemodialysis conduits. Dialy Transplant 1990; 19:486-89.
10. Rabiner SF. In: Uremic bleeding. Progress in hemostasis and thrombosis. New York & London: Grune & Stratton, 1972; 233.

11. Kaegi A, Pineo GF, Shimizu A. Arteriovenous shunt thrombosis. N Engl J Med 1974; 290:304–06.
12. Bouhoutsos J, Morris T, Chavatzas D, Martin P. The influence of haemoglobin and platelet levels on the results of arterial surgery. Br J Surg 1974; 61:984.
13. Dormandy JA, Edelman JB. High blood viscosity: An etiological factor in venous thrombosis. Br J Surg 1973; 60:187.
14. Paganini EP, Latham D, Abdulhadi M. Practical considerations of recombinant human erythropoietin therapy. Am J Kidney Dis 1989; 2419:19–25.
15. Zins B, Brueke T, Zingraff J. Erythropoietin treatment in anaemic patients on hemodialysis. Lancet 1986; 2:1329.

8

TREATMENT OF ANGIOACCESS ISCHEMIC STEAL BY REVASCULARIZATION

Harry Schanzer, M.D., Milan Skladany, M.D., and Moshe Haimov, M.D.

CONSTRUCTION OF AN ARTERIOVENOUS (A-V) FISTULA for hemodialysis access frequently results in reduction of blood flow to the hand.[1] Although in most cases a clinical problem does not result, symptomatic ischemia is by no means rare.[2-4] Manfestations range from intermittent claudication to severe pain at rest with neurologic deficits and digital gangrene. Bearing in mind the need for preservation of potential A-V fistula sites in patients requiring life-long hemodialysis, we have devised a physiologic approach to the treatment of ischemia occurring after A-V fistula creation that improves distal perfusion without endangering the angioaccess.[5] This work presents our expanded experience with this technique over the past five years.

Materials and Methods

Fourteen patients with end-stage renal disease (ESRD) requiring hemodialysis developed severe ischemia in the extremity carrying the angioaccess. Twelve patients had polytetrafluoroethylene (PTFE) bridge A-V fistulas, one had a brachiocephalic A-V fistula, and one had a radiocephalic A-V fistula. All patients had very severe ischemia with a threat of loss of function and tissue in the hand (figure 8-1). Five of the extremities already had gangrenous changes. Ten patients had symptoms immediately following construction of the access. The remaining four had late onset of ischemia. The surgical technique used to treat

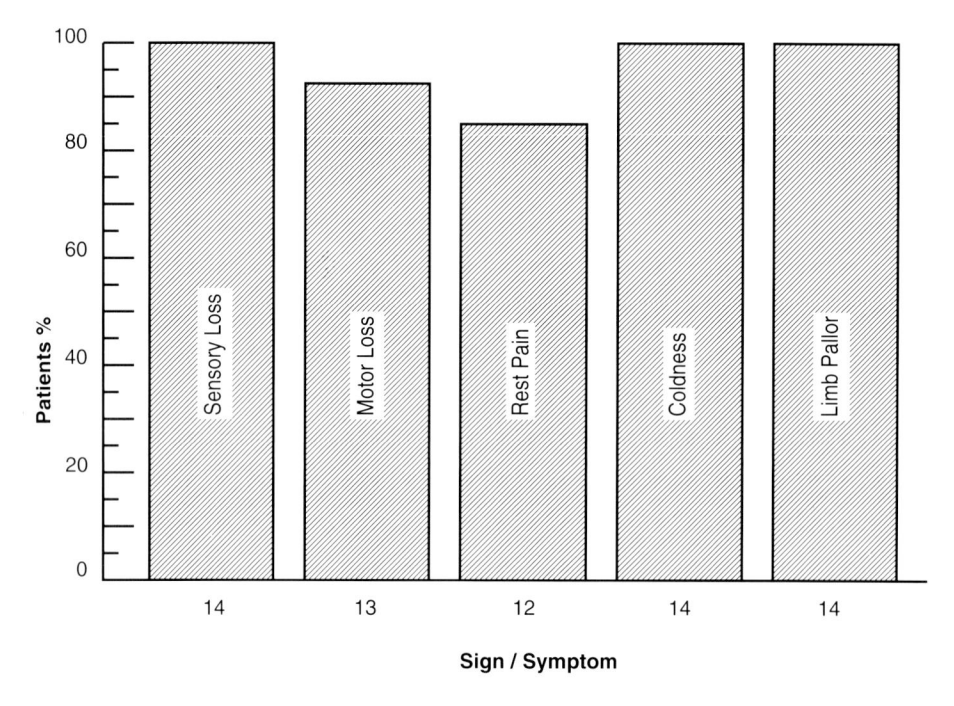

Figure 8-1. Clinical manifestation of ischemic steal.

these patients consists of ligation of the artery most distal to the takeoff of the fistula and arterial bypass from the artery proximal to the takeoff of the fistula to the artery distal to the ligation (figure 8-2). The intent of the ligation is to abolish the reversal of flow in the distal artery, and the bypass reestablishes normal arterial flow to the distal extremity.

The material used for bypass was saphenous vein in 13 cases and PTFE in one case. Patency of the arterial bypass was estimated by palpation of distal pulses and confirmed by Doppler arterial pressure measurements. Function of the access was assessed by palpation of a thrill and auscultation for a bruit.

Results

All 14 cases treated with this technique showed immediate signs of improvement after surgery. One patient with advanced gangrenous changes at the time of the corrected procedure required a forearm amputation 13 months later. The remaining 13 patients had complete resolution of the fistula and healing of the gangrenous lesions. The two patients with A-V fistulas requiring revascularization had the access patent at 11 and 17 months of follow-up. Patency of the bridge A-V fistula was 81.7% at one year, and no episodes of thrombosis were found in the arterial bypasses (figure 8.3).

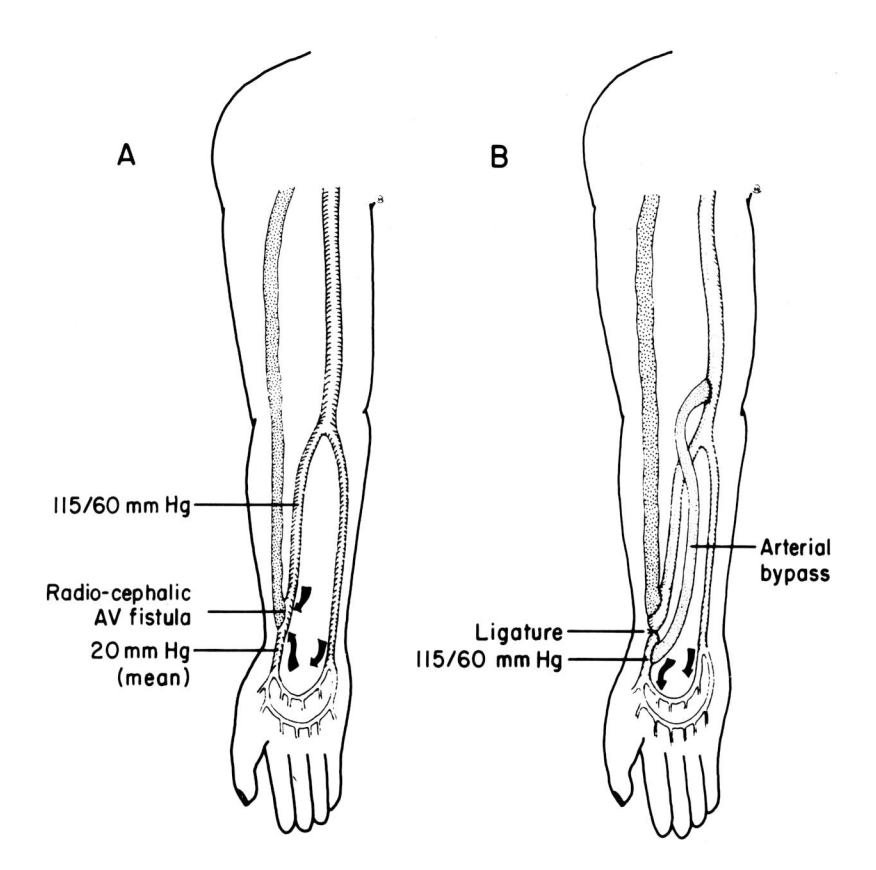

Figure 8-2. Surgical procedure performed on a 28-year-old diabetic patient who developed gangrene of the index finger two years after construction of radiocephalic A-V fistula. (A) Diagram with pressures obtained before doing corrective procedure. (B) Diagram of corrective procedure with ligation of the artery distal to the fistula, and bypass, with changes in pressures.

Discussion

Construction of an A-V fistula, either by direct A-V anastomosis or graft interposition, provides reliable vascular access for long-term hemodialysis. A recognized complication of this procedure is ischemia of the limb distal to the fistula site. In the bridge fistula, the incidence varies between 2.7% and 4.3%, while the incidence in radiocephalic A-V fistulas is less than 1%.[6-9] In our experience, more than 80% of patients complaining of ischemic symptoms early after the construction of the A-V fistula will show significant improvement after the first postoperative month. Patients who have an early severe ischemic limb with associated neuromuscular deficit or those having persistent symptoms require treatment of the steal phenomenon. The selection of a treatment modality re-

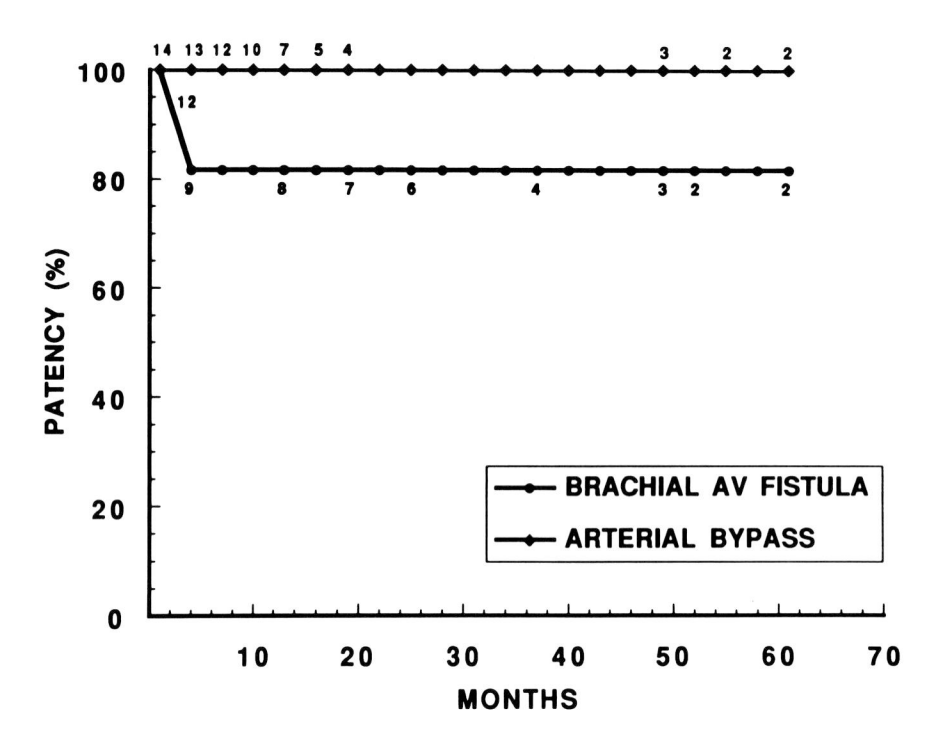

Figure 8-3. Cumulative patency rate for bridge A-V fistulas and arterial bypasses.

quires sound physiologic understanding of the hemodynamic changes that the A-V fistula produces and the mechanism of ischemia. The underlying pathophysiologic mechanism responsible for this condition is the reversal of flow in the portion of the artery distal to the fistula, induced by the low-pressure system present at the outflow side of the A-V connection. This alteration in flow has been labeled *steal;* when it is of sufficient magnitude and cannot be compensated by collateral flow, steal results in clinical ischemia.

Various methods have been devised for treatment of distal ischemia after A-V fistula construction. The simplest means to improve distal perfusion is ligation of the venous outflow of the fistula.[10] This procedure provides immediate improvement in perfusion, but eliminates a site for angioaccess and requires the immediate construction of another angioaccess. Other techniques have been described that do not sacrifice the fistula and yet improve distal perfusion. Ligation of the artery distal to the origin of the fistula will prevent retrograde flow and therefore will eliminate the steal phenomenon.[2] The efficacy of this procedure depends on the quality of the collateral arteries. In the distal radiocephalic A-V fistula where collateral vessels are abundant, this procedure will usually suffice. In the more proximal A-V fistula such as the brachial-axillary bridge fistula, this procedure may not be adequate. In this situation, other techniques have been tried. Narrowing (often called "banding") of the interposition graft will reduce flow and improve distal perfusion.[11,12] The problem with this procedure is the difficulty in determining the required amount of stenosis. A small degree of stenosis will not be enough to reverse steal, and too much stenosis may result in thrombosis of the access site. Another technique that has been used for the same purpose consists of adding extra length to the interposition graft, increasing resistance to the A-V fistula and thereby decreasing steal.[13] The same problems described for the banding procedure are encountered in this technique. The technique described herein provides an added collateral artery, which improves distal perfusion significantly without affecting the function of the A-V fistula. In our view, it is the procedure of choice for the correction of fistula-induced ischemic steal.

References

1. Kwun KB, Schanzer H, Finkler BA, Haimov M, Burrows L. Hemodynamic evaluation of angioaccess procedures for hemodialysis. Vasc Surg 1979;13:170–177.
2. Storey BG, George CRP, Stewart JH, Tiller DJ, May J, Sheil AGR. Embolic and ischemia complications after anastomosis of radial artery to cephalic vein. Surgery 1969; 66:325–27.
3. Russell JA, Abbott JA, Lim RC. A radial steal syndrome with arteriovenous fistula for hemodialysis: Studies in seven patients. Ann Intern Med 1971;75:387–94.
4. Kinnaert P, Struyven J, Mathieu J, Vereestraeten P, Tousaint C, Van Geertruyden J. Intermittent claudication of the hand after creation of an arteriovenous fistula in the forearm. Am J Surg 1980;139:838–43.
5. Schanzer H, Schwartz M, Harrington E, Haimov M. Treatment of ischemia due to "steal" by arteriovenous fistula with distal artery ligation and revascularization. J Vasc Surg 1988;7:770–73.
6. Munda R, First R, Alexander W, Linnenman C, Fidler J, Kittur D. Polytetrafluoroethylene graft survival in hemodialysis. JAMA 1983;249:219–22.
7. Merickel J, Anderson R, Knutson R, Lipshulz M, Hitchcock C. Bovine carotid artery shunts in vascular access surgery. Arch Surg 1974;109:245–50.
8. Haimov M, Burrows L, Schanzer H. Experience with arterial substitutes in the construction of vascular access for hemodialysis. J Cardiovasc Surg 1980;21:149–154.
9. Haimov M. Vascular access for hemodialysis. Surg Gynecol Obstet 1975;141:619–625.
10. Corry RJ, Patel NP, Natvarlal P, West JC. Surgical management of complications of vascular access for hemodialysis. Surg Gynecol Obstet 1980;151:49–54.
11. Ebeid A, Saranchak HJ. Banding of a PTFE hemodialysis fistula in the treatment of steal syndrome. Clin Exp Dialy & Aphresis 1981;5:251–57.
12. Dally P, Brantigan, C.O. Plethysmography and the diagnosis of the steal syndrome following placement of arteriovenous fistulae and shunts for hemodialysis access. J Cardiovasc Surg 1987;28:200–03.
13. West JC, Evans RD, Kelley SE. Arterial insufficiency in hemodialysis access procedures: Reconstruction by an interposition polytetrafluoroethylene graft conduit. Am J Surg 1987;53:300–01.

9

EARLY EXPERIENCE WITH ADJUNCTIVE ANGIOSCOPY IN THROMBECTOMY OF PTFE A-V FISTULAS

D.J. Wright, M.D.; R.G. Netzley, M.D.; and K.G. McAree, M.D.

THROMBOSIS CONTINUES TO BE a significant complication of angioaccess surgery.[1] Factors contributing to thrombosis include technical defects, inadequate outflow vein, recurrent needle trauma, hypotension, dehydration, compression at puncture sites or by hematoma, aneurysmal dilation, and venous anastomotic stenosis. Thrombectomy to achieve secondary patency of polytetrafluoroethylene (PTFE) fistulas has reported success rates of 40–70%.[2,3] When combined with revision or segmental graft replacement, secondary patency rates of up to 80% have been achieved.[2] However, every patient does not require graft revision following thrombectomy. Intraoperative angiography, as well as intraoperative assessment with dilators and Fogarty catheter balloons, has been advocated as a means of determining which patients require revision.[4]

In this study, we used intraoperative angioscopy to assess the results of thrombectomy. The diagnostic value of angioscopy has been well described over the past several years.[5-7] In our series, special emphasis was given to evaluating the ability of the angioscope to define intraluminal defects that might lead to recurrent thrombosis following thrombectomy. To date, this technique has not enjoyed widespread popularity, prompting this review of our early experience.

Materials and Methods

Between Feb. 1, 1991 and May 1, 1992, 13 patients had angioscopy-assisted thrombectomy performed on previously placed PTFE arteriovenous (A-V) fistulas. This review begins with the first such procedure and includes the most recent one. Follow-up was complete on all patients and was conducted using hospital, office, and dialysis unit records. Patency status at time of death was established on all patients who had expired.

Technique

This procedure was performed under local or regional anesthetic in the majority of patients, however, several patients required general anesthesia. In each case, the PTFE graft was exposed near the venous anastomosis. Incision was made in the graft after adequate proximal and distal graft control was obtained. A Fogarty embolectomy catheter was then passed and thrombectomy was performed for completion. This was defined as passage of the catheter until no residual thrombus was obtained. Presence of good flow through the graft was the second criterion used to determine when "blind" thrombectomy was terminated. At this point, a 2.3 mm Intramed angioscope was passed into the opening in the graft. Digital pressure over the arterial inflow was used to minimize blood loss during angioscopy. The examination included inspection of the entire course of the PTFE graft, the arterial and venous anastomoses, and the outflow vein.

When residual thrombus was identified, the Fogarty catheter was passed to remove the residual clot. If the clot could not be retrieved blindly, thrombectomy was performed under direct visualization using the angioscope. While the thrombus was visualized with the angioscope proximal to the clot, the Fogarty catheter was passed alongside the angioscope. The Fogarty catheter was then advanced beyond the thrombus, and the balloon was inflated. The catheter and angioscope were then withdrawn as a unit, keeping the engaged thrombus in sight as it was extracted. If the Fogarty catheter failed to remove the thrombus, a grasper was used in a similar fashion to retrieve the clot.

Results

A total of 13 thrombectomies were performed using adjunctive angioscopy. In 11 of 13 patients (85%), residual thrombus was identified within the graft or at the anastomosis. Five of these were noted to extend into the outflow vein, and another five patients required angioscopic-assisted thrombectomy. In five patients, angioscopy prompted either patch angioplasty[3] or segmental graft revision.[1] One patient had no adequate outflow vein available, and that fistula could not be salvaged. The remaining eight cases were treated by thrombectomy alone.

Of the 13 grafts, 12 (92%) were patent following this procedure. The previously described case of severe stenosis of the outflow vein and lack of an adequate alternate vein required placement of a new fistula. Of the 12 remaining grafts, four remained patent until the patient's death. Six of the eight remaining grafts (75%) remain patent at the time of this report, with an average patency of 2.75 months (range: 0.25-12.75 months). No mortalities or complications were associated with this procedure.

Discussion

This early experience with adjunctive angioscopy appears to support the value of this technique in the thrombectomy of PTFE A-V fistulas. Angioscopy has previously been found to be an excellent technique in evaluating the completeness of arterial thrombectomy. Residual thrombus has been identified in more than 75% of cases in some series. When angioscopy has been used to evaluate thrombectomy sites, both intraluminal thrombus and intimal defects have been readily identified.[8] In addition, angioscopy is being promoted by some as the technique of choice to be used at the completion of arterial bypass grafting.[5-7,9] The angioscope is believed to be more sensitive than either angiography or duplex scanning in these patients. Endoluminal inspection of these arterial bypasses has led to early correction of anastomotic and graft problems, which in turn has led to improved patency.

At least one other report has described angioscopy of PTFE A-V fistulas.[10] Koga et al. described using percutaneous angioscopy to monitor the changes in A-V fistulas following balloon and laser angioplasty. They observed that in addition to monitoring the site of angioplasty, they were able to clearly identify intraluminal thrombus, mural irregularities, and circumferential stenoses. They felt that "angioscopes provide extremely valuable additional information on hemodialysis A-V access fistulae".

In our experience, the most useful aspects of adjunctive angioscopy in the thrombectomy of A-V fistulas would appear to be the detection of unsuspected residual thrombus and intraluminal defects. We have seen residual thrombus of all varieties; these have ranged from relatively small mural thrombi to large nearly occlusive thrombi and to thrombi that appeared to have a ball valve effect at the anastomoses. Any of these could serve as the nidus for recurrent thrombosis. In addition, previous angioscopy studies have shown that passage of embolectomy catheters is often associated with disruption of the pseudointima of grafts and possibly the intima at the anastomoses. These catheter-induced injuries may lead to the failure of an otherwise successful thrombectomy if not repaired. The ability to identify and correct such problems at the time of the original thrombectomy should enhance both short- and long-term patency rates.

The identification of residual thrombus in so many patients (11 of 13) raises questions as to the significance of this clot. As previously mentioned, the sensitivity of angioscopy is quite high for thrombus and intraluminal defects, exceeding that of angiography. Obviously large, near-obstructive thrombi are at high risk of causing recurrent thrombosis. Smaller thrombi may be less impressive in appearance, but at this juncture we are aggressively removing these as well in order to eliminate the possible nidus for recurrent thrombosis.

Another useful aspect of adjunctive angioscopy is the ability to directly visualize the anastomoses and the outflow vein. In studies on completion angioscopy at the time of arterial bypass grafting, anastomotic problems have been identified in 2-10% of cases.[5] Because outflow obstruction due to stenosis at the site of venous anastomosis is a common cause of PTFE A-V fistula thrombosis, one would expect these rates to be even higher when endoluminal inspection is performed at the time of thrombectomy. Of the fistulas examined in our series, 38% had significant venous stenoses. This information is quite beneficial in deciding which fistulas to revise. In our current group of patients, we chose only to revise the graft (patch angioplasty, segmental graft replacement) when a well-defined angioscopic defect was noted. We believe that this reserves further revision for tertiary procedures and may enhance cumulative graft patency.

Another possible cause for recurrent thrombosis identified with the angioscope was thrombus extending into the outflow vein. Retained thrombi within this vein could understandably lead to early failure following thrombectomy. Once this clot was removed, the vein was inspected to assure adequate outflow. When the outflow vein appears inadequate, attempts can be made to "jump" the venous anastomosis to a better outflow vein.

Perhaps the most exciting aspect of angioscopic-assisted thrombectomy is the ability to perform procedures that have previously been done blindly. The range of instrumentation available to use through angioscopes remains rather limited, but passage of instruments and catheters alongside the angioscope has worked quite well in our experience. Many instruments designed for cutting and grasping through other larger endoscopes work well in this setting. Whatever instrumentation is used, the angioscope allows direct observation of the procedure; thus, immediate assessment of the results is made possible. It is this dynamic quality of adjunctive angioscopy that in our opinion makes it clearly superior to other methods currently available.

This experience is quite limited, but the early results are encouraging. We believe that angioscopy has thus far been a safe and effective adjunct to thrombectomy. It provides valuable information about residual thrombus, allows inspection of arterial and venous anastomoses, and assesses the outflow vein. It has also proven to be clearly advantageous in retrieving residual thrombus where "blind" thrombectomy has failed. Further study and more widespread use appear to be indicated in order to evaluate the long-term benefits of this procedure.

References

1. Wilson SE. Hemodialysis and vascular access. In: Moore WS. Vascular surgery: a comprehensive review. New York: Grune & Stratton, 1991.
2. Bone GE, Pomjzl MJ. Management of dialysis fistula thrombosis. Am J Surg 1979; 138:901–06.
3. Etheridge EE, Haid SD, Maeser MN, Sicard GA, Anderson CB. Salvage operations for malfunctioning polytetrafluoroethylene hemodialysis access grafts. Surgery 1983; 94:464–70.
4. Bell DD, Rosental JJ. Arteriovenous graft life in chronic hemodialysis. A need for prolongation. Arch Surg 1988; 123:1169–72.
5. Gilbertson JJ, Walsh DB, Zwolak RM, et al. A blinded comparison of angiography, angioscopy and duplex scanning in the intraoperative evaluation of *in situ* saphenous vein bypass grafts. J Vasc Surg 1992; 15:121–29.
6. Miller A, Stonebridge PA, Jepsen SJ, et al. Continued experience with intraoperative angioscopy for monitoring infrainguinal bypass grafting. Surgery 1991; 109:286–93.
7. Miller A, Campbell DR, Gibbons GW, et al. Routine intraoperative angioscopy in lower extremity revascularization. Arch Surg 1989; 124:604–08.
8. White GH, White RA, Kopchok GE, Wilson SE. Angioscopic thromboembolectomy: preliminary observations with a recent technique. J Vasc Surg 1988; 7:318–25.
9. Miller A, Jepsen SJ, Stonebridge PA, et al. New angioscopic findings in graft failure after infrainguinal bypass. Arch Surg 1990; 125:749–55.
10. Koga N, Sato T, Baba T, et al. Angioscopy in transluminal balloon and laser angioplasty in the management of chronic hemodialysis fistulae. Trans Am Soc Artif Intern Organs 1989; 35:193–96.

10

PRELIMINARY EXPERIENCE WITH A NEW PTFE GRAFT FOR VASCULAR ACCESS

Ingemar Dawidson, M.D., Ph.D., and Denise Melone, R.N.

Introduction

THE PURPOSE OF THIS STUDY was to evaluate the intraoperative performance of the new expanded polytetrafluoroethylene (ePTFE) vascular graft in patients requiring vascular access for hemodialysis. A second objective was to determine the feasibility of cannulating this graft in the early postimplantation period, prior to tissue attachment and incorporation.

The GORE-TEX Stretch Vascular Graft is the latest addition to ePTFE vascular grafts. This graft is constructed in the same manner as standard GORE-TEX Vascular Grafts. It consists of the same two basic components, a tube of ePTFE surrounded by a thin reinforcing film of open-structured ePTFE. The added physical property of this graft is longitudinal stretch.

The graft possesses memory, so that once moderately tensioned and released, it retracts slightly. The longitudinal extensibility of the graft can be characterized as "micro-crimping" of the fibril structure. When the graft has been moderately extended, the fibril length between the nodes of PTFE is identical to any standard GORE-TEX Vascular Graft, with a nominal internodal distance of 25 microns.[1]

Materials and Methods

Grafts were implanted over a six-month period (Nov. 1, 1991 to May 1, 1992) in 48 consecutive patients requiring vascular access for dialysis. The follow-up

Table 10-1. Type of Anastomosis

Arterial	
Brachial artery	32
Radial artery	16
Total	48
Venous	
Cephalic/superficial vein	37
Concomitant vein	11
Total	48

ranged from two weeks to six months. There were 32 females and 16 males, with a mean age of 50 years.

During the study period, the GORE-TEX Stretch Vascular Graft was used without exception in all patients for whom a forearm graft placement was indicated. The anastomoses, always located in the antecubital fossa, were performed with running sutures using either 6-0 Prolene suture (Ethicon) on a BV-1 needle or a CV-6 GORE-TEX suture (W.L. Gore and Associates) on a TT-9 needle. The arterial end of the graft was anastomosed to the distal brachial artery in 32 patients and to the proximal radial artery in 16 patients. The preferred location of the venous anastomosis was to a superficial antecubital vein (37 patients). Where no suitable superficial vein was available (11 patients), a deep concomitant vein was used (table 10-1). A 6 mm tunneling device was used, onto which the graft was tied and pulled through the tissue tunnel. A single counterincision at the apex of the loop was used.

Results

At the time of this report, 31 of 48 (65%) of the grafts had been cannulated for hemodialysis. Of these 31 grafts, 12 were cannulated within seven days of implantation. Eight of these 12 were cannulated within 24 hours after implantation. None of the patients cannulated between 24 hours and seven days after implantation experienced any acute problems. Of the eight patients whose grafts were cannulated within 24 hours, one experienced an episode of bleeding following removal of the venous return needle. The bleeding was noted at the antecubital incision. Pressure was applied over the needle puncture site and the bleeding ceased; no further intervention was required. None of the early cannulated grafts developed problems related to their cannulation. One of the early cannulated grafts thrombosed at week 21 during a transplant nephrectomy, and a second graft thrombosed at the fifth week (table 10-2). Both grafts were successfully thrombectomized.

Of the 48 grafts, six thrombosed, ranging from three days to 21 weeks after implantation. All six were successfully thrombectomized. One graft required two thrombectomies, and one graft required three. Both patients whose grafts developed multiple thromboses subsequently experienced wound infections ne-

Table 10-2. Early Cannulation

Patient no.	Day	Complications	Thrombosis
3	1	None	Week 21
4	1	None	....
12	1	None	....
14	1	None	....
30	1	None	....
39	1	Bleeding	....
45	1	None	....
48	1	None	....
16	7	None	Week 5
19	4	None	....
27	4	None	....
40	4	None	....

Table 10-3. Thrombosis in Six Patients

Patient no.	Time to event	Comments
3	wk 21	After nephrectomy
16	wk 5	Inadequate vein
17	wk 6 wk 10	Hyperplasia, infected?
24	day 3	Inadequate vein
35	day 6	Inadequate vein
37	day 2, day 10, wk 3	Obese, infected

cessitating graft removal. Of the six patients with thrombosed grafts, four had anatomically compromising factors, usually a small vein or marginal venous outflow at the time of initial graft implantation (table 10-3).

The conformability of the graft at the anastomotic sites was seen to be improved compared to standard ePTFE vascular grafts. Once moderately tensioned, the graft retracts slightly, making suturing easier. The longitudinal extensibility may also decrease the tendency for kinking at the antecubital fossa.

The comments from hemodialysis nurses have been uniformly positive. The graft feels softer and is easier to cannulate. However, the differences are very subtle. Many dialysis technicians cannot tell the difference between the new graft and the standard ePTFE vascular grafts when performing cannulation.

Summary and Comments

The GORE-TEX Stretch Vascular Graft offers improved anastomotic conformability during implantation. Additionally, this study demonstrates that the graft can be safely cannulated for hemodialysis 24 hours after implantation. Routine cannulation within 24 hours after surgery may be feasible, but requires further study. Early graft usage may be related to the graft's longitudinal extensibility and retraction properties, surgical implantation, or hemodialysis needle puncture techniques. Although others have reported cannulation of conventional ePTFE grafts in the early postimplantation period, there have been no randomized studies comparing this new graft to conventional ePTFE grafts.[2,3] Therefore, at this time, there are insufficient data to determine if the stretch graft offers improved safety in early cannulation for hemodialysis. The early cannulation of the GORE-TEX Stretch Vascular Graft should be performed with caution.

A vascular graft that could facilitate early cannulation would be highly desirable. Such a graft would avoid the necessity of using central venous catheters, with their attendant risks.[4,5,6] Both subclavian and femoral dual-lumen catheters carry a significant morbidity. Our results indicate that it is possible to cannulate the GORE-TEX Stretch Vascular Graft in the early postimplantation period in order to avoid the risks that may occur from the use of central venous catheters.

References

1. Boyce B. Physical characteristics of expanded polytetrafluoroethylene grafts. In: Biologic and synthetic vascular prostheses, Stanley JC, ed. New York: Grune & Stratton, 1982; 553–61.
2. Haag BW, Paramesh V, Roberts T, et al. Early use of polytetrafluoroethylene grafts for hemodialysis access. In: Vascular access for hemodialysis. Sommer BG, Henry ML, eds. Chicago: WL Gore and Precept Press, 1991;173–78.
3. Taucher LA. Immediate, safe hemodialysis into arteriovenous fistulas created with a new tunneler. Am J Surg 1985;150:212–15.
4. Schwab S, Quarles D, Middleton J, et al. Hemodialysis-associated subclavian vein stenosis. Kidney Int 1988;33:1156.
5. Van Holder R, De Clippelé M, De Cubber A, et al. Subclavian catheter as a vascular access for single needle hemodialysis. In: Access surgery. Kootstra G, Jorning PJG, eds. Lancaster: MTP Press, 1983;309.
6. Sherertz RJ, Falk R, Huffman K, et al. Infections associated with subclavian Uldall catheters. Arch Intern Med 1983;143:52.

PANEL DISCUSSION

Moderator:
  Mitchell L. Henry, M.D.
Incidence of Vascular Access Thrombosis in Patients Treated with Recombinant Human Erythropoietin
Presenter:
  George Carty, M.D.

Moderator: It seemed as if the end point of your EPO therapy was relatively low. The hemoglobins at the end point of the therapy were only around 8.5. Do you think that has an impact on the fact that the group did not seem to be more thrombogenic?

Dr. Carty: The change between pretreatment and post-treatment was relatively small. However, that is in line with the data reported from the U.S. Renal Service for 1991, which is only 2.5 percentage points different. So yes, the ideal increase has not been accomplished, and that might be a significant fact.

Discussant: As you stated, your hematocrit didn't change much. Approximately how many units of erythropoietin are the patients receiving?

Dr. Carty: They were given 50 to 100 U/kg. It changed their hematocrits by 12% and the hemoglobin by 10%.

Treatment of Angioaccess Ischemic Steal by of Revascularization
Presenter:
  Harry Schanzer, M.D.

Discussant: I understood you to say that all the GORE-TEX fistulas you had were brachial artery to axillary vein. To many, that procedure would seem to be a procedure for use in someone who had a failed forearm graft. Had all of these patients had previous forearm grafts, or was this the primary graft?

Dr. Schanzer: That is a rather controversial issue that I don't think is worthwhile to go into now. In our experience, the best patency we obtain is with this particular straight graft; we leave the loop graft as a secondary procedure.

Discussant: Were these 14 patients diabetic? If this is the case, would you be inclined to use a 4 mm to 7 mm graft as the primary procedure?

Dr. Schanzer: As I pointed out, 13 of the 14 patients (93%) were diabetic. I may anticipate the presence of ischemia in cases in which the patient is diabetic, has signs of poor flow to the fingers, has pale fingers, lower index, etc. In those cases, I would construct a GORE-TEX fistula between the axillary artery and the brachial vein—if there is a good brachial vein—and a reverse graft or a loop into the axillary vein. In our experience, the brachial artery has very good collateral circulation and it is not affected by steal as much as more distal arteries. The experience with the tapered graft is similar to that with banding. It's true that we are going to reduce the flow through the graft. The problem is that we are potentially obtaining more thrombosis from it.

Discussant: On a theoretical basis, the incidence of steal should be higher in cases in which there is either proximal arterial stenosis or perhaps stenosis at the artery-to-graft anastomosis. Did you have angiograms in these cases, and if so, was the angiogram consistent with steal, either proximally or distally? In those cases, was the steal perhaps secondary to a proximal problem?

Dr. Schanzer: It's true that a stenosis proximal to the takeoff of the fistula is a situation that favors the production of steal. The way we work this up preoperatively is to measure pressures and PVRs in the hand and radial artery, with and without occlusion of the fistula. If the pressure with occlusion is the same as the contralateral arm, then we assume that there is no proximal stenosis. We have not routinely done angiography in these cases. All cases have responded to this treatment with a bypass procedure.

Discussant: Since the central draining axillary vein is a very low-resistant system, do you think that a forearm loop graft might provide a higher venous resistance and therefore decreased potential for ischemia?

Dr. Schanzer: If you have steal, that means that the outflow still has lower resistance and is encouraging the production of reversal of flow that is pathological. This procedure will still be effective. In terms of how much more resistance you have at the venous site at the elbow or the axilla, I don't know if it makes a difference. We are talking about degrees of centimeters of water, which really is minimal when we consider all of the hemodynamic characteristics of the fistula.

Discussant: In your study, did you notice any correlation with size of the donor artery? The corollary of that question is, is it important to originate the bypass graft from a large donor artery?

Dr. Schanzer: I can only give you anecdotal information. When I have a very small donor artery, I worry because I think that is conducive to clinical steal, especially if it is in a diabetic. In those cases, I have decided to do the reverse graft, using the axillary artery as takeoff of the fistula.

Discussant: Have you attempted ligation of the distal artery without bypass, or are you aware of any studies done regarding the outcome?

Dr. Schanzer: Yes, ligation of the artery distal to the fistula definitely improves the pressure distal to the fistula. Actually, we routinely—and still do for academic purposes—measure pressures before ligation, after ligation, and after construction or opening of the bypass. We measure pressure with the bypass closed and the fistula open. There can be a proximal systemic pressure mean of 80, and distal to the fistula of 20. If the artery is ligated, increased pressure of 40 can be obtained. This seems paradoxical, because by ligating the artery, we are really stopping steal. When the bypass is performed, the pressure gets closer to systemic. When dealing with GORE-TEX A-V fistulas to a more proximal artery, I think it is safer to alter flow with the bypass.

Early Experience with Adjunctive Angioscopy in Thrombectomy of PTFE *A-V Fistulas*
Presenter:
   D. J. Wright, M.D.

Discussant: This looks like a nice technique, and you have some good thoughts about it. What is the cost of this so-called "disposable device" that you use? In our hospital, it is about $500 or $600. Second, in the lower-arm grafts, it is easy to get vascular control with a tourniquet, but what do you do up in the axilla? It is technically more difficult to get venous vascular control so you can get a good look.

Dr. Wright: You have to do more of a dissection in the upper-arm fistulas. In this series, only two of these were upper-arm fistulas. Three of them were loop forearm grafts, and the remainder were straight grafts in the forearm. The first question about cost is a very good one; the scopes that we are using are costing in between $400 and $500. Currently under development is a scope of about half the size of the standard angioscopes. If it is as effective as the standard scope, it is predicted that the cost will be about $200 per scope.

Discussant: Angioscopy requires continuous saline infusion for vision. Is this a problem in these anuric patients?

Dr. Wright: No. As a matter of fact, because we have control of the venous outflow, most of the liquid goes on our lap. We believe that the use of the pump mechanism shortens the necessary time interval, because we can rapidly infuse high volume under pressure in a very short time. One of the other advantages of a pump device is the fact that it also allows us to set volume limitations so that we are warned as soon as we've used a certain volume of infusate.

Air-Plethysmography: An Investigation of Its Use for the Detection of Upper-Extremity Venous Obstruction
Presenter:
   G. P. Gardner, M.D.

Discussant: The application of this technique ultimately would be in preoperative assessment for graft placement. Do you have any thoughts on how some of these values might change in people who either had grafts in the arm at the time that you studied them or may have had grafts that have failed, obviously having some change in their previous venous outflow?

Dr. Gardner: Interestingly enough, because there is a bypass with a patent fistula, we cannot conduct air-plethysmography because we can't occlude the venous outflow. So, if we have a patent graft, basically all bets are off. If it is a clotted graft, we can assess the outflow because we don't have a bypass of the venous system. In terms of the exact effect of the clotted fistula, all I can say is it is just the patency rate or the degree of collaterals or the degree of recanalization that affects the outflow. I don't think the clotted graft would have a great impact on this tool.

Discussant: In the chronic situation, where collateral circulation is already established or there has been prior recanalization, this most likely will be insensitive. However, I would suggest that this is the situation where we have greatest need for information. The real value for the test might be to do the same test with exercise. The same thing that we do in the legs should be done in the arm.

Dr. Wright: That's a very good question, and it really gets to the crux of the matter. Patients we have studied who had prior subclavian vein thrombosis were all asymptomatic when we studied them. Eight out of 10 had intermittent upper-extremity edema. However, when they were studied they were asymptomatic, yet they all had abnormal NBOs. In terms of the collateralization, it really doesn't matter whether a subclavian vein or a collateral vein provides the outflow as long as the outflow is adequate. I think it is pretty well known that all of the collateralization in the world is not enough for the prior patent subclavian vein, but what we want to know is whether the collateral provides enough outflow to support the graft. Duplex is very insensitive, because if there is a large collateral vein, this can be misinterpreted as a patent subclavian vein.

A Prospective Study—Evaluation from Permanent Vascular Hemodialysis Access 1986-90
Presenter:
G. B. Zibari, M.D.

Discussant: I have a question about your infection rates with Vancomycin. Is that an immediate postoperative infection rate?

Dr. Zibari: In 10 patients, it occurred within four weeks of surgery. The other infection occurred at about eight weeks. So four occurred after a month, but the first 10 infections were within a month from the time of surgery.

Preliminary Experience with a New PTFE Graft for Vascular Access
Presenter:
Ingemar Dawidson, M.D.

Discussant: When we attempted early use of standard PTFE several years ago on different occasions, our biggest problem with it was collapse of the graft during hemodialysis. I would like to ask what sort of flow rates were being used in this first week after the graft was implanted.

Dr. Dawidson: The flow rates were 300 cc/min.

Discussant: In some cases, we have used grafts early and in fact reported on our experience a couple of years ago. The only problem we have had is that the patient presented to the dialysis unit clotted. The patient came for thrombectomy and the graft had been lacerated. We had all kinds of bleeding, dissecting along the graft, and bleeding out where we made the incision. So if you use the grafts early, not only is it important that you let your inpatient unit know, but you also have to inform your outpatient unit. They need to be sure that if the graft is clotted, they must not stick it again and again because the graft will be lacerated.

Dr. Dawidson: I tend to agree that the way you stick these grafts is perhaps the deciding factor as to whether it is going to work.

Discussant: Is the stretch graft reinforced with the standard outer wrap of GORE-TEX?

Dr. Dawidson: Yes, it is reinforced.

Discussant: When you are doing a thrombectomy, is there any difficulty in declotting it because it is more "stretchy"?

Dr. Dawidson: We have had no problems. Had I not known this was a stretch graft, I couldn't tell the difference from a regular GORE-TEX graft.

Discussant: We have been using early cannulation of standard GORE-TEX quite often. The important technical maneuver is to make sure you have a single-wall puncture and that you don't go through the back wall. Otherwise, you get bleeding around the catheter or around the GORE-TEX.

Discussant: I have been most fully satisfied with the 4–7 mm GORE-TEX, and we used those the same day, going directly from the operating room to the dialysis unit.

Discussant: What are the theoretical advantages to this over standard GORE-TEX? It wasn't entirely clear to me that it was new, but new isn't necessarily better, and why is this better?

Dr. Dawidson: It's easier to handle, it's easier to sew, and it conforms better at the anastomosis site. There is potential for it to bleed less than standard material.

Moderator: There clearly is interest in very early use of these grafts. Let's take a little informal poll here. How many use PTFE grafts in the forearm in the first 24 hours after they are put in? Two of you. How many wait a week? How many two weeks or more? The attendees here certainly don't use PTFE grafts early. Is that by experience or by invention? How many have had experience with using GORE-TEX early? It looks like about 60% of the room. That would suggest that you can't do it. You must be doing something very different from what the rest of us here do.

Dr. Dawidson: I want to make it very clear that this isn't my standard practice. We have done this on several occasions. My preference obviously is to leave them alone and let them mature.

11

USE OF 6 mm STRETCH PTFE GRAFTS FOR EARLY USE IN HEMODIALYSIS

*Eugene J. Simoni, M.D., F.A.C.S., F.I.C.S.,
Krishna M. Jain, M.D., F.A.C.S., and John S. Munn, M.D.*

OVER THE PAST FOUR YEARS, polytetrafluoroethylene (PTFE) has become the most commonly used graft for hemodialysis. One of the drawbacks of this graft has been the delay required between implantation and use.[1] Occasionally, the graft has been used soon after the operation, but usually a delay of one to three weeks is required for ingrowth of tissue around the graft. One of the main reasons for this delay in use is the amount of time it takes to stop needle-hole bleeding from the grafts. With the introduction of the stretch PTFE graft, consideration was given to using the grafts within the first 24 hours after implantation because of its new physical characteristics.

This graft consists of two components, a tube of expanded PTFE surrounded by a thin film of PTFE. The longitudinal extensibility—the stretch feature of the graft—can be characterized as a microcrimping of the fibrils. The graft is not distensible in a radial direction, but maintains a small amount of longitudinal elastic recoil. Early experience with this graft in arterial reconstructive surgery showed a marked reduction in needle-hole bleeding.

We undertook this study to see if cannulation of the stretch PTFE within 24 hours of implantation for dialysis would have excessively high complication rates.

The authors wish to acknowledge assistance of Virginia Keith, Carmen Moncure, Jackie Jordan, and Elouise Farrar in preparation of this manuscript.

Table 11-1. Follow-up Scan at 1-2 Weeks

	Perigraft hematoma	Pseudoaneurysm
Forearm loop	0/7	0/7
Upper arm straight	0/7	0/7
Abdominal wall (loop)	0/1	0/1

Table 11-2. Follow-up Scan at 4-6 Weeks

	Perigraft hematoma	Pseudoaneurysm
Forearm loop	0/7	0/7
Upper arm straight	0/5	0/5
Abdominal wall (loop)	0/1	0/1

Patients and Methods

Between Nov. 20, 1991, and May 1, 1992, all patients requiring prosthetic grafts for long-term hemodialysis had a 6 mm stretch PTFE graft placed. These grafts were placed in one of three positions: (1) loop forearm, (2) straight upper arm, or (3) loop abdominal wall.[2] All of these grafts were then punctured within 24 hours and used for routine hemodialysis.

All grafts were followed at one to two weeks, and at four to six weeks, with color flow Doppler imaging (CFD) to assess the grafts for perigraft hematomas, pseudoaneurysms, or other graft complications.

The bleeding time from the puncture sites after needle removal was also recorded for the first three dialysis treatments.

During this time period, 15 grafts were placed. Seven were in the forearm location (loop), seven were in the upper arm location (straight), and one was in the abdominal wall (loop).

Results

All of the grafts were imaged at one to two weeks after placement. No perigraft hematomas or pseudoaneurysms were noted at this time (table 11-1). At four to six weeks after insertion, 13 of 15 grafts were imaged. Again, no perigraft hematomas or pseudoaneurysms were seen (table 11-2).

Five grafts underwent seven thrombectomies—six in the forearm location and one in the upper-arm location. Two of these grafts were lost after thrombectomies due to small venous outflow tracts. In these patients, upper-arm

Table 11-3. Complications

	Forearm loop	Upper arm straight	Abdominal wall
Thrombosis	6 (4 patients)	1	0
Grafts lost	2	0	0
Steal syndrome	1	1	0
Infections	0	0	0
Bleeding	0	1	0

grafts were placed that functioned normally. The other three patients suffered idiopathic thrombosis and had successful thrombectomies.

Other complications of the grafts during the first six weeks included two steal syndromes (one upper-arm graft and one forearm graft). These were corrected by tapering the graft with the aid of CFD.[3,4]

There was one episode of bleeding from the incision site of an upper-arm graft. This occurred at the first dialysis run. When the graft was operatively explored, it was found that the venous needle had punctured both sides of the graft. The puncture sites were not actively bleeding. The returned venous blood from the dialysis machine was tracking from the needle along the graft to exit at the incision (table 11-3). During the first three dialysis treatments, bleeding was noted to cease in 5–7 minutes at both the arterial and venous needle puncture sites.

Discussion

In our series, early use of the stretch PTFE graft for hemodialysis has had favorable results. During the first two weeks while the graft was incorporating, no pseudoaneurysms or perigraft hematomas were noted in any of the 15 grafts. Also, after four to six weeks of use, no pseudoaneurysms or perigraft hematomas were seen in the 13 grafts that had been followed to that point. Bleeding from the puncture sites was easily controlled by the dialysis staff after needle removal.

The two grafts that occluded and could not be restored to function were found to have small venous outflow tracts and high venous pressures. These grafts were replaced with upper-arm grafts that remained patent past the six-week period. The other three patients had successful thrombectomies that resulted in normally functioning dialysis grafts. Thrombosis could not be attributed to early graft use or a specific graft problem in these cases. One bleeding complication occurred, but this was secondary to faulty needle placement.

In conclusion, we believe that the stretch PTFE graft can be successfully cannulated within 24 hours of implantation without an excessive complication rate.

References

1. Rapaport A, Noon G, McCollum C. Polytetrafluoroethylene (PTFE) graft for haemodialysis in chronic renal failure: Assessment of durability and function at three years. Aust NZ J Surg 1981; 51:562-67.
2. Raju S. PTFE grafts for hemodialysis access. Technique for insertion and management of complications. Ann Surg 1987; 206:666-73.
3. Rosental J, Bell D, Gaspar M, Movius H, Lemire G. Prevention of high flow problems of arteriovenous grafts. Am J Surg 1980; 140:231-33.
4. Jain KM, Simoni EJ, Munn JS. A new technique to correct vascular steal secondary to hemodialysis grafts. Surg Gynecol Obstet 1992; 175:183-84.

12

DIALYSIS ACCESS USING PTFE-COATED WOVEN GRAFTS

Ralph Didlake, M.D., Edna Curry, R.N., B.S.N., Ed Rigdon, M.D., Seshadri Raju, M.D., and John Bower, M.D.

POLYTETRAFLUOROETHYLENE (PTFE)-COATED woven polyethylene terephthalate (PET) was introduced as an experimental vascular prosthetic by Yeh et al.[1] and by Hoffman et al.[2,3] It was found to combine the low thrombogenicity of a polymerized PTFE surface with the well-documented strength of a woven PET wall. This combination of materials, in its externally supported configuration (Plasma TFE, Medtronics, Inc., Minneapolis, MN), was first used in human arterial bypass applications by Bauer and for vascular access by Jendrisak.[4,5] In contrast to expanded PTFE (ePTFE), such as Gore-Tex (W.L. Gore & Associates, Flagstaff, AZ) and Impra (Impra, Tempe, AZ), Plasma TFE (pl-TFE) can be cannulated for dialysis within the first week following implantation.

This report compares our experience with 93 consecutive pl-TFE hemoaccess devices to that with a cohort of ePTFE access grafts.

Materials and Methods

The study population consisted of 93 consecutive patients with end-stage renal disease (ESRD) who underwent prosthetic vascular access placement between January 1990 and February 1991. This cohort represents all patients referred for placement of a prosthetic vascular access device during this period.

The authors wish to acknowledge assistance of Virginia Keith, Carmen Moncure, Jackie Jordan, and Elouise Farrar in preparation of this manuscript.

Only candidates for creation of autogenous arteriovenous (A-V) fistulas were excluded from this study. All surgical protocols, consent forms, and methods of data collection were approved by the institution's Human Investigation Committee. In each case, the access was constructed using 6 mm, externally supported, untapered pl-TFE graft material. These conduits consist of non-crimped woven PET wall with an ultrathin PTFE coating that is applied using a glow-discharge process.[2,3] A helical polypropylene support is applied to the exterior of the conduit.

The external surface of the graft was preclotted using 25 ml of the patient's blood mixed with 1,000 units of liquid thrombin (Thrombostat, Parke-Davis, Morris Plains, NJ). Whenever possible, grafts were placed in a straight configuration between the radial artery at the wrist and the antecubital venous complex. Loop grafts were created if the patient had a previous radial artery anastomosis, a history of significant atherosclerosis or diabetes mellitus, a diminished radial artery pulse, an exceptionally short forearm, or no intact palmar arterial arch. A subcutaneous tunnel was created using the Gore tunneling device. Vascular anastomoses, performed under systemic heparinization, were fashioned using running PTFE suture (CV-6, W.L. Gore & Associates, Flagstaff, AZ). Systemic heparinization was seldom reversed.

All pl-TFE access grafts were made available for immediate cannulation. An early access protocol was established that dictated cannulation with 17-gauge needles and limitation of dialyzer pump speed to 150 ml/min for the first 45 minutes of therapy. Pump speed was slowly advanced to a maximum of 250 ml/min over the course of the dialysis session. This protocol was followed for the first three dialyses, after which routine dialysis procedures were followed.

Grafts in the ePTFE cohort were constructed using 6 mm untapered, standard-wall reinforced ePTFE (GORE-TEX, W.L. Gore & Associates, Flagstaff, AZ). Selection of graft configuration, placement technique and anastomosis were the same as those described for pl-TFE grafts except that no preclotting was performed. Cannulation of ePTFE grafts was delayed for a minimum of seven days, and the early cannulation protocol was not employed.

Patients in both groups were reviewed for age, sex, race, graft configuration, and interval (days) between placement and cannulation. The pl-TFE and ePTFE groups were then reviewed for the number of postoperative infections, unanticipated admissions, and early thromboses, and for event-free patency (EFP). A postoperative infection was defined as any perigraft infection that occurred within 14 days after operation and required antibiotic therapy or surgical intervention. An unanticipated admission was defined as any nonelective hospitalization that occurred within 72 hours of an outpatient access procedure and was related to a problem that was unresolved by outpatient surgery or a complication of the surgery performed. Early thrombosis was defined as any occlusion of a new graft that occurred within 14 days after surgery. EFP, a parameter of long-term graft outcome, was defined as the interval (in days) between graft placement and the patient's death, loss of follow-up, or any event requiring surgical therapy (e.g., thrombosis, infection, pseudoaneurysm formation, recirculation, or excessive venous pressure).

The frequency of complications was compared between groups by the Fisher exact test.[6] Median EFP was estimated by probit.[7] For the purpose of this calcu-

Table 12-1. Demographic Data for 93 Patients Undergoing Placement of pl-TFE Access Grafts

Age (mean ± SD)	51.4 ± 15.6 yr
Age range	16 to 85 yr
Male (%)	53 (56.4%)
Female	41 (43.6%)
African-American	82 (87.2%)
Native American	2 (2.2%)
White	10 (10.6%)

Table 12-2. Location and Configuration of 93 Consecutive pl-TFE Dialysis Access Grafts

Configuration	Right	Left	Total
Forearm straight	19	30	49
Forearm loop	19	16	35
Leg loop	3	2	5
Upper arm loop	1	2	3
Upper arm straight	0	1	1
Total	42	51	93

lation, actual event-free survival times were defined as the time between graft placement and thrombosis, infection, or revision. If a graft was event-free at the time of analysis, the patients' death, or loss of follow-up, that time was accepted as a censored event-free survival time. EFP was compared between groups using the Cox proportional hazards model.[8] EFP was expressed graphically as described by Kaplan and Meier.[9]

Results

Demographic data for 93 patients undergoing placement of pl-TFE grafts, given in table 12-1, show a predominance of black male patients. This group reflects the demographics of the dialysis population of the Deep South.[10] In table 12-2 are shown the location and configuration of all 93 pl-TFE grafts placed, demonstrating the preference of our group for straight grafts placed in the nondominant forearm.

The mean interval to cannulation of pl-TFE access grafts was 3.9 days (range: 0–112 days). Thirty-three grafts (35.5%) were cannulated on the day of placement (day 0). An additional 34 grafts were cannulated on the first postoperative day, and another 15 were cannulated prior to the seventh postoperative day.

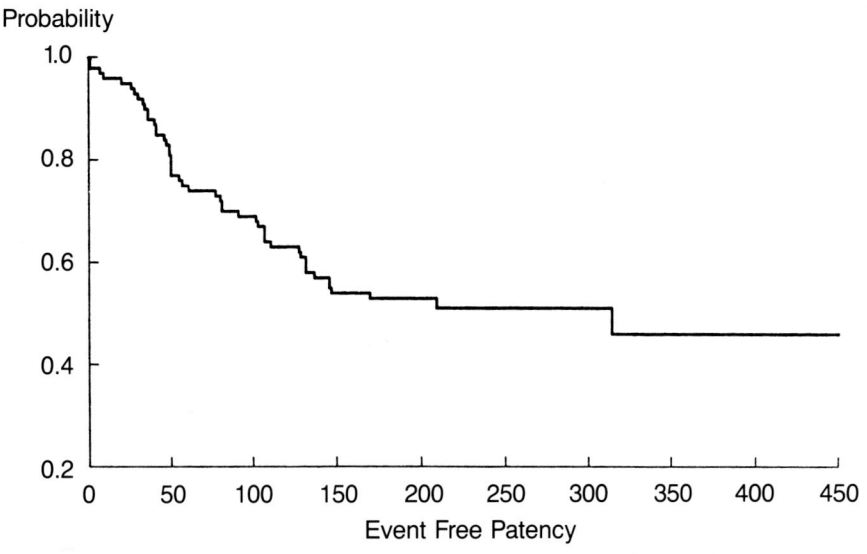

Figure 12-1. Actuarial analysis of event-free patency (EFP) for 93 pl-TFE hemodialysis access grafts. This analysis includes all graft configurations.

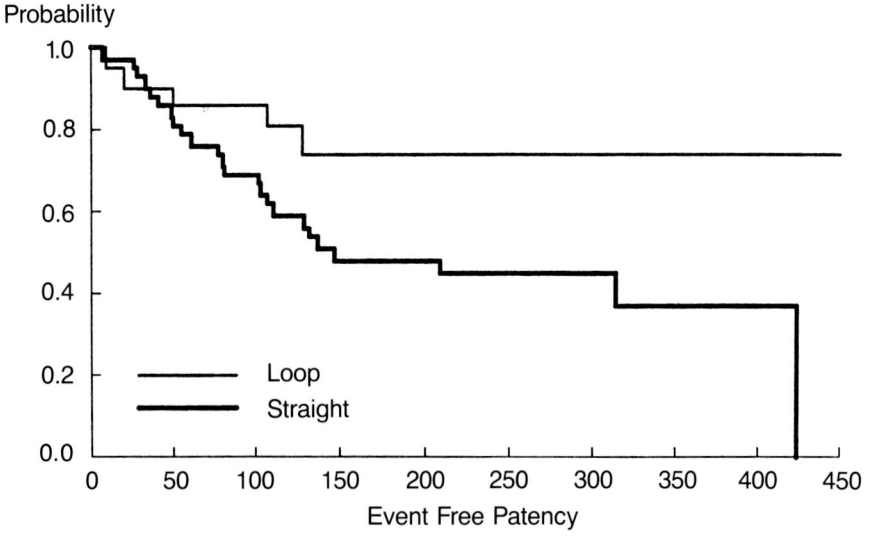

Figure 12-2. Actuarial analysis of EFP for pl-TFE grafts placed in previously unoperated forearms stratified by graft configuration reveals significantly better patency in access devices fashioned in a loop configuration.

A total of 74 grafts (79.6%) were cannulated during the first 72 hours and 82 (88.2%) during the first week. No complications of early cannulation were encountered in any of the pl-TFE grafts.

An actuarial survival curve based on EFP for all 93 pl-TFE grafts is shown in figure 12-1. The median EFP for this group was 130.5 days, with a one-year primary patency of 50%. Patency for the pl-TFE group was stratified by graft con-

Table 12-3. Events Occurring in 93 pl-TFE Hemodialysis Access Grafts

Event	No (%)	Time to event* (days)
None	39 (41.9)	—
Infection	4 (4.3)	117.8 ± 74.2
Pseudoaneurysm	2 (2.2)	181.5 ± 187.4
Thrombosis	41 (44.1)	83.1 ± 80.2
Death	7 (7.5)	74.6 ± 60.1
Total	93 (100.0)	—

* Mean ± standard deviation

Table 12-4. Patient Demographics and Configuration of 68 pl-TFE and 83 ePTFE Grafts Placed in Previously Unoperated Forearms

	pl-TFE	ePTFE	p value
Age (years) (mean ± SD)	52 ± 17.1	53 ± 17.2	0.729*
Straight	45	62	0.282†
Loop	23	21	
Right	32	26	0.064†
Left	36	57	
Male	30	32	0.599†
Female	38	51	
Total	68	83	—

* Compared by Student's *t*-test
† Compared by Fisher exact test

figuration; chi-square comparison of logistic analysis of the subgroups using a proportional hazards model reveals no statistically significant difference in EFP among the four graft configurations (p >0.05).

Events occurring in the pl-TFE group during the follow-up period are shown in table 12-3. Thrombosis was by far the most common event, and infection and pseudoaneurysm formation were relatively rare. Sixty-eight of the 93 pl-TFE grafts were placed in previously unoperated forearms. Configuration and demographics of these grafts are given in table 12-4. Our preference for straight hemoaccess grafts is again evident.

Actuarial analysis of EFP for grafts placed in unoperated forearms stratified by graft configuration (figure 12-2) demonstrates that loop pl-TFE access grafts remained event-free longer than straight pl-TFE grafts (p 0.045). The events seen in these 68 patients are given in table 12-5. Only two perigraft infections

Table 12-5. Events Occurring in 68 pl-TFE and 83 ePTFE Grafts Placed in Previously Unoperated Forearms

Event	pl-TFE n[1]	pl-TFE I[2] (days)	ePTFE n	ePTFE I (days)	p-Value n[3]	p-Value I[4]
Thrombosis	29	91 ± 45	40	214 ± 127	0.516	0.008
Perigraft infection	2	115 ± 8	3	346 ± 197	1.0	0.489
Pseudoaneurysm	1	314	2	479 ± 269	1.0	___[5]
Death	6	65 ± 30	11	234 ± 144	0.447	0.105
None	30	___	27	___	0.178	___

[1] n = number of events observed
[2] I = interval between graft placement and event ± standard deviation
[3] Frequency of events (n) compared by Fisher exact test (two-tailed)
[4] Interval means compared by Student's *t*-Test (unpaired)
[5] Valid statistical comparison not possible

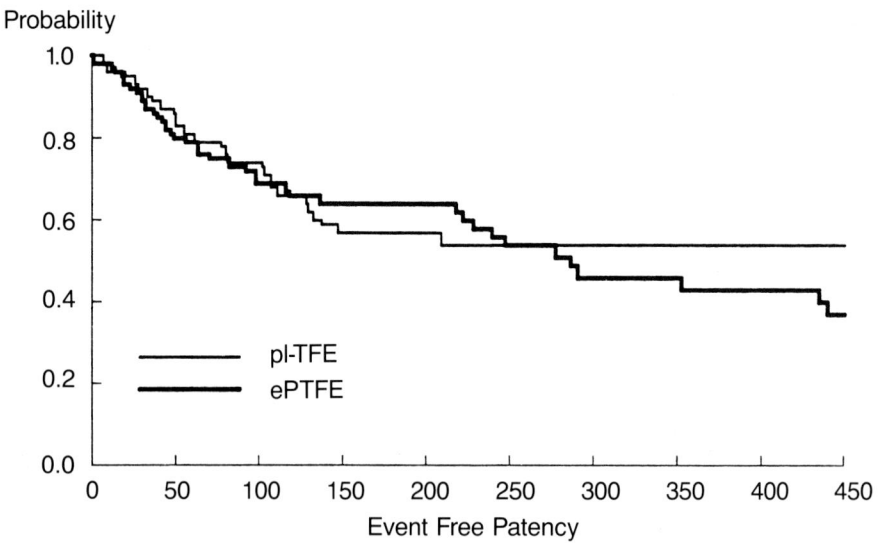

Figure 12-3. Comparison of 68 pl-TFE and 83 ePTFE access grafts placed in previously unoperated forearms shows no difference in overall primary patency.

were seen in this group and occurred late (103 and 128 days). No perioperative infections (i.e., < 14 days) occurred in the pl-TFE group. Pseudoaneurysm formation was also uncommon, occurring only once during the follow-up period. Thrombosis occurred in 29 of these grafts at a mean interval of 91.9 ± 90.7 days. Three of these thromboses occurred in nine days or less and each was related to problems of hypotension or hypovolemia. Thirty pl-TFE grafts remained event-free during the period of observation.

Tables 12-4 and 12-5 also show the comparison of the 68 initial pl-TFE grafts with 83 ePTFE grafts that were also placed in previously unoperated forearms.

Table 12-4 demonstrates that these two populations were no different in terms of age, sex, and graft configuration. Events occurring in the ePTFE control cohort are shown in table 12-5, and the frequency of and mean time interval to these events are compared to the pl-TFE group. Although the frequency of thrombosis was no different between the two groups (p 0.625), the mean interval to the initial thrombosis was shorter in the pl-TFE group (91 ± 45 days vs. 214 ± 127 days, p 0.008). The frequency of and interval to perigraft infection, pseudoaneurysm formation, and death were no different between the two groups. Actuarial analysis of EFP for initial pl-TFE and ePTFE grafts is displayed graphically in figure 12-3. Median EFP was 272.9 days for initial pl-TFE grafts and 283.1 days for initial ePTFE grafts. Cox proportional hazards model reveals no significant difference between these patency rates (p 0.676). In contrast to the pl-TFE group, stratification of ePTFE grafts revealed no difference in EFP between straight and loop graft configurations.

Survival following an initial thrombosis was significantly lower in the pl-TFE group than in grafts constructed of ePTFE (p 0.003). Median survival following an initial thrombotic episode was 41 days for the pl-TFE group and 132 days in the ePTFE group. More pl-TFE grafts were also abandoned at the initial thrombectomy as compared with ePTFE grafts (8 vs. 3, p 0.044).

Discussion

A high-flow vascular access device is an essential component of effective dialysis therapy for patients with ESRD. At present, there is little question that the autogenous A-V fistula, as described by Brescia et al,[11] is the access device of choice. When creation of such a fistula is possible, its resistance to infection, its low thrombogenicity, and its long-term durability make it clearly superior to prosthetic hemoaccess devices. Unfortunately, the anatomy and condition of the veins in many patients prevent the construction of an autogenous fistula of adequate caliber and flow.

Time constraints may also make creation of an autogenous fistula impractical if the patient needs to begin chronic dialysis prior to fistula maturation. Although temporary access devices may be placed during the four- to six-week maturation period, there are hazards of infection and venous stenosis, especially in the long-term management of the chronic hemodialysis patient. We are particularly concerned about subclavian vein complications that can impair venous hemodynamics in the upper extremity and complicate maintenance of high-flow vascular access. Spinowitz et al. and Barrett et al., in a prospective study of the subclavian veins of patients who had previously undergone placement of subclavian dialysis catheters, found that about half of the patients had radiographic evidence of subclavian vein stenosis on the cannulated side.[12,13] Schwab et al. found subclavian vein stenosis in 12 of 47 patients undergoing venography for fistula dysfunction. All 12 had a prior history of subclavian vein cannulation for temporary dialysis access. These investigators also showed that stenosis can recur following ostensibly successful transluminal angioplasty. The internal jugular approach has subsequently been shown to be the route of choice for temporary access placement.[15]

The issue of avoiding placement of temporary access devices is of particular concern in our region, where rural dwellers, who frequently have limited resources and are often undereducated, often must travel long distances for dialysis. This population also has many barriers to renal transplantation as renal function replacement therapy. Therefore, we feel it is prudent to assume that these patients are likely to need long-term vascular access and that using temporary access catheters carries some added risk. In this setting, the ability to access a prosthetic graft immediately is very attractive.

Expanded PTFE, both in its reinforced (Gore-Tex) and its nonreinforced (Impra) configuration, has proven to be useful in the construction of hemoaccess devices because of its durability, low thrombogenicity, biocompatibility, and ability to undergo thrombectomy. Although cannulation of these materials within 72 hours of placement has been reported,[16] our experience has shown that a seven- to 10-day maturation period is necessary in order to keep cannulation and decannulation complications at an acceptable level. Again, temporary access devices are frequently required in this setting.

PET, originally marketed as Dacron by Du Pont, continues to have great utility as a vascular prosthetic for arterial bypass and replacement applications.[17] Woven PET conduits have demonstrated exceptional durability and wall strength, but their surfaces are known to be more thrombogenic than PTFE.[9] Hoffman et al. and Yeh et al. demonstrated that an ultrathin layer of PTFE could be covalently bound to woven PET.[1,2] Such conduits were shown to be less thrombogenic than uncoated Dacron in an ex vivo baboon shunt model[3] and a canine carotid replacement model.[18] Jendrisak, who reported the first clinical use of commercially available PTFE-coated PET (Atrium, Medtronics, Minneapolis, MN) in a vascular access application, found that this type of conduit could be accessed immediately without excessive bleeding.[5]

Although the general procedure for placement of pl-TFE access grafts and ePTFE grafts is similar, certain nuances must be appreciated by the operator. Woven PET materials traditionally have not required preclotting, but some form of preclotting is recommended both by the manufacturer and by our experience. This may be achieved in a number of ways either prior to tunneling or *in situ*. We chose to preclot the graft prior to tunneling and to preclot only the exterior surface of the conduit. In this manner, preclotting prevented blood loss through the graft wall into the tunnel and obviated the need to clear the lumen of any clots before establishing flow. The ends of the graft must be tailored for anastomosis using a thermal cautery that melts and fuses the cut ends of PET fibers, thereby preventing unraveling of the woven graft wall. A disposable, battery-operated thermal cautery device for this purpose is provided with each graft marketed by Medtronics. In order to prevent creation of a bead of melted PET along the cut edge, the cut must be made as quickly as the heat of the cautery will allow. This bead renders the graft orifice somewhat ridged and makes both conformation of the orifice to the native vessel and passage of the needle and suture through the graft wall more difficult.

The manufacturer recommends that the graft be placed under slight tension in order to "lock" the weave. The recommended stretch of 5% is difficult to determine precisely in the clinical setting, but did appear to improve hemostasis following decannulation. Placement of the graft in its resting state was found to be detrimental for a second reason. Three grafts placed early in our series thrombosed owing to graft redundancy that allowed the conduit to become acutely angulated at the venous end. Each of these grafts was placed without the recommended stretch, and, over time, the exceptional axial compliance characteristics of pl-TFE caused the conduit to elongate effectively in response to the energy of arterial pulse waves. This elongation over the fixed venous anastomosis resulted in angulation and thrombosis.

Our experience indicated that safe access and effective dialysis therapy can be achieved immediately after graft placement, even as early as 30 minutes after implantation. No complications of early needle puncture were encountered in any of the pl-TFE grafts, even though 33 (35.5%) were cannulated on the day of placement and 74 (79.6%) within 72 hours of placement. In no instance was postoperative insertion of a temporary access device necessary. The early access cannulation protocol was designed to reduce the size of needle holes and to protect the graft and anastomosis from the jet effects of blood returning from the dialyzer pump. Our experience does not allow comment on the necessity of this protocol because it was not compared to standard dialysis technique. We can state, however, that adequate dialysis therapy was achieved in all patients who underwent early cannulation of pl-TFE access using the protocol described.

Patency of the 93 pl-TFE grafts compared favorably with one-year primary patency rates reported by others,[20] but it must be acknowledged that comparison of hemoaccess patency rates between studies is fraught with statistical hazard. In order to make a meaningful comparison between pl-TFE and ePTFE materials, we chose to compare EFP in forearm grafts placed in virgin extremities. This avoids the variables of reoperation and anatomic location as potential pitfalls in the analysis.

Comparison of primary forearm pl-TFE and ePTFE grafts reveals no statistically significant difference in the interval from placement to an initial event (p 0.598). If the initial event was a thrombosis, it tended to occur earlier in the pl-TFE group, but the frequency of this complication was no different between the groups. In the primary forearm graft population, stratification of EFP for pl-TFE grafts by configuration revealed that loop grafts exhibited substantially better patency than straight grafts. No difference in patency was found between loop and straight configurations in ePTFE grafts. The origins of this disparity, currently under investigation in our laboratory, may be related to the biomechanical properties of the pl-TFE conduit, its efficiency in transmitting energy to the venous anastomosis, and the relationship between energy dissipation and pseudointimal hyperplasia at the venous anastomosis. Such a difference in biomechanical properties may also relate to the shorter interval between placement and thrombosis seen in pl-TFE grafts. Loop graft configuration of pl-TFE access devices may allow more energy to be dissipated before the pulse wave reaches the venous anastomosis.

Differences in cumulative patency between straight and loop ePTFE graft configuration have been reported, but are difficult to compare to primary patency data.[21] A pseudointimal hyperplasia-like reaction at the venous end of the graft was the most common cause of pl-TFE access thrombosis and was universally more exuberant than that seen in ePTFE grafts. Determination of the exact histologic nature of this hyperplastic reaction and its comparison to the pseudointimal hyperplasia seen in ePTFE grafts are the focus of ongoing investigations in our laboratory.

Another clear difference between pl-TFE and ePTFE is the relative difficulty encountered in thrombectomy of pl-TFE grafts. Thrombus is easily delivered from the graft lumen using standard balloon-tipped catheter techniques, but the moderately adherent pseudointimal cast of collagen, macrophages, and fibroblasts must also be removed in order to achieve successful thrombectomy. If portions of this cast remain in the lumen, they tend to embolize and cause rethrombosis. The intense hyperplastic reactions seen at the venous anastomosis of pl-TFE grafts have required that a larger number of these grafts undergo revision or abandonment at the initial thrombectomy. The functional interval between an initial thrombotic episode and a second event was also shorter in the pl-TFE group. Second and subsequent thromboses also were usually the result of venous hyperplastic reactions that recurred or progressed following initial thrombectomy or revision.

Our experience with the pl-TFE hemoaccess devices has demonstrated that immediate cannulation of this material is possible without fear of perigraft hematoma formation during dialysis, and that bleeding from this material following decannulation is not different from that from mature ePTFE. Although overall patency of pl-TFE grafts was similar to ePTFE access devices, they are significantly more difficult to thrombectomize. The biomechanical properties of pl-TFE that allow safe early cannulation and that may be responsible for the exuberant hyperplastic reactions merit additional study.

References

1. Yeh YS, Iriyama Y, Matsuzawa Y, Hanson SR, Yasuda H. Blood compatibility of surfaces modified by plasma polymerization. J Biomed Mater Res 1988; 22:795–818.
2. Hoffman AS, Garfinkle AM, Ratner BD. Surface modification of small diameter Dacron vascular grafts after a tetrafluoroethylene glow discharge treatment. Trans Soc Biomater 1984; VII:337.
3. Garfinkle AM, Hoffman AS, Ratner BD, Reynolds LO, Hanson SR. Effects of tetrafluoroethylene glow discharge on patency of small diameter Dacron vascular grafts. Trans Am Soc Artif Intern Organs 1984; 30:432–39.
4. Bauer R, Salem G. Erste Erfahrungen mit der neuen Plasma-TFE-Prothese. Angio Archiv Bd 1986; 11:115–16.
5. Jendrisak M, Bander S, Windus D, Delmez J. Early cannulation of plasma tetrafluoroethylene (Plasma-TFE) grafts for dialysis. Kidney Int 1990; 37:303.
6. Zar J. Biostatistical analysis. II. Englewood Cliffs, NJ: Prentice-Hall, 1984; 390–395.
7. Finney DJ. Probit analysis. 2nd ed. New York: Cambridge University Press, 1962.
8. Cox DR. Regression models and life-tables. J Royal Stat Soc 1972; 34:187–220.
9. Kaplan EL, Meier P. Nonparametric estimation from incomplete observations. J Am Statist Assoc 1958; 53:457–81.
10. ESRD Network 8, Jackson, MS.
11. Brescia MJ, Cimino JE, Appel K, Hurwich BJ. Chronic hemodialysis using venipuncture and a surgically created arteriovenous fistula. N Engl J Med 1966; 275:1089–92.

12. Spinowitz BS, Schechter L. Subclavian vein stenosis as a complication of subclavian catheterization for hemodialysis. Arch Intern Med 1987; 147:305-07.
13. Barrett N, Spencer S, McIvor J, Brown EA. Subclavian stenosis: A major complication of subclavian dialysis. Nephrol Dial Transplant 1988; 3:423-425.
14. Schwab SJ, Quarles LD, Middleton JP, Cohan, RH, Saeed M, Dennis VW. Hemodialysis-associated subclavian vein stenosis. Kidney Int 1988; 33:1156-59.
15. Cimochowski GE, Worley E, Rutherford WE, Sartain J, Blondin J, Harter H. Superiority of the internal jugular over the subclavian access for temporary dialysis. Nephron 1990; 54:154-61.
16. Taucher LA. Immediate, safe hemodialysis into arteriovenous fistulas created with a new tunneller, an 11 year experience. Am J Surg 1985; 150:212-15.
17. Mitchell RS, Miller DC, Billingham ME, Mehigan JT, Olcott C IV, Stinson EB. Comprehensive assessment of the safety, durability, clinical performance, and healing characteristics of a double velour knitted Dacron arterial prosthesis. Vasc Surg 1980; 14:197-212.
18. Sauvage LR, Davis CC, Smith JC, et al. Development and clinical use of porous Dacron prostheses. *In*: Sawyer PN, ed. Modern vascular grafts. New York: McGraw-Hill, 1987; 225-255.
19. Greisler HP, Dennis JW, Schwarcz TH, Klosak JJ, Ellinger J, Kim DV. Plasma polymerized tetrafluoroethylene/polyethylene terephthalate vascular prostheses. Arch Surg 1989; 124:967-72.
20. Mehta S. Statistical summary of clinical results of vascular access procedures for hemodialysis. *In:* Sommer BG, Henry ML, eds. Vascular access for hemodialysis. II. Chicago: WL Gore and Precept Press, 1991:145-57.
21. Rizzuti RP, Hale JC, Burkart TE. Extended patency of expanded polytetrafluoroethylene grafts for vascular access using optimal configuration and revisions. Surg Gynecol Obstet 1988; 166:23-27.

13

A PROSPECTIVE RANDOMIZED COMPARISON OF BOVINE HETEROGRAFTS VERSUS IMPRA GRAFTS FOR CHRONIC HEMODIALYSIS

*Jeffrey C. Reese, M.D., Robert Esterl, M.D.,
Lisa Lindsey, P.A.-C, Della Aridge, R.N., M.S.N.,
Harvey Solomon, M.D., Ralph B. Fairchild, M.D.,
and Paul J. Garvin, M.D.*

THE CONTINUED GROWTH of the end-stage renal disease (ESRD) program in the last decade—more than 100,000 patients are currently on chronic hemodialysis—has resulted in a progressive increase in the number of primary and secondary vascular access procedures performed.[1] With a disproportionate number of diabetic and elderly patients comprising the current ESRD population, creation and maintenance of vascular access in these patients presents an increasing challenge for surgeons involved in vascular access. A primary arteriovenous (A-V) fistula remains the ideal angioaccess in patients undergoing chronic hemodialysis. However, when an autologous fistula has failed or cannot be created, a prosthetic bridge A-V fistula is indicated. Historically, numerous materials have been used successfully in this setting. There is a recent trend toward the use of expanded polytetrafluoroethylene (PTFE) grafts in most institutions.

Although numerous retrospective reviews have reported higher patency rates and decreased complications in PTFE versus bovine heterografts,[2,3,4] few prospective trials comparing these grafts have been performed, and the results are conflicting.[5,6] At our institution, the bovine heterograft was used exclusively for vascular access until December 1985, with results comparable to published series with PTFE grafts.[7] To address the issue of whether one graft material was superior to the other, a prospective randomized trial was designed to compare PTFE (Impra, Tempe, AZ) and bovine heterografts (Johnson & Johnson, New Brunswick, NJ).

Patients and Methods

Between Jan. 1, 1986, and Dec. 31, 1989, a randomized prospective trial comparing bovine heterografts versus Impra dialysis accesses was conducted at Saint Louis University Hospital and John Cochran Veterans Administration Medical Center (both Saint Louis). During this interval, 138 bovine and 153 Impra grafts were implanted. In this same period, 36 successful primary radiocephalic fistulas were constructed. Descriptions of our surgical technique and criteria for inflow and outflow have been described, as well as our treatment for clotted and aneurysmal grafts.[7,8,9] Briefly, all patients undergoing insertions and revisions received a cephalosporin antibiotic. Most of the procedures were performed under local anesthesia. Our preference is to insert a straight forearm graft. Lower-arm loop grafts, upper-arm grafts, and thigh grafts were used in decreasing frequency. This policy preserves the greatest number of access sites and should also favor limb salvage if complications arise.

Fistulograms were done at the end of all procedures. Grafts were not used for at least two weeks. An aggressive standardized approach to the management of access complications was carried out. Thrombosed grafts were thrombectomized, and venous outflow obstructions were corrected with patch angioplasty or interposition grafting to the more proximal vein or a new vein. Arterial inflow problems were corrected, if possible, by interposing to a more proximal artery. Infected graft aneurysms were ligated and excised. Noninfected aneurysms were revised only for impending rupture or if they interfered with graft function; they were treated by excision with placement of an interposition graft. All infected bovine grafts were removed. Infected Impra grafts were removed if the infection did not resolve with antibiotics and dressing changes.

The following variables were analyzed in all patients: age, gender, presence of diabetes, primary versus secondary access, and graft configuration. A comparison of the results between the two groups was accomplished using the Student's t-test. In both groups, the incidence of infection, thrombosis, and aneurysm was then determined. Infections were further subdivided into operative (<30 days) and dialysis-associated infections (>30 days). Last, cumulative patency between the groups was analyzed with regard to actual graft survival and incidence of revisions (reported as number of revisions per 100 graft-months). Patients were followed until their death, transplantation, transfer to units where adequate follow-up was unavailable, graft abandonment, or through December 1990.

Table 13-1. Patient Characteristics

	Bovine	Impra
Mean age (years)	57	57
% Older than 60 years	61	57
% Older than 70 years	21	17
% Diabetic	32	35
% First access	50	41
% Female	25	39

Table 13-2. Graft Configurations

	Bovine	Impra
% Forearm straight graft	91	86
% Forearm loop graft	5	4
% Upper arm graft	3	8
% Thigh graft	1	2

Results

The mean age, as well as the percentage of patients older than 60 and older than 70, was not significantly different in the two groups. In addition, the incidence of diabetes, male/female ratio, and number of primary versus secondary accesses was similar (table 13-1). The distribution of various graft configurations is shown in table 13-2. The high incidence of straight forearm grafts in both groups reflects our policy of reserving more proximal vessels until distal sites are exhausted.

The incidence of infections leading to graft loss, although not statistically significant, was greater in the group with bovine heterografts (13% vs. 9%). Most of these infections occurred >30 days after insertion and were probably related to breaks in technique during dialysis (table 13-3). Few grafts were lost or needed to be revised for complications secondary to aneurysm formation (table 13-4). Late complications were seen, with aneurysmal bovine grafts lost at 20, 29, and 47 months, and aneurysmal Impra grafts lost at 5, 20, 32, and 41 months, respectively. About 25% of the patients in each group expired or were transplanted with functioning accesses in less than one year. Throughout the

Table 13-3. Graft Infections

	Bovine	Impra	p Value
Graft loss due to infection	18/138 (13.0%)	14/153 (9.2%)	NS
<30 days	4/18	3/14	
31-365 days	10/18	8/14	
>365 days	4/18	3/14	

Table 13-4. Aneurysmal Complications

	Bovine	Impra	p Value
Graft loss due to aneurysm	3/138 (2.2%)	4/153 (2.6%)	NS
Grafts revised due to aneurysm	2/138 (1.4%)	2/153 (1.3%)	NS

Table 13-5. Follow-up of Patients with Functioning Accesses

	Bovine	Impra
Total no. patients	138	153
Transplant with functioning access (<1 yr)	11 (8.0%)	9 (5.9%)
Transfer with functioning access (<1 yr)	6 (4.3%)	6 (3.9%)
Death with functioning access (<1 yr)	29 (21.0%)	27 (17.6%)
Transplant with functioning access (all)	16 (11.6%)	12 (7.8%)
Transfer with functioning access (all)	9 (6.5%)	12 (7.8%)
Death with functioning access (all)	47 (34.1%)	47 (30.7%)

Table 13-6. Actual Graft Survival

	Bovine	Impra	p Value
Early graft survival (<1 mo)*	132/136 (97.1%)	135/142 (95.1%)	NS
One-year graft survival†	58/98 (59.2%)	71/107 (66.4%)	NS

* Patients transplanted, transferred, or expired with functioning accesses (<1 mo) were excluded
† Patients transplanted, transferred, or expired with functioning accesses (<1 yr) were excluded

study, >40% of the patients expired or were transplanted with functioning accesses (table 13-5). Early graft survival is the same in both groups.

One-year actual graft survival was better in the Impra grafts (66% vs. 59%), but the difference was not significant (table 13-6). Patients with functioning accesses who expired, were transplanted, or were transferred before one year were

Table 13-7. Revisions (Incidence per 100 Graft-Months)

	Bovine	Impra	p Value
No. revisions (grafts functioning <1 yr)	6.5	5.0	NS
No. revisions (grafts functioning >1 yr)	4.4	4.2	NS

excluded from the one-year graft survival analysis. The revision rate, calculated as number of revisions per 100 graft-months, was not statistically different between the two grafts. For grafts functioning less than a year, the trend was toward fewer revisions in the Impra grafts; for well-functioning grafts (>1 year), no trend could be seen (table 13-7). All grafts are included in this analysis until thrombosed and not salvageable, removed for infection or aneurysm, patient transplanted, transferred, or death.

Discussion

With the progressive growth of the ESRD program since its inception, vascular access procedures have become commonplace in most institutions. Although significant advances have been made in surgical technique, graft materials, and dialysis technology, long-term maintenance of vascular access continues to be problematic. Contributing to this problem are the advancing age of the dialysis population and the increasing number of diabetic patients. The result is a high incidence of cardiac disease associated with hemodynamic instability and of peripheral vascular disease, creating problems with adequate inflow.

The primary A-V fistula continues to be the access of choice, whenever technically feasible. However, in the current dialysis population, it is usually not an option. This is evident in our patient population, in which only 11% of patients were candidates for the procedure. Over the past 20 years, numerous conduits have been used to create interposition A-V fistulas. These have included autogenous,[10] allogeneic saphenous vein,[11] umbilical vein graft,[12] bovine heterografts,[13] and PTFE grafts. The most frequently used material for vascular access was the bovine heterograft, with excellent patency rates reported from several centers.[4,7] Proposed advantages of the PTFE grafts include less thrombogenicity, decreased incidence of aneurysm formation, and greater resistance to infection. After early clinical trials, a gradual trend has been seen toward the use of PTFE grafts. Numerous retrospective reviews using one type of graft or the other, or both, have demonstrated better patency, with fewer revisions and complications seen in PTFE grafts.[2,3,4] Conversely, Brems et al. showed patency and complication rates of bovine grafts comparable to the best results of PTFE grafts.[7] Only two prospective trials comparing these graft types have been conducted. Hurt et al. could not demonstrate any difference in two groups in terms of patency rates and complications, whereas Sabanayagam et al. showed a 20% greater patency rate with fewer revisions in PTFE grafts.[5,6] These conflicting data provided the impetus for our randomized trial.

Historically, infected bovine grafts had to be removed,[6,7] although some centers reported maintaining infected PTFE accesses with conservative treatment.[15,16] In our study, graft loss was not statistically different between the two groups. Most of the infections were late, probably related to the handling of the graft after initiation of its use, as opposed to postoperative infections. All bovine grafts were removed without a trial of conservative management. Although conservative management was attempted in some PTFE grafts, all were eventually removed.

True aneurysms do not occur in PTFE grafts as they do in bovine grafts, but the overall graft loss due to aneurysms is similar in both groups. Most aneurysms are false and are handled similarly.[9,17] This was true in our study as well, and few grafts in either group needed to be revised or ligated due to aneurysm formation.

In our study, one-year graft patency rates were not statistically significantly different, although the trend was toward better patency in PTFE grafts. Early graft loss was the same in both groups. This would be expected, because early graft losses are usually secondary to technical errors, judgment errors, infections, or death, not graft type. The revision rates for short-term functioning accesses (<1 year) or long-term functioning accesses (>1 year) were similar in the two groups. These rates are comparable to previously published pooled data accumulated by Mehta.[4] Significant differences in graft survival of more than one year cannot be answered by our study because so many patients were lost to death, transplant, or transfer.

Finally, the patient cost of an Impra graft was about $650, compared to about $1,030 for a bovine graft (1989). This represents a substantial savings, considering the number of dialysis accesses created.

Conclusion

Our prospective randomized trial confirmed our retrospective trial that there is very little difference in the complication rate, revision rate, and graft survival between the two types of grafts studied. Because of the lower cost and the generally better familiarity with handling of PTFE grafts in dialysis units, we now prefer PTFE grafts.

References

1. U.S. Renal Data System: 1991 annual report.
2. Butler HG, Baker LD, Johnson JM. Vascular access for chronic hemodialysis: Polytetrafluoroethylene (PTFE) versus bovine heterografts. Am J Surg 1977;134:791-93.
3. Sicard GA, Allen BT, Anderson CB. Polytetrafluoroethylene grafts for vascular access. In: Sommer BG, Henry ML, eds. Vascular access for hemodialysis. Chicago: WL Gore and Pluribus Press, 1989;51-64.
4. Mehta S. Statistical summary of clinical results of vascular access procedures for hemodialysis. In: Sommer BG, Henry ML, eds. Vascular access for hemodialysis II. Chicago: WL Gore and Precept Press, 1991;145-57.
5. Sabanayagam P, et al. Angio-access—A decade of experience. In: Sommer BG, Henry ML, eds. Vascular access for hemodialysis II. Chicago: WL Gore and Precept Press, 1991;52-59.
6. Hurt AV, et al. Bovine carotid artery heterografts versus polytetrafluoroethylene grafts—A prospective randomized study. Am J Surg 1983; 146:844-47.
7. Brems J, Castaneda MA, Garvin PJ. A five year experience with the bovine heterograft for vascular access. Arch Surg 1986;121:941-44.
8. Garvin PJ, Codd JE. An aggressive approach to late thrombosis of bovine heterografts. Arch Surg 1979;190:743-45.
9. Garvin PJ, Castaneda MA, Codd JE. Etiology and management of bovine graft aneurysms. Arch Surg 1982;117:281-84.
10. Girardet RE, Hackett RE, Goodwin NJ, et al. Thirteen month experience with the saphenous vein graft arteriovenous fistula for maintenance hemodialysis. Trans Am Soc Artif Intern Organs 1970;16:285-91.
11. Adar R, Segal A, Bogokowsky H, et al. The use of arteriovenous autograft and allograft fistula for chronic hemodialysis. Surg Gynecol Obstet 1973;136:941-44.
12. Dardik H, Ibrahim IM, Dardik I. Arteriovenous fistulas constructed with modified human umbilical cord vein graft. Arch Surg 1976;111:60-62.
13. Rosenthal JJ, Spigelman A, Gaspar MR, et al. Problems with bovine heterografts for hemodialysis. Am J Surg 1975;130:182-88.
14. Tellis VA, Kohlberg WI, Bhat DJ, et al. Expanded polytetrafluoroethylene graft fistula for chronic hemodialysis. Ann Surg 1979;189:101-105.
15. Bhat DJ, Tellis VA, Kohlberg WI, Driscoll B, Veith FJ. Management of sepsis involving expanded polytetrafluoroethylene grafts for hemodialysis access. Surgery 1980;87:445-50.
16. Tellis VA, Weiss P, Matas AJ, Veith FJ. Skin flap coverage of polytetrafluoroethylene vascular access graft exposed by previous infection. Surgery 1988;103:118-21.
17. Halstuk K, Bern A. Aneurysmal disease and puncture site complication in vascular access. In: Sommer BG, Henry ML, eds. Vascular access for hemodialysis II. Chicago: WL Gore and Precept Press, 1991;75-84.

PANEL DISCUSSION

Moderator:
Ronald M. Ferguson, M.D., Ph.D.

Use of 6 mm Stretch PTFE Grafts for Early Use in Hemodialysis
Presenter:
Eugene T. Simoni, M.D.

Moderator: I haven't yet heard a theoretical reason why you can stick a stretch graft within 24 hours, when the entire audience, save two, don't stick regular PTFE grafts early.

Dr. Simoni: Our study was started out of pure coincidence. We had a patient who was 16 years on dialysis, with no access available at all. We had used loop necklaces, legs, arms. She was a diabetic, blind female, right above-knee amputation, and had a PermCath in her right external iliac vein, which she pulled out and almost bled out from it. She was in hypovolemic shock from that and was taken back to the operating room. We started using stretch grafts for aortic surgery and noticed that the needle holes either didn't bleed or had very minimal bleeding. We had a limb of aortic graft that was unused and sterile, and we placed a loop abdominal wall access from the external iliac artery to the external iliac vein, and were able to stick it early out of necessity. This patient started the study.

Moderator: We have also used this. Dr. Henry just brought to my attention that one theoretical advantage is the way this is constructed; it collapses much more readily around the needle. Have you looked histologically at the needle holes in these in fresh sticks? Do they seal more quickly?

Dr. Simoni: We haven't studied that.

Discussant: I have implanted the stretch graft, and I punctured the graft directly in view and it bled massively. I think that these kinds of conclusions have to be taken with a grain of salt. When a patient cannot be cannulated in any other way, we will use early puncture in PTFE grafts. If a highly trained nephrologist or nurse is available, it can be done. My question is that I am a little bothered by the patency rate. You have about six or seven grafts that clotted. How do you rule out that all of those thromboses were not due to the fact that you had a graft hematoma or that compression by the nurses was done with too much vigor?

Dr. Simoni: We believe that the two that were lost were secondary to the small venous outflow. Also, it was documented by color flow imaging that the venous outflow tracts were extremely small. These grafts did function for six weeks, although they were thrombectomized twice. The third time they clotted, we went ahead and placed upper-arm accesses on them. In two of the other grafts that clotted, the patient slept on his forearm and woke up with a clotted graft. The last one clotted as a result of excessive pressure applied at one of the dialysis units outside the institution.

Discussant: I have a technical question. I have placed a couple of these grafts, and I would like to ask how much tension you place this graft under when you are putting it in—full stretch, half stretch, no stretch?

Dr. Simoni: I pull it out to almost full stretch until the longitudinal lines are usually the same size and the cross lines are smaller. When you put it on enough tension, they actually end up being the same diameter across. Not full stretch, but close.

Discussant: Did you notice any difference between the stretch graft and the regular graft in terms of tissue reaction and skin edema?

Dr. Simoni: We used the Gore tunneler on these grafts, which really facilitated their placement, and we really didn't see much perigraft edema or any kind of reaction around the graft after placement. They were easily palpated and cannulated by the dialysis staff.

Discussant: After the placement of a GORE-TEX Graft, you normally get significant fibrosis around the graft. Do these stretch grafts maintain their "stretchiness"? If they don't, what is the advantage of using this material?

Dr. Simoni: They do lose their stretch once they are incorporated. The handling of the graft in the operating room is much more precise and conforms more at the anastomotic site. In my opinion, there is a big difference in reduced bleeding, and I think it may be because of the longitudinal extensibility of this graft.

Dialysis Access Using PTFE-Coated Woven Grafts
Presenter:
Ralph Didlake, M.D.

Discussant: I had an experience with this graft previously, but because it really isn't easier to handle, I stopped using it. The inner and outer capsule adherence is very poor, and when the graft is thrombectomized early, you can end up pulling out the whole inner capsule. The problem is that if you don't remove all of the longitudinal stretchability, and you blow up the thrombectomy balloon a little bit too much, you can move the graft inside the outer capsule. You then have a sieve in the forearm with arterial pressure in it and the predicted major problems.

Dr. Didlake: That is exactly our experience. Another pitfall of not putting the appropriate stretch on this graft is that with time and the lack of true tissue ingrowth, the residual stretch can walk down the tunnel. We've had two dialysis accesses kink over at the distal end and one femoral-popliteal bypass that were placed under inappropriate stretch.

Discussant: A couple of comments. The graft seems to be poorly incorporated, so that it is very easy to move it; also, it is very difficult to thrombectomize it. I previously have done a study comparing these grafts to PTFE to see if energy transfer could be limited by these grafts. I implanted this graft on one side and PTFE on the other, and found that there was no benefit in the energy transfer that occurred. In fact, if anything, these grafts developed just as much hyperplasia. In addition, they developed a pseudointima within the graft that, as you mentioned, was much more impressive, about 10 times thicker. In the course of three months, in fact, it became so thick that it began to become flow-limiting within the graft. Our experimental and clinical results have indicated that this is not a very good graft.

Dr. Didlake: There are other aspects about the biomechanics of this type of graft. We have implanted this graft in ballistic gelatin and measured not only the pulse wave velocity down the graft, but the actual mechanical energy transmitted down the wall of the graft. The graft just sits there and oscillates because it stretches with each impulse. There is not only the kinetic energy pulse wave but also a hammer effect at the end.

A Prospective Randomized Comparison of Bovine Heterografts versus Impra Grafts for Chronic Hemodialysis
Presenter:
Jeffery C. Reese, M.D.

Moderator: What happens if you immediately stick a bovine graft?
Dr. Reese: You can't do it. Bovine grafts get infected and you have to take them out.
Moderator: Based on this study, what graft material are you going to use in the future?
Dr. Reese: Currently, we use only PTFE grafts, because the trend is toward better patency. I think the complications are a little easier to deal with and the product is much cheaper.

SECTION IV

14

SALVAGE SURGERY FOR ARTERIOVENOUS CONDUITS: DOES IT MAKE SENSE?

Stephen B. Leapman, M.D., Mark D. Pescovitz, M.D., J. Vincent Thomalla, M.D., Martin Milgrom, M.D., and Ronald S. Filo, M.D.

CHRONIC ACCESS TO THE VASCULAR SYSTEM has been the most vulnerable aspect of chronic hemodialytic therapy. Since the introduction of Silastic shunts by Quinton et al. in 1960, many devices and techniques have been introduced into the realm of "access surgery."[1] None, however, has been as effective as the endogenous arteriovenous (A-V) fistula described by Brescia and co-workers in 1966.[2] Although the fistula continues to enjoy the highest patency rates and the fewest complications, this type of access cannot be placed in many individuals because of their venous or arterial anatomy, underlying vasculopathy, exhausted peripheral vessels, or the size of the arm. Therefore, it was not surprising that biologically altered, autogenous, or synthetic materials might provide a viable alternative to the preferable Brescia-Cimino A-V fistula.

The patency rates and success of A-V conduits depend on the prevention or treatment of many complications. These include technical misplacement of the grafts, subintimal hyperplasia resulting in stenosis and subsequent thrombosis, infection, aneurysm and pseudoaneurysm formation, steal syndromes resulting in ischemia, lymphoceles, chronic edema of the extremity, cardiac failure, and venous hypertension. Most of these serious complications are reversible and correctable, and, if treated aggressively, will result in restoration of a functional graft. Four reasons to restore grafts are: (1) the graft will be immediately available as access for hemodialysis, (2) the operation is not technically difficult, (3) it can be done on an outpatient basis or with minimal hospitalization, and (4) it will save precious autogenous vessels for future use if necessary.

Since 1974, we have pursued an aggressive policy toward the salvage of all A-V conduits. This report summarizes our experience with 420 patients. We have examined all of the revisions of these grafts, seeking to answer the question of whether salvage therapy is a useful, practical alternative to graft abandonment and establishment of new graft in a different location.

Materials and Methods

From July 1974 through June 1989, 512 A-V conduits were created in 420 patients with end-stage renal disease (ESRD) at the Indiana University Medical Center and the Roudebush Veterans Medical Center (both Indianapolis). These consisted of 397 polytetrafluoroethylene (PTFE) conduits, 99 bovine heterografts, and 12 saphenous vein autografts. During this same time period, 926 radiocephalic A-V fistulas were constructed at these institutions. Saphenous vein grafts were placed from 1974 to 1977, and bovine grafts were used from 1974 until 1984. Expanded PTFE has been the main conduit material used since 1977. There were 292 (57%) males and 220 (43%) females; their age ranged from 12 to 83 years. More whites (n = 291, 57%) received conduits than blacks (n = 221, 43%).

Vascular procedures were performed by the authors either as the primary surgeon or assisting surgical resident. Primary conduits were generally placed in a loop configuration in the nondominant forearm. The arterial anastomosis was end-to-side to the distal brachial artery, and the venous limb was anastomosed to the basilic or the antecubital vein (usually end-to-side). Occasionally, the grafts were inserted in the proximal thigh, using the superficial femoral artery and the proximal saphenous vein as the arterial and venous insertion sites, respectively. When PTFE was used, a 6 mm diameter conduit was preferred. The operations were generally performed under local or regional anesthesia, but occasionally, either because of complexity, length of the operation, or patient preference, a general anesthetic was employed.

Revisional salvage surgery was employed if the graft became nonfunctional or if the attending nephrologist noted an anatomic abnormality (such as aneurysm) or a physiologic abnormality (such as increasing venous pressures or decreasing arterial flow rates compared to previous readings). Salvage procedures included thrombectomy, angioplasty of a stenosis (usually with a PTFE patch), PTFE interposition grafts, or partial excision of the graft if it was infected. The last was possible only with PTFE grafts; bovine grafts required total excision, as the entire graft was usually infected. Partial revision of the infected PTFE or autogenous conduit was limited to either the arterial or the venous limb. The ends of the remaining PTFE were oversewn and buried in the subcutaneous tissue until the infection had cleared and the wound was closed. An interposition graft was used to restore continuity. Only 8% of the salvage procedures had subtotal excisions. The type of revision was always at the discretion of the operating surgeon, but stenoses of 2–4 cm in length generally were repaired by angioplasty, whereas longer stenotic irregular native vessels or graft segments required an

Table 14.1. Salvage Procedures for Arteriovenous Conduits

Procedures	Alone No. (%)	With thrombectomy No. (%)
Thrombectomy	261 (29)	— —
Angioplasty	105 (12)	213 (43)
Interposition grafts	207 (23)	256 (52)
Angioplasty + interposition	213 (24)	25 (5)
Partial excision	69 (8)	— —
Total excision	41 (4)	— —
Total	896 (100)	494 (100)

interposition graft. In a few instances (n = 3), ultrasensational anatomic bypass interposition grafts were created from the arm to the internal jugular vessels.

Patency rates were analyzed by actuarial techniques using the Kaplan-Meier life table analysis. Vascular access failure was defined as follows: (1) complete abandonment of the graft because it could no longer be repaired, (2) the patient received a renal transplant, (3) the patient switched modes of dialytic therapy from hemodialysis to peritoneal dialysis, or (4) the patient died.

Results

The salvage procedures employed in this review are noted in table 14-1. Thrombectomy usually accompanied patch angioplasty or interposition grafting because the patients presented with thrombosis of the graft. Early in our experience, the first procedure employed was a thrombectomy alone. Arteriography was used as a follow-up study to identify any critical lesions; if found, the lesions were repaired at a second operation. That experience resulted in a new approach in which thrombectomy would be performed as the initial stage of the operation, and the definitive repair (angioplasty or interposition) would be done at the same time. Intraoperative arteriography was employed at the discretion of the operating surgeon.

Although revisions were necessary in most conduits (table 14-2), 36% of all grafts placed never required operative intervention and continued to function until the graft was exhausted or the patient died, changed dialytic techniques, or underwent transplantation. Half of the saphenous vein grafts required revisions, whereas 62% of the bovine and 66% of the PTFE grafts required revision. The time from initial placement of the graft until the first revision and the number of revisions per graft to maintain patency is noted in table 14-3. The long interval noted in the saphenous vein grafts is explained by an outlier and is noted by the large standard error. PTFE grafts required fewer revisions than

Table 14-2. Conduit Revisions

Conduit	Conduits inserted	Revisions	%
Saphenous vein	16	8	50
Bovine	99	60	62
PTFE	397	261	66
Totals	512	329	64

Table 14-3. Initial Revision Times and Number of Revisions per Life of Graft

Conduit	Time from insertion until first revision (mo) n	Time from insertion until first revision (mo) mean +/- SE	No. revisions per life of graft mean +/- SE
Saphenous vein	8	25.8 +- 14.4	2.1 +- 1.8
Bovine	60	10.7 +- 1.6	6.8 +- 3.9
PTFE	261	10.5 +- 0.8	1.9 +- 0.4

did the saphenous or the bovine conduits (1.9 revisions per graft versus 2.1 and 6.8 revisions per graft, respectively).

The life table analysis for graft survival is shown in Figure 14-1. There is a marked difference between the saphenous grafts and the other two conduits. Patency rates between the bovine heterograft and the PTFE conduits are different at all time intervals examined. The one-year patency rate for PTFE grafts was 93%; it fell to 74% at five years. The same time intervals for the bovine heterograft were 71% and 42%, respectively. Actuarial survival for the entire revised group was 89% at one year, 66% at five years, and 56% at 10 years. Mean graft survival for all 329 revised grafts regardless of material was 3.4 ± 0.2 years with a range from 0 to 15 years.

Discussion

Data from this 15-year study have led to several conclusions regarding aggressive salvage attempts to prolong A-V conduits. The overall revision rate of this series was 65%, and the mean time from insertion of a graft until the first repair was 10 months. Although 35% of patients never required revisions, an equal number of patients (35%) required one or two operative procedures; 31% required three or more procedures to maintain patency. A small cohort of conduits (1.4%) were revised 14–22 times to maintain flow.

Despite the large number of procedures, the patients were spared additional surgery on the contralateral upper extremity by maintaining patency in the original graft. The overall patency rate of all conduits was 89% at one year and

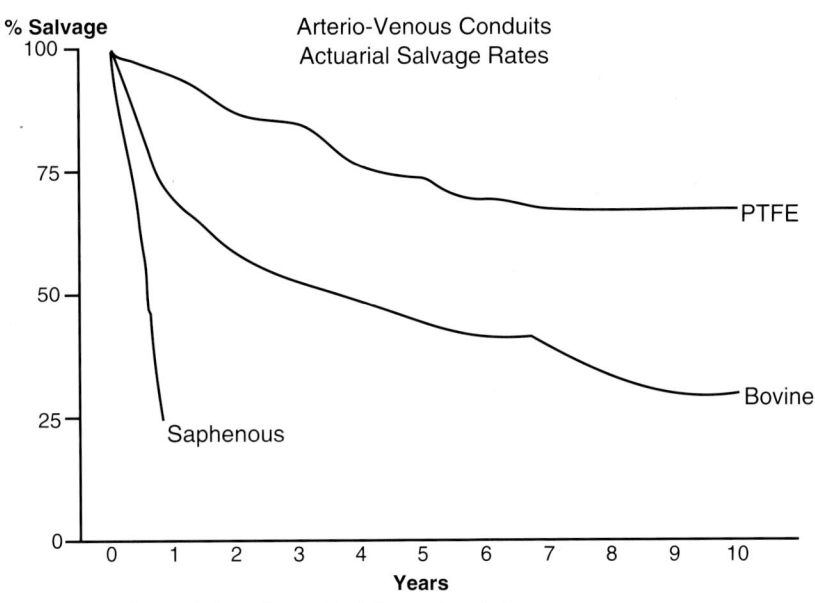

Figure 14-1. Actuarial graft survival for revised saphenous vein, bovine, and PTFE grafts are compared. Patency rates for PTFE at one, five, and 10 years are 93%, 74%, and 68%, respectively.

56% at 10 years. The actuarial graft survival of PTFE grafts was 95% and 68% at one and 10 years, respectively; survival of the bovine conduits was 71% and 29%. The PTFE grafts proved easy to use, easy to revise and repair, had a long shelf life, and could withstand the rigors of dialytic cannulations and surgical repairs for many years. PTFE grafts also could withstand infectious complications by segmental resection with eventual restoration. Bovine grafts required total excision to cure the infection.

Contraindications to restoring patency of an A-V conduit were few. These included chronic edema, steal syndromes so threatening to the extremity or hand that only total excision or ligation of the conduit would be acceptable, exhaustion of peripheral vessels, and repeated thromboses without anatomic abnormalities as determined by arteriography. Only severe steal syndromes have prevented us from attempting a revision at least once.

This aggressive approach to maintaining patency is also used by others. Etheredge et al. reported a series of 214 grafts (all PTFE), of which 74 were salvageable.[5] In this series, 140 patients never required revision or clinically could not be revised. These investigators reported that 78.7% of the grafts were functional at one year compared to 53.7% of the salvaged (repaired) grafts. The time interval between the first and second revision was 7.9 months. Tellis et al. also reported a series of PTFE conduits that had a nonrevision rate of 31%, but a cumulative one-year patency rate of 62.4%.[6] Sabanayagam et al. noted one-year patency rates by life table analysis of 90.5% for 225 grafts that required secondary procedures.[7] Lilly et al. compared bovine heterografts with PTFE grafts.[8] PTFE one-year patency rates were 85% versus 73% for the bovine grafts. This is similar to our series, in which the patency rates were 93% for PTFE and 71% for bovine. In addition, the incidence of infected grafts in the Lilly study was identical to ours. Butler and colleagues, who also compared bovine and PTFE graft patency, noted patency rates similar to ours.[9]

Polo and co-workers reported on 16 patients whose peripheral veins had been exhausted and whose axillar or subclavian veins were stenotic or occluded.[10] They created brachial-jugular conduits and were able to maintain patency for eight to 26 months in all but two patients. We have used this ultrasensational anatomic bypass interposition in three patients to salvage conduits that had no venous runoff. Two of the patients currently have functioning grafts more than 12 months after the original conduit was revised.

In conclusion, 64% of all conduits placed for A-V access will require revision. The revision usually will not be necessary for 10 months after insertion. Aggressive salvage therapy resulted in 93% and 68% patency rates for PTFE conduits at one and 10 years, respectively. The salvage procedures of choice included partial excision with eventual reconstitution, angioplasty, and interpositions (sometimes as ultrasensational bypass grafts). Salvage rate was better for PTFE than for bovine grafts or saphenous vein grafts. These data support the hypothesis that aggressive salvage procedures for A-V conduits is a practical alternative to graft abandonment and subsequent placement of a new conduit in another extremity.

References

1. Quinton WE, Dillard D, Scribner BN. Cannulation of blood vessels for prolonged hemodialysis. Trans Am Soc Artif Intern Organs 1960; 6:104.
2. Brescia MJ, Cimino JE, Appel K, Hurwich BJ. Chronic hemodialysis using venipuncture and a surgically created arteriovenous fistula. N Engl J Med 1966; 275:1089.
3. Chivitz JL, Yokoyama T, Bower R, Swartz C. Self sealing prosthesis for arteriovenous fistula in man. Trans Am Soc Artif Intern Organs 1972; 18:452.
4. Johnson JM, Baker LD, Williams T. Expanded polytetrafluoroethylene: A subcutaneous conduit for hemodialysis. Dialy and Transpl, April 1976.
5. Etheredge EE, Hard SD, Maeser MN, Sicard GA. Salvage operations for malfunctioning polytetrafluoroethylene hemodialysis access grafts. Surgery 1983; 94:464.
6. Tellis VA, Kohlberg WI, Bhat DJ, et al. Expanded polytetrafluoroethylene graft fistula for chronic hemodialysis. Ann Surg 1979; 189:101.
7. Sabanayagam P, Schwartz AB, Soricelli RR, et al. Experience with one-hundred reinforced expanded PTFE grafts for angioaccess in hemodialysis. Trans Am Soc Artif Intern Organs 1980; 26:582.
8. Lilly L, Nghiem D, Mendez-Picon G, Lee HM. Comparison between bovine heterografts and expanded PTFE grafts for dialysis access. Am Surg 1980; 47:694.
9. Butler HG, Baker LD, Johnson JM. Vascular access for chronic hemodialysis: polytetrafluoroethylene (PTFE) versus bovine heterograft. Am J Surg 1977; 134:791.
10. Polo JR, Sanabra J, Garcia-Sabrido J, et al. Brachial-jugular polytetrafluoroethylene fistulas for hemodialysis. Am J Kidney Dis 1990; 16:465.

15

4–7 mm TAPERED EXPANDED PTFE ACCESS GRAFTS: TECHNIQUES OF CONSTRUCTION AND PRESERVATION OF GRAFT LIFE

Leonard H. Hines, M.D., F.A.C.S.,
G. Randolph Turner, M.D., F.A.C.S.,
William Scott King, M.D., F.A.C.S.,
Carter E. McDaniel III, M.D., F.A.C.S.,
and David J. Dodd, M.D.

RECORDS OF 278 EXPANDED POLYTETRAFLUOROETHYLENE (ePTFE) 4–7 mm Tapered GORE-TEX Vascular Grafts (W.L. Gore & Associates, Flagstaff, AZ) implanted in 248 hemodialysis patients were analyzed to determine primary and secondary patency rates as well as the factors that influence successful chronic hemodialysis. Revision and thrombectomy were shown to prolong graft survival 2.5 times over the primary patency rate. The overall incidence of complications was acceptable, and the ePTFE graft material was shown to be especially durable and resistant to infection. On the basis of our experience, when autogenous fistulas are not feasible, the 4–7 mm tapered ePTFE graft is the best alternative for arteriovenous (A-V) access. The loop configuration in the forearm is preferred because of its distal location and because the added length of the loop offers more sites for cannulation, thus extending the life of the graft.

Although the use of autogenous tissue, as in the Brescia-Cimino fistula, is the preferred procedure for establishing A-V access for long-term hemodialysis, most patients require multiple synthetic grafts to establish and continue vascular access over the course of their dialysis treatments. To conserve potential access sites and prolong graft life, several important factors must be considered

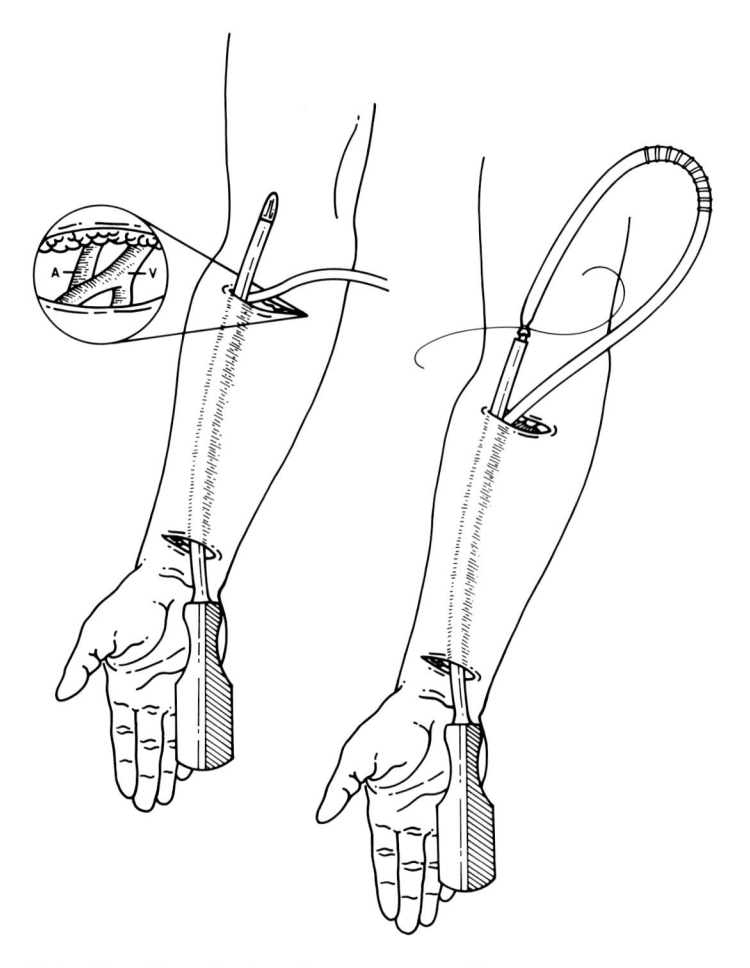

Figure 15-1. Gore Tunneler in subcutaneous position with graft attached to stylet (A-artery, V-vein).

before implanting the initial graft, including hemodynamic effects, convenience of access, and avoidance of contamination during access. The prosthetic device must be durable, resistant to infection, and easily incorporated into the host tissue during the healing process.

This report describes our experience with the ePTFE 4–7 mm Tapered GORE-TEX Vascular Graft implanted in the upper extremities, with emphasis on techniques of implantation and data concerning primary and cumulative patency.

Materials and Methods

The grafts were implanted using the standard technique described below and shown in figures 15-1 and 15-2, with minor variations determined by the particular situation. The adequacy of arterial flow to the hand is assessed by physical

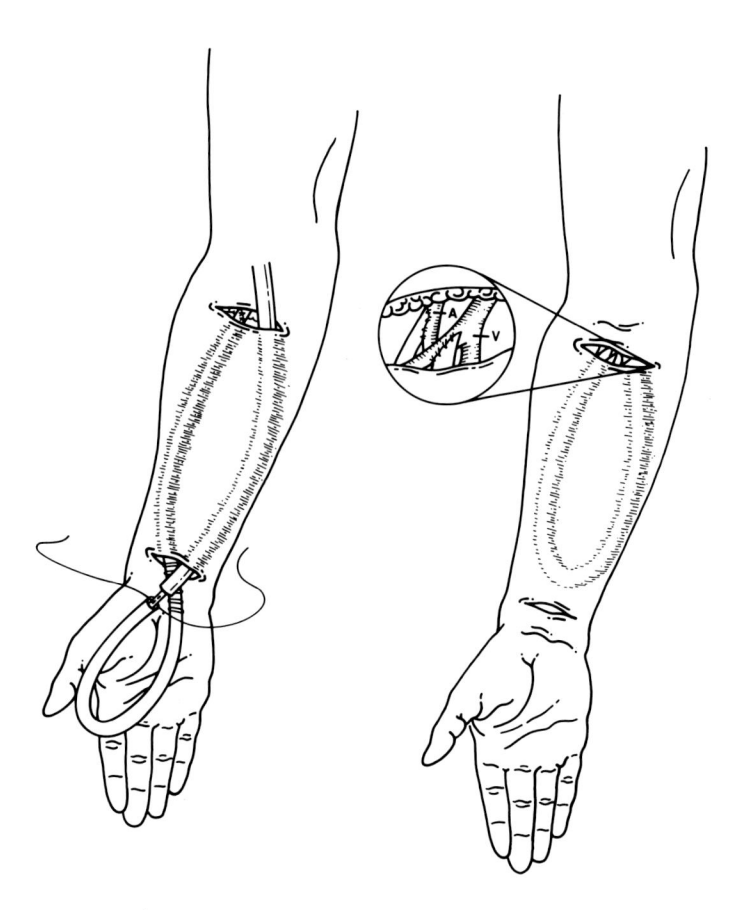

Figure 15-2. Graft placed in final position with anastomoses completed (A-artery, V-vein).

examination and Doppler evaluation to avoid the possibility of compromise as a result of arterial steal. All patients receive prophylactic antibiotic coverage and, depending on the risk to the patient, either local or general anesthesia. Our preferred site is the volar surface of the nondominant forearm, with the graft placed in a loop configuration to provide more sites for cannulation. A transverse incision is made just distal to the antecubital fossa and the caliber of the veins is measured. A lumen diameter of at least 3–4 mm is usually adequate, but a confluence of veins individually at least 2–3 mm in diameter may also provide satisfactory outflow. If venous outflow is determined to be inadequate, a straight brachioaxillary graft in the upper arm is chosen.

For the loop configuration, the brachial artery is exposed in the area of its bifurcation, and a longitudinal arteriotomy (no greater than 1.5 times the diameter of the vessel) is made. Dilute heparin (100 U/cc) is injected proximally and distally, and the 4 mm end of the 4–7 mm tapered ePTFE vascular graft is sewn end-to-side using CV-7 Gore-Tex Suture. The heparin solution is instilled into the graft at intervals to prevent blood from clotting before flow is established. The course of the graft is plotted on the skin and a counter transverse

```
          53.6
```

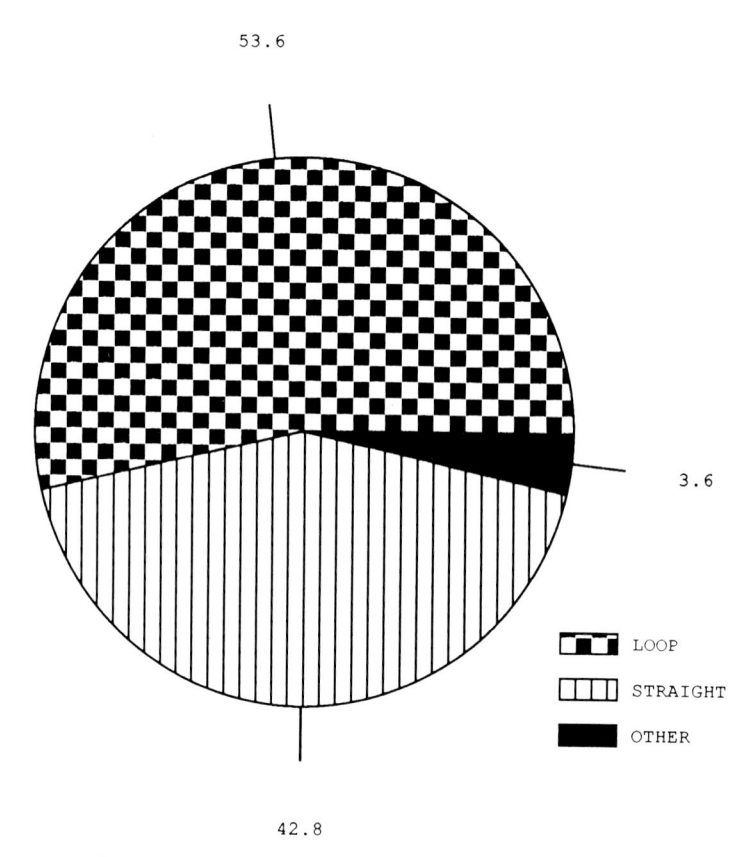

```
              LOOP
              STRAIGHT
              OTHER
```

```
    3.6
    42.8
```

Figure 15-3. Graft configuration (percentage).

incision is made about 2 cm distal to the end of the proposed loop. To avoid devascularizing the skin proximally, the incision is carried to the prefascial level. The proximal limit of the curved course of the graft is then created by subcutaneous dissection.

The Gore Tunneler using the 8 mm sheath is then passed subcutaneously from the distal incision proximally. Care is taken to avoid devascularizing the skin or, in the obese patient, placing the graft too deep for easy access. The bullet tip of the tunneler is removed, the graft is sewn to the stylet, and the arterial limb is pulled into position. The venous limb track is created in similar fashion, and the appropriate tension is used to create a gentle curve of the loop, taking care to avoid kinking or twisting the graft. The externally ringed graft has been used more recently to avoid these technical misadventures. Heparin solution is used again to distend the graft, assuring the appropriate positioning. The venous anastomosis is then performed with CV-7 ePTFE suture. Satisfactory flow produces a thrill over the graft. With the exception of constructing the loop, the techniques for implanting the straight brachioaxillary graft are similar to those described above.

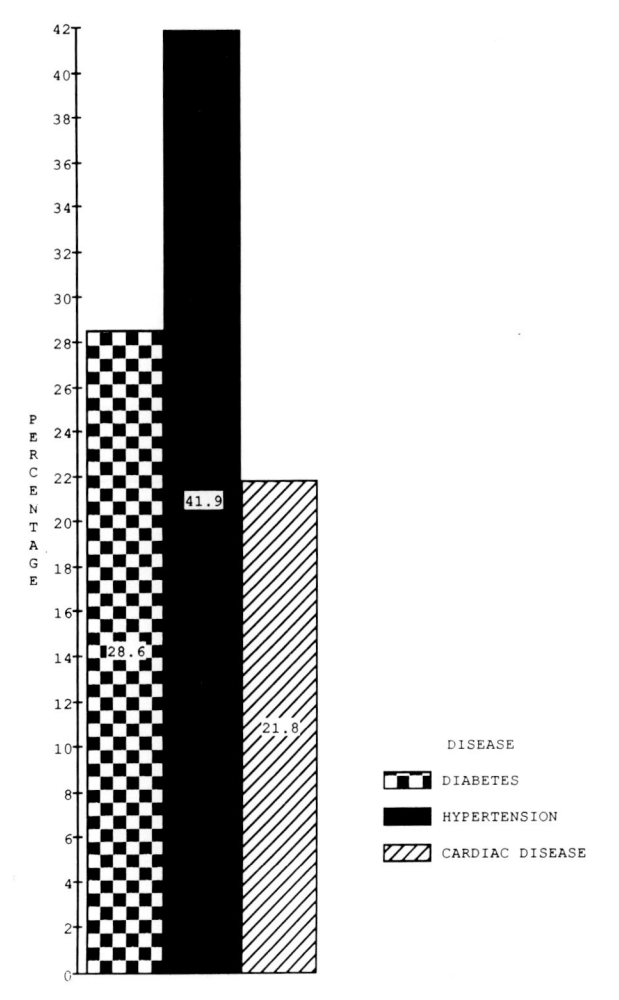

Figure 15.4. Percent of most frequent concurrent diseases in study group.

Results

Sixty percent of the patients in this group were over 55 years old, and 37% were over 65. Patient sex was evenly matched: 50.4% were male and 49.6% were female. Age and sex were not correlated to site location or graft configuration. The graft site selections were also similar, with 50.7% of the grafts inserted into the forearm and 46.4% in the arm. Graft configuration was not as evenly distributed throughout the population: 53.6% of the grafts were placed in a loop configuration and 42.8% were straight (figure 15-3). Associated medical conditions (figure 15-4) included diabetes (28.6%), cardiac disease (21.8%), and hypertension (41.9%).

Thrombosis of the graft was the most common complication, occurring in the 131 (47%) of the 278 grafts, translating into 4.29 incidents of thrombosis

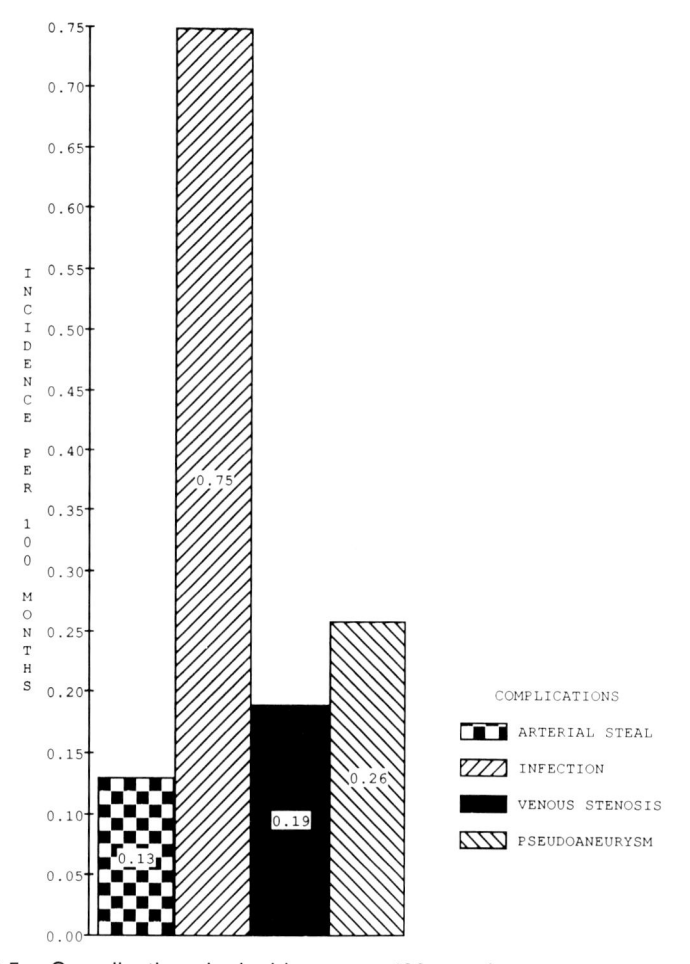

Figure 15-5. Complications by incidence per 100 months.

per 100 months of graft life for the entire study population. Neointimal hyperplasia appears to be the most common cause of graft thrombosis necessitating revision. Seventy-four grafts (26%) required revision, for a rate of 2.42 revisions per 100 months of graft life. The incidence of other complications was relatively low in this group. Infection, which was seen in 23 (8.2%) of the 278 grafts, was treated by antibiotic therapy, usually with partial or complete graft removal. This incidence of infection translated into 0.75 per 100 months of graft life. Pseudoaneurysm occurred in eight cases (2.8%), translating into a rate of 0.26 per 100 months, and arterial steal was seen in five cases (1.8%), for a rate of 0.13 per 100 months of graft life. Figure 15-5 is a graph of the rates of complications in this study population.

Primary and secondary patencies of all grafts were compiled using life table analysis. Primary patency, which refers to graft life from initial insertion to the first thrombosis, occlusion requiring revision, or graft excision, was 48% at 12 months and 15% at 48 months (figure 15-6). Cumulative or secondary patency includes total graft life from initial insertion to any nonsalvageable failure after revision. Secondary patency was about 72% at 12 months, 55% at 24 months, 46% at 36 months, and 37% at 4 years postoperatively (figure 15-6). These data compare favorably with data reported by others.[1]

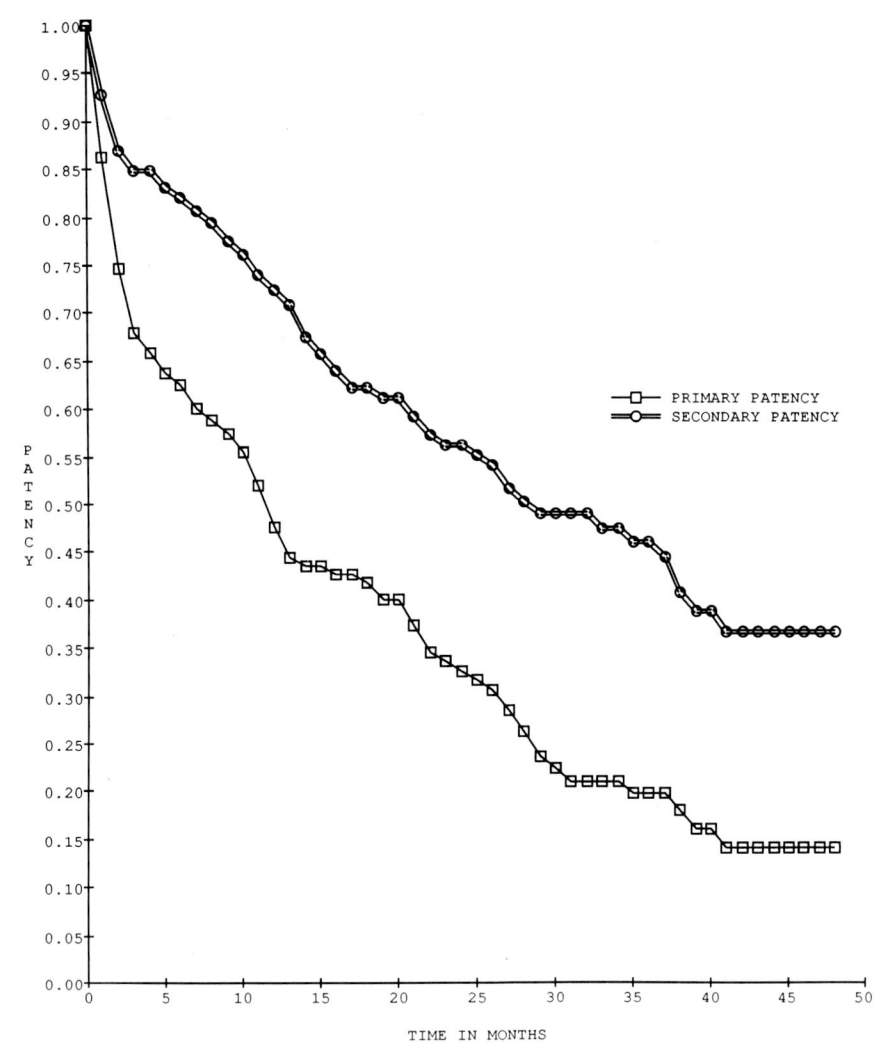

Figure 15-6. Primary and secondary patency of 4-7 mm Tapered GORE-TEX Vascular Grafts for hemodialysis access.

Discussion

An increasingly elderly hemodialysis population and frequent concomitant peripheral vascular disease challenge the vascular surgeon's technical expertise and imagination to provide continuous, effective, and complication-free access to the circulatory system. This capability has evolved over many years since Dr. Willem Kolff developed the first artificial kidney machine in the Netherlands in 1940.[2] However, patients were not able to be maintained adequately on hemodialysis until a means of long-term cannulation became available.

The development of the Scribner A-V shunt in 1960 provided the first relatively safe and easy continuous access.[3] This and other specialized external shunts were widely adopted as the acceptable means of supporting patients with end-stage renal disease (ESRD). High rates of infection, frequent thrombosis, bleeding, and restriction of the patient's daily activities have reduced the use of these shunts.

In 1966, the development of the Brescia-Cimino autogenous A-V fistula was a major advance in the support of chronic hemodialysis.[4] It was originally described as a side-to-side anastomosis joining the cephalic vein to the distal radial artery, and several variations in the type of anastomosis and location of these fistulas have been used with good success. Although many weeks of "arterialization" are required before repeated venipunctures can be tolerated, the Brescia-Cimino fistula has proved the most complication-free, durable, and dependable of all types of long-term vascular access techniques. Unfortunately, because successful long-term management of ESRD is frequently associated with the need for several access routes, and because many patients have inadequate veins, only about 15% of patients are candidates for construction of an autogenous A-V fistula.[5] As a result, the use of both biologic and prosthetic materials for constructing bridge fistulas has evolved in an effort to establish the ideal vascular access.

A variety of grafts has been used, including autogenous saphenous vein, preserved saphenous allografts, tanned bovine heterografts, glutaraldehyde-tanned human umbilical vein, and Dacron velour (Du Pont). Each of these has advantages and disadvantages, and some are still used routinely in certain areas. However, because of frequent complications such as infection, nonanastomotic aneurysm, and thrombosis, the search for a better graft has continued.[6-10]

In 1976, ePTFE was reported as an alternative prosthetic material[11] and rapidly became the most commonly used material for A-V bridge fistulas, if only because it was the most recent prosthesis to be developed with at least comparable performance to its predecessors. Since that time, it has proved easy to handle, resistant to the spread of infection, and durable, tolerating repeated punctures with a reported low incidence of nonanastomotic pseudoaneurysms when compared with bovine heterografts.[12-14] Thrombectomy is accomplished quite readily, and ePTFE holds sutures securely even after multiple procedures. Although complications do occur, our experience confirms that these complications frequently can be treated without sacrificing the graft, allowing the possibility to resume dialysis access immediately. For example, an interposition graft can be implanted around a pseudoaneurysm, stenotic site, or focally infected segment.

Patency of ePTFE grafts is acceptable. Several reports have indicated 24-month patency of >70%, and some have shown a decided advantage when compared with bovine heterografts.[15-17] Long-term patency is the most significant indicator of access success and is directly related to the results of graft revision and secondary patency. Bell and Rosental report an average length of primary patency for tapered ePTFE grafts of about one year.[5] Although they state that 70% of A-V graft procedures performed over a five-year period were revisions and thrombectomies, they maintain that the variability in their study group precluded analysis of secondary patency.

Our graft population allowed us to collect and consider data concerning secondary patency. Life table analysis of these data prove that thrombectomy and revision greatly enhance cumulative graft patency and increase group secondary patency by 2.5 times over primary patency. This increased patency not only correlates with access site conservation, but allows the salvaged graft to be used immediately for dialysis.

The final step in the evolutionary process to present-day dialysis access has been primarily in the direction of preventing the potentially devastating sequelae of arterial steal caused by the shunting of retrograde arterial flow into the graft. Early symptoms of arterial steal include decreased temperature, pain, and pallor of the hand, with or without neurological deficit and dampened or absent distal pulses. If left untreated, arterial steal can lead to permanent neuromuscular impairment, necrosis, and possible loss of the hand.

Most patients handle shunting of blood into the low-pressure venous system with either transient ischemia or the absence of clinical symptoms of hypoperfusion in the distal extremity. However, diabetics and patients with severe, distal vascular disease seem more predisposed to the steal phenomenon. Symptomatic steal has been reported in as many as 7% of cases in which either 8 mm or 6-8 mm tapered ePTFE grafts were used.[18] Efforts to preserve the graft site and diminish flow without precipitating thrombosis have consisted of banding techniques,[18] suture tapering of the arterial limb hood,[19] arterial ligation distal to the graft with revascularization,[20] and suture tapering of the arterial end of ePTFE grafts to a diameter of 4 mm before insertion.[21] The last technique prompted the development of perhaps the most widely used prosthetic graft for A-V access, the 4-7 mm tapered ePTFE 40 cm graft and, more recently, a 45 cm version with 10 cm of removable rings for the loop configuration. Our experience confirms that the 4-7 mm tapered graft was associated with a very low incidence of arterial steal. Cases noted were in patients of advanced age (>68 years) and may have been more closely related to significant concurrent peripheral vascular disease. The 4-7 mm tapered ePTFE graft not only provides satisfactory A-V access but also appears to be the most successful available prophylaxis against the steal phenomenon.

Several authors have indicated a correlation between outflow intimal hyperplasia and graft thrombosis, with the association being present in more than 50% of occluded grafts. Many hemodynamic theories have been advanced in an effort to explain this phenomenon.[1,5,13,22] Fillinger et al., using a reproducible canine A-V loop graft model of intimal-medial hyperplasia, postulate that the kinetic energy generated by flow turbulence causes vibration in perivascular tissue that is directly related to intimal-medial hyperplasia.[22] These studies show that the 4-7 mm tapered graft in loop configuration causes less flow disturbance than a nontapered graft in the same configuration. Although Fillinger was unable to show a flow difference between the 4-7 mm tapered graft and the 6 mm graft, suspected lower flow and increased flow stability at the venous outflow site conceivably would reduce the incidence of intimal hyperplasia. Also, the additional length of the loop configuration may allow the perivascular tissue to absorb some of the pulsatile energy over a broader area and help stabilize blood flow before it reaches the venous outflow site.

Although we did not correlate graft configuration with cumulative patency rates, perhaps the aforementioned considerations explain how Rizzuti et al.[1]

showed a better patency rate in loop grafts than in straight grafts. Certainly, the loop configuration allows for more access sites and is essentially as easy to thrombectomize or revise as the straight graft.

Conclusion

The success of long-term hemodialysis largely depends on conserving access sites and preserving established dialysis grafts. Satisfactory long-term patency correlates with graft preservation and involves an aggressive effort to successfully thrombectomize and revise grafts when necessary. The 4–7 mm tapered ePTFE vascular graft, preferably placed in loop configuration in the forearm, has proven to be a viable alternative when autogenous fistulas are not feasible. The graft is durable and easy to revise, with an acceptable rate of complications, and the lower rate of inflow appears especially to reduce the incidence of arterial steal.

References

1. Rizzuti RP, Burkart TE. Extended patency of expanded polytetrafluoroethylene grafts for vascular access using optimal configuration and revisions. Surg Gynecol Obstet 1988; 160:23–27.
2. Teschan PE. Historical perspectives on dialysis. In: Vascular Access for Hemodialysis, Sommer BG, Henry ML, eds. Chicago: WL Gore and Pluribus Press, 1989; 1–7.
3. Quinton WE, Dillar D, Scribner BH. Cannulation of blood vessels for prolonged hemodialysis. Trans Am Soc Artif Intern Organs 1960; 6:104–13.
4. Brescia MJ, Cimino JE, Appel K, et al. Chronic hemodialysis using venipuncture and a surgically created arteriovenous fistula. N Engl J Med 1966; 275:1089–92.
5. Bell DD, Rosental JJ. Arteriovenous graft life in chronic hemodialysis. J Vasc Surg 1989; 9:277–85.
6. Chinitz JL, Yokoyama T, Bower R, et al. Self-sealing prosthesis for arteriovenous fistula in man. Trans Am Soc Artif Intern Organs 1972; 18:452–56.
7. Garvin PJ, Cateneda MA, Codd JE. Etiology and management of bovine graft aneurysms. Arch Surg 1982; 117:281–84.
8. Hertzer NR, Beven EG. Venous access using carotid bovine heterograft—techniques, results, and complications in 75 patients. Arch Surg 1978; 113:696–701.
9. Lilly L, Ngheim D, Mendez-Picon G, et al. Comparison between bovine-heterografts and expanded PTFE grafts for dialysis access. Am Surg 1980; 46:694–96.
10. Oakes DD, Specs EK, Light JA, et al. A three-year experience using modified bovine arterial heterografts for vascular access in patients requiring hemodialysis. Ann Surg 1978; 187:423–29.
11. Baker LD, Johnson JM, Goldfarb D. Expanded polytetrafluoroethylene (PTFE) subcutaneous arteriovenous conduit: an improved vascular access for chronic hemodialysis. Trans Am Soc Artif Intern Organs 1976; 22:382–87.
12. Rossi G, Munteau FD, Padula G, et al. Nonanastomotic aneurysms in venous homologous grafts and bovine heterografts in femoropopliteal bypasses. Am J Surg 1976; 132:358–62.
13. Connolly JE, Brownell DA, Levine EF, McCart PM. Complications of renal dialysis access procedures. Arch Surg 1984; 119:1325–28.

14. Anderson CB, Sicard GA, Etheridge EE. Bovine carotid artery and expanded polytetrafluoroethylene grafts for hemodialysis vascular access. J Surg Res 1980; 29:184-88.
15. Bone GE, Pomajzl MJ. Prospective comparison of polytetrafluoroethylene and bovine grafts for hemodialysis. J Surg Res 1980; 29:223-27.
16. Jenkins AM, Buist TAS, Glover SD. Medium-term follow-up of forty autogenous vein and forty polytetrafluoroethylene (Goretex) grafts for vascular access. Surg 1980; 88:667-72.
17. Haimov M, Burrows L, Baez A, et al. Experience with arterial substitutes in the construction of vascular access for hemodialysis. J Cardiovasc Surg 1980; 21:149-54.
18. Mattson WJ. Recognition and treatment of vascular steal secondary to hemodialysis prosthesis. Am J Surg 1987; 154:198-201.
19. Khalil IM, Livingston DH. The management of steal syndrome occurring after access for dialysis. J Vasc Surg 1980; 7:572-73.
20. Shanzer H, Schwartz M, Harrington E, et al. Treatment of ischemia due to "steal" by arteriovenous fistula with distal artery ligation and revascularization. J Vasc Surg 1988; 7:770-73.
21. Rosental JJ, Bell DD, Gasper MR, Movius HJ, Lemire CG. Prevention of high flow problems of arteriovenous grafts. Am J Surg 1980; 140:231-33.
22. Fillinger MF, Resetarits DE, Brendenberg CE. Graft geometry and venous intimal medial hyperplasia in arteriovenous loop grafts. J Vasc Surg 1990; 556-66.

16

GRAFT CURETTAGE

*John W. Puckett, M.D., F.A.C.S., and
Stephen F. Lindsay, M.D., F.A.C.S.*

DIALYSIS PATIENTS WHO CANNOT HAVE autogenous vein fistulas depend on functioning polytetrafluoroethylene (PTFE) dialysis grafts for ongoing life support. Maintenance of the patency of these grafts by durable and reliable salvage operations is of critical importance.

It is universally accepted that during PTFE dialysis graft salvage procedures, venous outflow stenosis due to intimal hyperplasia must be investigated, and if present, corrected. Arterial stenosis is an uncommon cause of graft failure.[1] At times, rethrombosis of dialysis grafts seems to occur without a definable anatomic cause.[2] It has been suggested that midgraft stenosis might account for premature rethrombosis of carefully salvaged dialysis grafts, but this has not been generally emphasized.[3]

It is our contention that midgraft stenosis secondary to fibrous tissue ingrowth, particularly in the areas of needle puncture sites, is a clinically important cause of dialysis graft thrombosis and premature failure after salvage attempts. Several years ago, cases of premature rethrombosis after thorough salvage procedures stimulated our interest in this area. These grafts exhibited both rough withdrawal of the Fogarty catheter during thrombectomy and angiographic evidence of midgraft fibrous tissue buildup (figure 16-1). At that time, a Kevorkian-Younge endometrial biopsy curette was used as a means of removing the fibrous tissue buildup in the midgraft, with favorable results. This readily available instrument has a rectangularly shaped back-cutting tip ideal for thorough, safe curettage of the PTFE graft lumen (figure 16-2). Routine use of the Kevorkian-Younge curette was adopted to definitively clean out

---

The authors would like to thank William E. Barlow, Ph.D., for statistical assistance and Carey Ware for assistance with manuscript preparation.

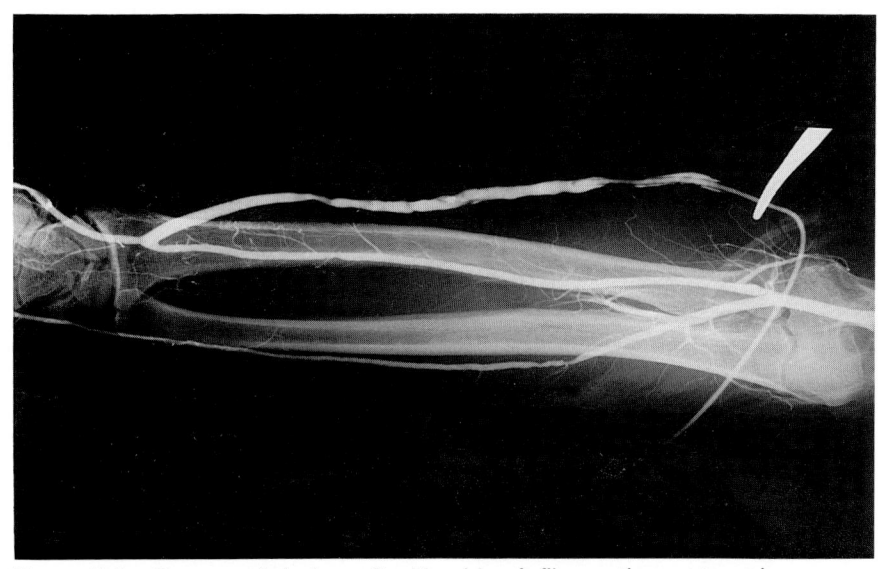

Figure 16-1. Forearm dialysis graft with midgraft fibrous tissue stenosis.

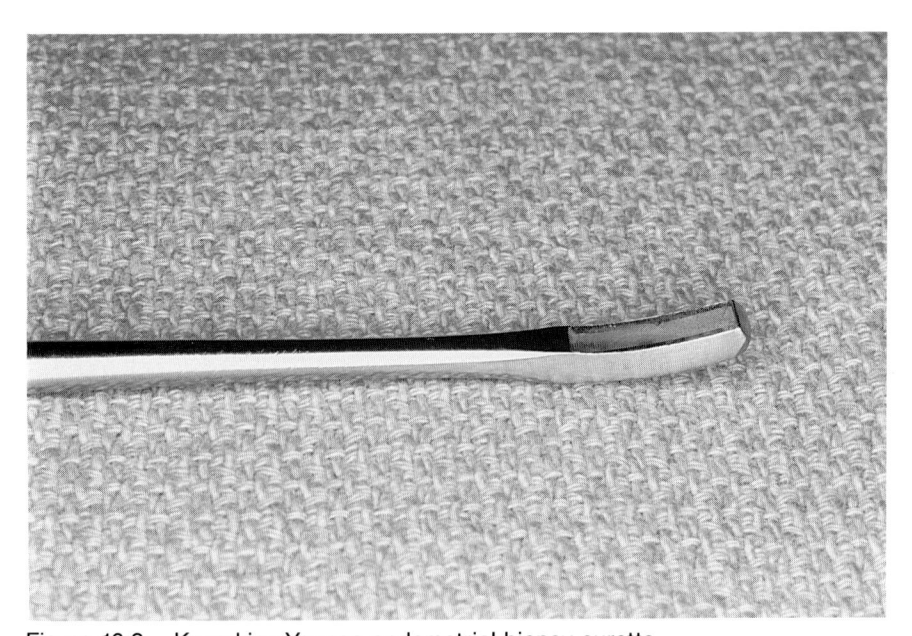

Figure 16-2. Kevorkian-Younge endometrial biopsy curette.

the entire length of the PTFE graft during salvage procedures. Following is a description of our simple midgraft curettage technique. In addition, the overall patency data of our PTFE grafts and specific results regarding the use of midgraft curettage techniques are detailed.

Patients and Methods

A retrospective review using office, hospital, and dialysis unit records was conducted for upper extremity PTFE dialysis graft procedures performed in our practice from January 1980 through December 1987. The patients were managed in four community hospitals in southern Orange County, California. A total of 127 grafts were placed in 118 patients. The 58 men and 60 women in the patient group had a mean age of 67 years (range: 25–91 years). The underlying renal abnormalities consisted of diabetes mellitus (21%), nephrosclerosis (50%), glomerulonephritis (10%), polycystic renal disease (7%), renovascular hypertension (5%), multiple myeloma, systemic lupus, analgesia overuse (2% each), and amyloid (1%). Primary and secondary patency rates of the grafts were expressed using life table analysis.[4] Primary patency was defined as patency during the period from installation of the graft to first thrombosis. Secondary patency was defined as patency during the period from installation to ultimate abandonment of the graft for a new access site. A total of 129 salvage operations were performed on 68 grafts in 64 patients, for a mean requirement of 1.9 salvage operations per graft. The mean follow-up period was 23.2 months (range: 1–94 months). During the follow-up period, six patients underwent renal transplantation, and 65 patients died.

The major goal of the report was to evaluate the effect of the Kevorkian-Younge curette on the patency rate of salvage operations. To do this, a nonrandomized historic control comparison of first salvage patency was carried out between the noncurettage patients treated 1980–82 and the curettage patients treated 1982–87. The comparability of the two groups for age and sex was made using chi-square analysis; no statistically significant differences emerged. In order to focus on anatomic flow disturbances leading to thrombosis, other factors precipitating graft revision led to exclusion of that particular patient. Therefore, graft thromboses due to chronic hypotension, defined hypercoagulable states, as well as graft revisions for infection, nonthrombosed stenosis, and pseudoaneurysm were excluded. Chronic hypotension was defined as systolic pressure below 100 mm Hg between dialysis runs. Of the remaining 52 grafts that underwent at least one salvage repair for thrombosis, 35 were treated with the Kevorkian-Younge curette and 17 were not. The patency rates of the curettage and noncurettage first salvage operations were analyzed using life table analysis. Comparison of the two curves was performed using Wilcoxon analysis.

All grafts placed were 4-7 mm Tapered GORE-TEX (W.L. Gore & Associates, Inc., Flagstaff, AZ).[5] Choice of the location in the upper extremity for the graft was based on quality of pulses, Allen test results, and presence of a usable antecubital vein. An attempt was made to stay as distal as possible in the upper extremity for graft placement in order to conserve graft sites. Of 127 grafts, 67 were straight forearm grafts between the distal radial artery and the antecubital vein, 17 were forearm loop grafts between the proximal radial artery and the antecubital vein, and 43 were arm grafts between the brachial artery and the axillary vein.

Graft placement was performed under either local or regional anesthesia. Prophylactic antibiotics used included cefazolin or a single dose of vancomy-

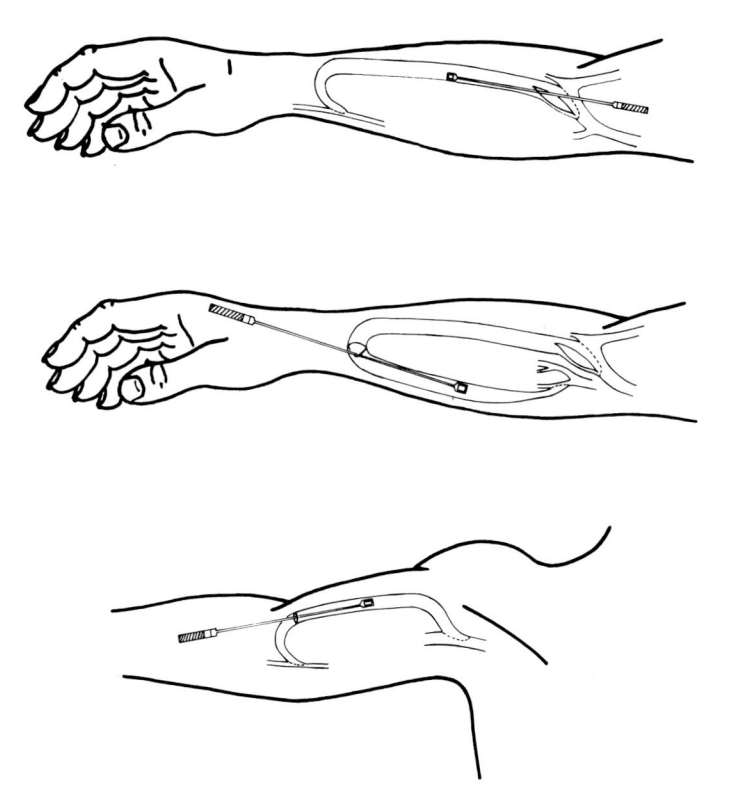

Figure 16-3 Technique of curettage using appropriate placed graftotomy. *(Top)* In the forearm straight graft, the curette is passed from the venous end graftotomy. *(Middle)* In order to curette both limbs of the forearm loop graft, an apical graftotomy is used. *(Bottom)* Because of the proximity of the chest wall, it is not possible to pass the rigid curette downward from the axillary vein end graftotomy in an arm graft. An additional graftotomy adjacent to the arterial end is used.

cin. Forearm straight and arm grafts were looped distally at the arterial anastomosis to allow gentle curving of the graft to the lateral aspect of the upper extremity. By having the graft curve into the artery in this way, retrograde passage of the balloon embolectomy catheter during thrombectomy was directed proximally in the artery, and an increased length of graft was obtained for needle placement. Hegar dilators were used to form the graft tunnels. Heparin (5,000 U) was used for anticoagulation, and anastomoses were sewn with 6-0 Prolene. Skin incisions were closed with interrupted subcutaneous and running subcuticular absorbable suture.

Graft salvage in a patient with normal blood pressure was approached with the expectation of finding an anatomic cause of graft thrombosis. Under local anesthesia, the venous end of the graft was dissected out, controlling the proximal and distal venous branches with small vessel loops. Systemic anticoagulation with heparin was used. A longitudinal (rather than transverse) graftotomy in the venous anastomotic hood was performed to visualize venous end intimal hyperplasia and to facilitate placement of a longitudinal patch angioplasty (if used). The venous end was opened and evaluated. After the thrombus was removed, the finding of spontaneous venous back-bleeding was a favorable sign. A thrombosed vein was bypassed to a more proximal patent level by adding a new PTFE graft segment. Attempts at thrombectomizing an extensively thrombosed vein were not made in the belief that the vein had intimal damage and would not remain patent if used. Thrombectomy of the graft itself was performed with a No. 4 balloon embolectomy catheter. Two centimeters of thrombus was intentionally left in the arterial end to avoid the need for establishing separate arterial control at this stage of the operation.

Next, the Kevorkian-Younge endometrial biopsy curette was used to thoroughly clean the midgraft segment. In the case of the forearm straight graft, the curette was passed directly from the venous graftotomy. With the forearm loop graft, a separate apical graftotomy was made to allow access to both limbs of the loop. For arm graft curettage, a separate graftotomy adjacent to the arterial end was needed to pass the curette proximally in the graft (figure 16-3). The rigid curette could not be used from the axillary venous graftotomy down the arm because of the proximity of the chest wall. By curetting the full length of the graft, it was possible to routinely evaluate the degree of fibrous tissue buildup in the graft and routinely clean the entire graft. The curettage technique involved passing the curette into the graft and then drawing it back with moderate outwardly directed force to engage the cutting tip to remove the fibrous lining of the graft. Passes were made in serial radial manner to curette all aspects of the graft. Curettage fragments were intermittently removed during the procedure, using the Fogarty catheter and a heparinized saline flush through a pediatric feeding tube. Care was taken to leave the arterial plug in place to avoid bleeding and embolization into the artery.

After thorough curettage, the arterial end was completely thrombectomized with additional passes of the balloon embolectomy catheter. It was thought necessary to retrieve a meniscus-shaped thrombus fragment to confirm complete arterial thrombectomy. If doubt arose as to the quality of arterial input or completeness of the arterial thrombectomy, a retrograde angiogram was obtained. Occasionally, direct exploration of the arterial end was needed. Venous end closure or revision with a patch or segment was completed, and flow in the graft was reinstituted. Flow was evaluated by the presence of a thrill in the graft and by palpating the graft with and without venous end occlusion. If venous outflow was adequate, the graft had minimal pulsation with the venous end open. If arterial inflow was adequate, the graft was noted to distend instantly upon gentle venous end occlusion with vascular forceps. Skin incisions were closed carefully with interrupted subcutaneous and running subcuticular absorbable sutures in order to avoid graft exposure and infection.

Results

The overall primary and secondary patency rates of the 127 grafts followed are summarized in figure 16-4. The one-year primary patency rate was 64%, whereas the one-year secondary patency rate was 95%. The outcome of the original 127 grafts included three infections and two pseudoaneurysms. Four

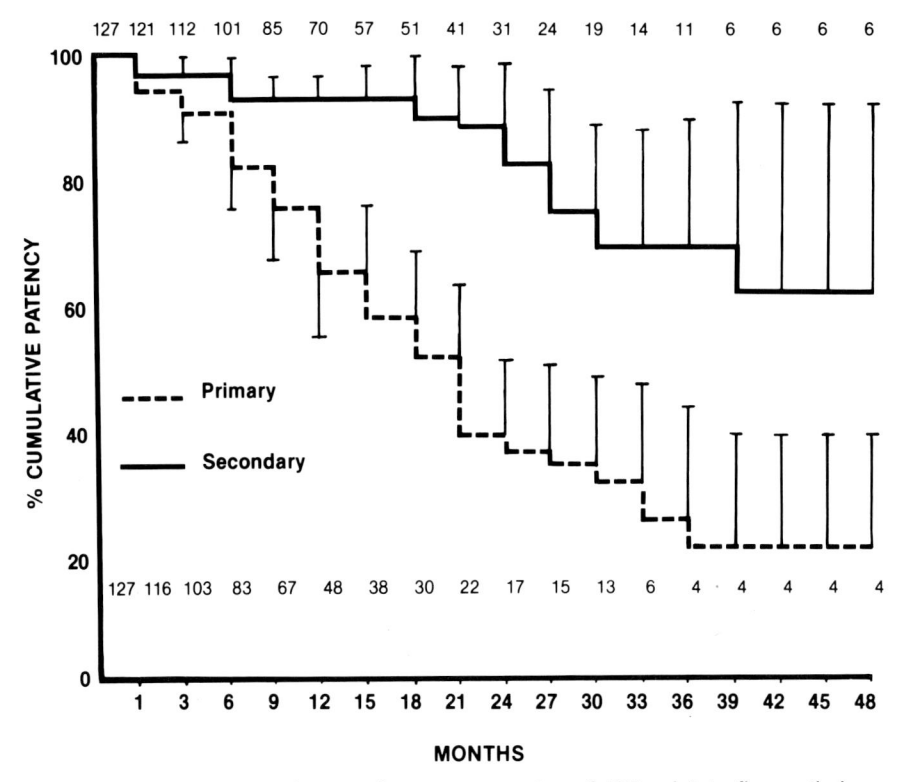

Figure 16-4. Primary and secondary patency rates of 127 polytetrafluoroethylene upper extremity dialysis grafts.

of the original grafts were not thrombosed, but required revision for venous outflow stenosis. Significant chronic hypotension associated with recurrent dialysis graft thrombosis developed in four patients, all of whom died within six months due to end-stage cardiac failure. Recurrent thrombosis of a graft occurred in one patient with an antithrombin III deficiency and in one patient with systemic lupus erythematosus with an increased anticardiolipin antibody titer.

Because the Kevorkian-Younge curette was helpful in evaluating the midgraft, it was possible to determine the primary cause of graft thrombosis in 35 patients who underwent curettage during salvage surgery. Venous end intimal hyperplasia was the primary cause of thrombosis in 18 grafts (51%), whereas significant midgraft fibrous tissue buildup was the most significant finding in eight grafts (23%). Additional causes of thrombosis were arterial end stenosis in three grafts (9%), temporary hypotension in two grafts (6%), and no documented cause of thrombosis in four grafts (11%).

Of the 35 grafts treated with curettage, two patients had significant midgraft bleeding during the surgery. One of these required direct suturing of the graft, and the other required replacement of the midgraft segment. Curettage was particularly difficult due to calcification in two patients with secondary hyperparathyroidism. In these patients, adequate curettage could not be performed, and segmental graft revision was required.

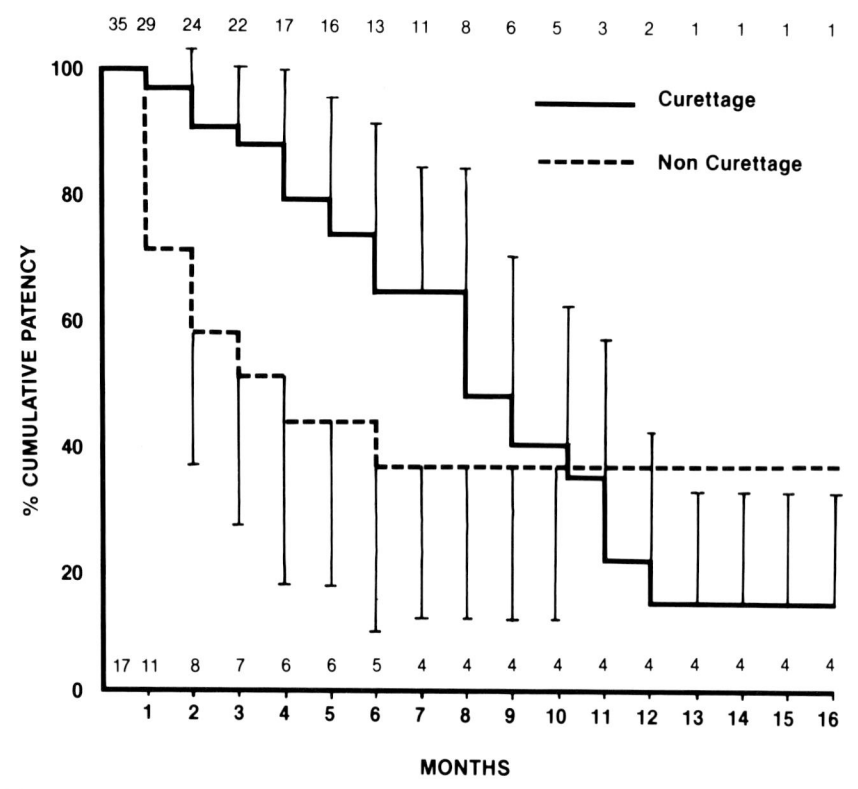

Figure 16-5. Patency rates of first salvage operations for thrombosis comparing 17 procedures without curettage with 35 procedures using curettage.

Microscopic examination showed the midgraft process to be a stratified organizing thrombus. The deep layers adjacent to the graft wall were well organized with fibroblasts and formed collagen matrix, with a gradual transition to fresh thrombus adjacent to the flowing blood. Nutrient vessels were observed in the deep layers inside the graft. These vessels appeared to enter the graft via the needle puncture sites. Microscopic examination also demonstrated evidence of mild chronic foreign body reaction with the finding of giant cells.

Figure 16-5 illustrates the results of the first graft revision patencies for graft thrombosis, contrasting the noncurettage group with the curettage group. Wilcoxon analysis showed that the difference in the curves was marginally statistically significant (p 0.053). The effect was most dramatic in the first six months, with apparent crossing of the two curves at 10 months. Statistical significance could not be demonstrated with the log-rank test.[17] Wilcoxon analysis is more powerful for detecting significant difference early in a study period and in the case of nondiverging curves, as seen here.[18] Technically, neither method is optimal for comparing crossing functions.

Comments

Most investigators reporting patency data for PTFE dialysis grafts have reported one-year secondary patency rates of 62-90%.[2,6-11] In addition, a primary patency rate of 77% at one year has been reported.[5,6] Our PTFE graft patency data are comparable to those in the literature.

The most common postoperative complication of dialysis grafts is thrombosis.[12] Early thrombosis after placement of a new graft is usually a technical problem stemming from an inadequate artery or vein, an anastomotic imperfection, graft kinking, or a perigraft hematoma causing localized graft compression. The major cause of late graft thrombosis is stenosis, usually involving the venous end. Skipped venous narrowings well above the venous anastomotic site may be detected.[12] Ideally, successful salvage procedures depend on accurate identification and definitive repair of all underlying stenotic problems. Late thrombosis is occasionally caused by hypotension or hypercoagulability.[10]

Inability to identify a specific cause of PTFE dialysis graft thrombosis followed by premature rethrombosis is a well-known occurrence.[3,13] Palder et al. reported that recurrent thrombosis accounted for 56% of all PTFE graft thromboses and that rethrombosis occurred at a mean of nine days after initial thrombosis.[2] In a normotensive patient with a thrombosed PTFE dialysis graft, it should be possible to identify a specific anatomic cause of the thrombosis. Midgraft stenosis secondary to fibrous tissue ingrowth is a cause of late thrombosis, which may go unrecognized during salvage surgery if the subtle snagging of the balloon embolectomy catheter is not appreciated.[3]

We believe that untreated midgraft stenosis accounts for most unexplained premature dialysis graft rethromboses. In the present series, midgraft stenosis was an important cause of thrombosis, accounting for 23% of graft thromboses. Midgraft stenosis has been attributed to the buildup of fibrin at needle puncture sites.[9] The development of a pseudointimal layer is known to occur in PTFE grafts and in bovine carotid heterografts.[10,14]

The use of angiography to examine the midgraft segment has been previously reported.[11,15] The literature is limited regarding techniques of managing the graft stenosis. The balloon embolectomy catheter cannot remove the fibrous midgraft buildup, and instead may raise flaps, ultimately making the midgraft area more thrombogenic and thus explaining instances of immediate graft rethrombosis.[11]

Local exploration with separate graftotomies has been advocated.[3] Segmental graft replacement is a more thorough approach, but has the disadvantage of additional incisions, new tunneling, and the need for temporary access while the midgraft is healing. Dilation using coronary dilators and dilatation balloons has been used for dialysis graft venous stenosis but has no known benefit in midgraft problems.[1,2,16]

Use of the Kevorkian-Younge curette to definitively clean out the full length of a PTFE dialysis graft has not been previously described. Routine use of the curette provides both direct assessment and simultaneous treatment of the midgraft stenosis. Difficulty in passing the curette and removal of large volumes of curetted fragments indicate significant midgraft fibrous buildup. Simply treating every thrombosed graft with curettage eliminates possible errors in judgment as to whether or not midgraft stenosis is significant. Our technique allows immediate use of the dialysis graft after surgery without the need for a temporary subclavian dialysis catheter.

Data comparing the first salvage patency rates in curettage and noncurettage patients revealed a superior patency rate in the curettage group that was marginally statistically significant. The fact that the superiority of the curettage group was demonstrated to be only marginally statistically significant is attributed to the small sample size, particularly in the noncurettage control group of only 17 patients. It is our strong clinical impression that early rethrombosis within one month has been virtually eliminated in normotensive patients by this technique. The 97% one-month patency rate in our curettage group is superior to the results of others. Two other reports without curettage include a one-month salvage patency of 65%,[3] and an 83% immediate patency rate, which decreased to 77% one month postoperatively.[8]

The safety of using the Kevorkian-Younge curette inside a PTFE dialysis graft appears to be quite acceptable. The strength of the incorporated PTFE graft prevents graft disruption. Bleeding due to reopening of previous needle puncture sites was rare. Frank perforation with the Kevorkian-Younge curette occurred once while negotiating a tight curve. Proper placement of the graftotomy is important to allow safe passage of the rigid curette.

We conclude that routine use of the Kevorkian-Younge curette during PTFE dialysis graft salvage for thrombosis eliminates midgraft stenosis as a factor in causing premature postsalvage rethrombosis. Combined with a thorough technique of venous end revision, complete arterial thrombectomy, and angiography, midgraft curettage helps ensure maximum reliability of PTFE dialysis graft salvage.

References

1. Weinbaum F, Riles T. Thrombosis of vascular access grafts and its management. In: Waltzer W, Rappaport F, eds. Angioaccess. Orlando, FL: Grune & Stratton 1984; 119–24.
2. Palder S, Kirkman R, Whittemore A, Hakim R, Lazarus J, Tilney N. Vascular access for hemodialysis. Ann Surg 1985; 202:235–39.
3. Etheredge E, Haid S, Maeser M, Sicard G, Anderson C. Salvage operations for malfunctioning polytetrafluoroethylene hemodialysis access grafts. Surgery 1983; 94:464–70.
4. Rutherford RB, Flanigan DP, Gupta S, et al. Suggested standards for reports dealing with lower extremity ischemia. J Vasc Surg 1986; 4:80–94.
5. Rosental JJ, Bell DD, Gaspar MR, Movius HJ, Lemire CG. Prevention of high flow problems of arteriovenous grafts. Am J Surg 1980; 140:231–33.
6. Sabanayagam P, Schwartz A, Soricelli R, Chinitz J, Lyons P. Experience with one hundred reinforced expanded PTFE grafts for angioaccess in hemodialysis. Trans Am Soc Artif Intern Organs 1980; 26:582–83.
7. Sabanayagam P, Schwartz A, Soricelli R, Lyons P, Chinitz J. A comparative study of 402 bovine heterografts and 225 reinforced expanded PTFE grafts as AVF in the ESRD patient. Trans Am Soc Artif Intern Organs 1980; 26:88–92.

8. Wilson SE. Complications of vascular access procedures. In: Wilson SE, Owen M, eds. Vascular access. Chicago: Year Book Medical, 1980; 185–207.
9. Butler H, Baker L, Johnson JM. Vascular access for chronic dialysis: Polytetrafluoroethylene (PTFE) versus bovine heterograft. Am J Surg 1977; 134:791–93.
10. Tellis VA, Kohlberg W, Bhat D, Driscoll B, Veith F. Expanded polytetrafluoroethylene graft fistula for chronic hemodialysis. Ann Surg 1980; 189:101–05.
11. Munda R, First MR, Alexander JW, et al. Polytetrafluoroethylene graft survival in hemodialysis. JAMA 1983; 249:219–22.
12. Haimov M. Construction of vascular access using vascular substitutes. In: Haimov H, ed. Vascular access: A practical guide. Mt. Kisco, NY: Futura, 1987; 72–85.
13. Steed DL, McAuley CE, Rault R, Webster M. Upper arm graft fistula for hemodialysis. J Vasc Surg 1984; 1:660–63.
14. Bone GE, Pamajzl MJ. Management of dialysis fistula thrombosis. Am J Surg 1979; 138:901–06.
15. Weiner SN. Complications of vascular access devices for hemodialysis. Angiology 1985; 36:275–84.
16. Jenkins AM, Buist TAS, Glover SD. Medium term follow-up of forty autogenous vein and forty polytetrafluoroethylene (Gore-Tex) grafts for vascular access. Surgery 1980; 88:667–72.
17. Peto R, Pike MC, Armitage P, et al. Design and analysis of randomized trials requiring prolonged observations of each patient. II. Analysis and examples. BR J Cancer 1977; 35:1–39.
18. Lawless JF. Statistical models and methods for lifetime data. New York: John Wiley, 1982; 425–27.

PANEL DISCUSSION

Moderator:
   Ronald M. Ferguson, M.D., Ph.D.
Panelists:
   Leonard Hines, M.D.
   Mark Pescovitz, M.D.
   John Puckett, M.D.

Discussant: Dr. Puckett, this concerns the timing of your surgery. If you get a graft that clots off on Saturday, do you feel comfortable waiting until Monday to take the patient to surgery? Do you feel that using the curettage technique obviates the need for angioscopy, since you are getting out everything?

Dr. Puckett: In terms of the timing, I don't think graft thrombectomy and salvage is necessarily an emergency operation. We try to do it as soon as reasonably possible, and I wait overnight on most instances if we hear about a graft thrombosis late in the day. I try to avoid taking action for several days; however, I don't have any real data to support this approach. I have seen instances in which I worry that the thrombosis propagates up the venous outflow. I have had no experience using angioscopy. It is an interesting adjunct to use of curettage, but it would not necessarily eliminate the value of endoscopy.

Discussant: Dr. Pescovitz, you had several illustrations showing that you had a looped forearm graft that extended up above the elbow up to even midarm. Do you do this very often?

Dr. Pescovitz: Our standard graft is actually one that plugs into the basilic vein. We always make a sigmoid incision that extends up the medial arm and routinely find the basilic vein just above the elbow. If that thromboses, then the advantage is that we can slowly walk up the basilic vein all the way to the axilla. We do not use ringed grafts in that instance.

Discussant: I was interested to see that the first two speakers put their loop grafts in the opposite configuration. I think it is important to get some sort of standardization of this and have either the artery medial or the artery lateral, because the dialysis units all over the country need to know which way to stick the grafts.

Dr. Hines: I don't know whether there was a mistake on the slide or not, but our artery is always medial, and the venous limb is always lateral.

Dr. Puckett: I agree, and that's the way I do it. I thought everybody did it that way until I saw that the first speaker did it the other way.

Dr. Pescovitz: The venous limb is always medial and the arterial limb is always lateral. Most of the patients we dialyze are dialyzed in our center and they are there from then on. I guess there are going to be patients who are going to travel to another institution where it might be reversed, but identifying the direction of flow is not difficult.

Discussant: Could we poll the room on that to see what the percentage is? I have the feeling that you are in the minority.

Moderator: We would be delighted to poll the room. Exactly what would you like polled? Why don't we say that we have a Memphis technique and an Indiana technique (Drs. Hines and Pescovitz)? How many do it like they do it in Memphis, where the artery is on the medial limb? Looks like about 40%. How many do it the other way? Looks like about 5%. How many do it both ways? About 30%. I guess your point is well taken. There isn't uniformity, but whether it is a problem, I don't know.

Discussant: Dr. Hines, I was wondering if you had any specific protocol as to how long you made the 4 mm part of the tapered grafts?

Dr. Hines: We end up cutting off a little bit of the 4 mm end. We haven't noticed any problems that we have had that are related to doing that.

Discussant: Dr. Pescovitz, you seem to have a lot of interposition revisions versus angioplasty. What are your indications for using one or the other? Do you have any experience with dilation of subclavian vein stenosis by angioplasty? Dr. Puckett, I noticed on your slides that the radial artery anastomosis is put in backward. I assume that that is a correct picture and it directs that Fogarty catheter upward. I thought you might want to comment on that. Finally, I would like the panel to tell us if they do any preoperative evaluation other than a clinical exam on these dialysis patients for primary graft placement.

Dr. Pescovitz: We have limited experience through our radiologists of dilation and endovascular stenting for central venous stenoses. My feeling is that it's not as effective as we'd like it to be. We generally do a lot of interposition grafts. The first thing we do is open up over the venous end, because that is usually where the problem is. If that is not the problem, we do an arteriogram on the table. If this is a midgraft stenosis, it is almost entirely due to multiple cannulation injury. In those instances, we simply excise that whole segment, usually either the venous or arterial limb. Because we use a loop configuration, the other half of the graft, either the arterial or the venous limb, is usable for immediate dialysis access until the new limb has had a chance to heal.

Dr. Puckett: We put our grafts in kind of backward at the arterial end, increasing the "shore line" so to speak, in order to attain a greater length of usable graft in either the forearm or upper arm position. The reason I like that technique, particularly for patients with small brachial arteries, is that I may want to use the full length of the 4 mm graft in order to get maximum flow attenuation. So using a lazy loop and positioning it in a convex arrangement allows the 4 mm and tapered portions to occupy that loop position. By the time you get into prime upper-arm position, you've got a 7 mm graft that the nurses can find and use.

Moderator: The third question related to evaluation of the hand prior to placing an access.

Dr. Puckett: I measure the blood pressure in both arms, talk to the patient about handedness, and look at the veins in the forearm to evaluate those ahead of time with a blood pressure cuff. I have not been using routine duplex scanning or more sophisticated Doppler analysis. If there are obvious pulse deficits, then I would have the patient go to the vascular lab and have finger pressures measured.

Dr. Pescovitz: In a primary A-V conduit when no one has operated on that arm before, we don't do anything to evaluate the venous outflow. As for the arterial flow, it is obviously a concern in diabetic patients. We have tried such things as arteriography, distal blood pressures, and Allen's tests, but we don't seem to be able to predict very well which patients are going to develop problems. We try to keep the patients well informed and keep a very close eye on them postoperatively for early signs of steal.

Dr. Hines: We don't do anything more in a routine case than what I mentioned in my talk. Clinical assessment is really as good as anything else, as far as duplex scanning is concerned. If the veins are not good where we are looking, we just dissect or crawl up the extremity in order to try to find a usable vein.

Discussant: Dr. Pescovitz, you listed decreased radial pulses as an indication for A-V conduits. What would your primary access site be for a 65-year-old diabetic with no palpable radial pulses and coronary disease and who is not a candidate for peritoneal dialysis?

Dr. Pescovitz: Generally, we would try to do an A-V conduit in the forearm, a loop A-V conduit. Obviously, in such a patient we would need to be concerned about steal.

Moderator: I would like to poll the audience. Dr. Hines, I believe you said there was a 1.8% incidence of steal in your series with a 4–7 mm tapered graft. How many here believe that using a 4–7 mm tapered graft decreases steal? How many believe it does not? Looks like it is split right in half. It looks like it is a matter of faith.

Discussant: I always draw a diagram after every case indicating whether the outflow vein is medial or lateral. One copy goes on the chart that goes to dialysis, one is for the inpatient chart, and one goes to the doctors. It is pasted right on the chart so that everyone knows which direction the flow is and can stick the vein accordingly.

Moderator: One more poll. How many in the audience use a curette technique of one kind or another? How many do not? About a third do and two thirds do not.

Discussant: I would like to make a comment about the loop configuration. Even if you don't have a drawing, all you need to do to see which end has arterial flow is to compress the graft. It's the simplest thing to do. I am one of the people who don't believe a 4–7 mm graft really decreases steal any more than the size of the anastomosis, the distal outflow, or the collateral circulation. Are there any prospective trials comparing the two?

Dr. Hines: I am not aware of any.

Discussant: Referring to Dr. Puckett's paper, we've routinely used the loop graft in the forearm and declot from the apex of the graft. We usually do routine angiography, and I have been impressed that the venous limb of the loop graft often will have narrowed areas, but the arterial limb almost never does. In view of the change from regular dialysis to high-flux dialysis, do you think we are going to see an increased incidence? I always assumed it was the return of blood to the venous limb and the turbulence that caused these injuries.

Dr. Puckett: I don't know the answer to that.

Discussant: I would like to ask Dr. Hines about those five patients who developed steal despite using the 4-7 mm graft. We have also seen that despite routine use of that graft, some patients with very small brachial arteries will still develop steal. Over the past year or so, we implanted 3-6 mm grafts made by Impra into four patients. We first did it with trepidation, thinking that there was no way a 3 mm graft would stay open, but none of them have clotted yet. The first one was put in about a year ago. So I would like to ask Dr. Hines what he did for those five patients with steal.

Dr. Hines: Those occurred over a period of a couple of years. In the patients who manifested significant symptoms, we simply removed the graft. I fear that trying to salvage the graft with banding will either not solve the ischemic problem or will cause thrombosis. However, your experience with a 3 mm graft may give us some encouragement in that respect.

Discussant: In terms of placement of the initial graft, my preference is always a loop in the forearm. If there is no visible superficial vein, I usually go to the upper arm. Should we first go to the deep veins of the forearm and then, if that is not suitable, make another incision in the upper arm?

Dr. Puckett: I prefer going to the forearm first. If I feel that I can examine the vein relatively effectively, and if the vein is not very good, I move directly to the upper arm. If the patient is obese, and the vein is difficult to evaluate, then I think one is obligated to make an antecubital incision and check the veins.

Dr. Pescovitz: As I mentioned, we nearly always make an antecubital incision that extends up a slight distance along the medial arm. If we see a large antecubital vein when we make a transverse incision, we plug into it. By and large, we go directly to the basilic vein just above the elbow, unless that arm has been used before.

Dr. Hines: We have tried to use the deep veins in the forearm, but those have not worked well at all. If you happen to get one to work for a while, you have your hands full when you have to thrombectomize or revise, so our tendency has been similar to the others.

Discussant: It seems that we are missing one important point. Instead of wasting time exploring the veins, why not do a venogram? It takes about a minute and a half to do a venogram on the table. After gaining access on the back of the hand and injecting a little dye, you can see exactly where the veins are and which ones are usable. It seems that we have been a little cavalier over the years about evaluating patients for access and treating them. At our lab, we fully evaluate them with duplex scanning, not only arterial but also venous. Within a couple of hours after the surgery, we also evaluate the arterial tree to see what kind of drop in pressure has occurred.

Discussant: That is not an efficient use of resources in our hands. We have found that a good physical exam and intraoperative exploration work the best.

Discussant: Does anyone use or construct antecubital A-V fistulas?

Dr. Puckett: I do it in selected cases. One thing I have found in using upper-arm fistulas is that the break-in period is more troublesome. The nurses have more trouble cannulating the vein, which seems to be thinner and produces more bleeding and more hematomas, so it is a little bit more stressful.

Discussant: If antecubital or upper-arm veins are used, I think it is important to ligate deep branches to encourage superficial flow into the cephalic system, thereby making cannulation easier.

Discussant: How do you treat recurrent seromas?

Dr. Puckett: One has to be aware that PTFE will form seromas. Some segments of PTFE will weep fluids, and if you simply drain that area, you will be faced with a recurrence. The segment that is weeping must be replaced. You can sometimes actually see the weeping of fluid through the pores of the PTFE at the time of surgery.

Discussant: It has not been my experience that one must ligate infected segments of PTFE and come back weeks later. I have been very successful putting interposition grafts around these areas immediately. I don't think you have to wait that long.

Dr. Pescovitz: Our group is perhaps a bit conservative. I am aware of the reports that describe what you have done, which is an immediate reconstruction of the graft. We have not tried that yet, but certainly the results are good. The advantage is that you can dialyze these patients immediately rather than find some sort of temporary dialysis.

Moderator: The key is to utilize an uninfected area to put a new tunnel for your new graft material.

Discussant: Dr. Pescovitz, at what size pseudoaneurysm do you decide to intervene, either at the anastomosis or at some point along the graft?

Dr. Pescovitz: I suppose the size would be somewhere around a centimeter. My experience is that if a pseudoaneurysm is forming somewhere on the graft, more than one area is involved. It usually is a sign that the graft is becoming worn out. The remedy is segmental repair over a fair length of that graft. Usually, once this is done the rest of the graft is fine. It may be a sign of deeper problems that require major revisions. When the nurses are having problems cannulating the graft, I use this as an indication for doing a definitive revision.

Discussant: If you have a single aneurysm, then we recommend rotation to another area. If the aneurysm is getting bigger, and if it looks as if the skin is thinning or is bleeding, we would excise it.

Dr. Puckett: An anastomotic aneurysm is different; I would repair it the minute I know it's there.

17

ENDOVASCULAR SALVAGE OF FAILING PTFE GRAFTS

Michael J. Verta Jr., M.D.

SINCE ITS USE AS A CONDUIT FOR VASCULAR ACCESS was first proposed in 1976, expanded polytetrafluoroethylene (ePTFE) has quickly become the most commonly used material.[1] Its popularity is understandable, for it is available in a wide variety of sizes and configurations, is easy to handle, does not need to be preclotted, and has good patency rates. Two-year and three-year patency rates of 60-70% have been reported, and are far superior to those for bovine heterografts.[2-5] However, thrombosis of PTFE grafts is a relatively common event, being reported in up to 55% of patients.[2-4,6] Although simple thrombectomy can restore immediate patency in up to 90% of cases, sustained patency is achieved in fewer than one-half.[4,7] Most patients with PTFE grafts will suffer repeated episodes of thrombosis and require multiple revisions to maintain long-term function.[4,7,8]

Causes of Graft Failure

The most common single cause of graft thrombosis in the literature is stenosis at the venous outflow anastomosis due to pseudointimal hyperplasia.[4,7,8] However, in a report by Etheredge et al., causes other than venous anastomotic stenosis accounted for nearly three out of four failures.[7] Intragraft accumulations of pseudointima, probably in response to repeated needle-puncture trauma (so-called "one-site-itis"), have been reported in several series.[7,9,10] They may help to explain not only the failure to achieve long-term patency after simple thrombectomy, but also cases of "persistent venous hypertension."

Management of Graft Failure

Although thrombectomy and direct surgical revision has long been the accepted means of restoring function to the failing access graft, the success of intraluminal methods for restoring patency in stenotic arteries has provoked a reexamination of treatment strategies in the failing PTFE access graft.

Venous stenosis is by far the most commonly reported cause of access graft failure. Because this lesion anatomically resembles segmental arterial stenosis, balloon angioplasty has been advocated for its treatment. The reported results, however, are quite variable, in most cases not approaching those achieved by surgical revision.[7-9,11-14] Furthermore, it has been pointed out by Brooks and associates[11] and by Tortolani and his group[8] that PTFE is not distensible and that hyperplastic pseudointima compresses poorly if at all. Thus, other techniques that rely on actual removal of obstructing material have drawn considerable interest. Chief among these methods is the Simpson Atherocath (Devices for Vascular Intervention, Redwood City, CA), a device shown to be effective in removing both atheroma and hyperplastic neointima in human arteries.[15] Both Zemel et al. and Gaylord have reported results in failing PTFE grafts that are clearly superior to those of balloon angioplasty and approach those of direct surgical revision.[10,16]

Directional Atherectomy

Device Description

The Simpson peripheral atherectomy catheter is a semiflexible catheter whose distal housing unit contains a cutter, retrieval chamber, and opposing balloon. A short floppy guidewire is attached to the tip to allow the operator to advance the unit through the residual lumen. Inflation of the opposing balloon causes the longitudinal side opening of the cutting chamber to engage the area to be treated. A cylindrical cutting blade driven by a battery-powered motor drive in the handpiece then slices off strips of atheroma or neointima. The removed material is pushed into the storage chamber in the distal tip. The cutting blade spins at about 2,000 rpm. The catheters are available in sizes 6 through 11 French, for vessel diameters of 4 through 10 mm, respectively.

Indications and Limitations

The optimal lesion for Simpson directional atherectomy is a short, discrete, eccentrically placed lesion. Stenotic lesions are more suitable than total occlusions, and concentric lesions also can be successfully treated. Pseudointimal hyperplasia is quite easy to remove with the Simpson catheter, but heavily calcified lesions can sometimes be rather difficult to clear. The directional capability of the Simpson catheter makes it possible to remove only hyperplastic pseudointima in stenotic anastomoses without damaging healthy neointima in the graft.

The major limitation of the Simpson catheter lies in the fact that it is somewhat stiff and bulky and is therefore difficult to use in tortuous or acutely angled vessels. Furthermore, large lesions can require a long time to clear completely because only small strips of material are removed with each passage of the blade.

Technique

When the Simpson catheter is used in PTFE access grafts, the usual arterial technique is slightly modified. All endovascular graft reconstructions are done under local anesthesia with fluoroscopic control. Loop grafts are usually entered at the nadir of the loop, and straight grafts are entered at midbody. Open Fogarty catheter thrombectomy is done at the outset of every procedure. Fluoroangiography after thrombectomy is used to assess the presence of anastomotic stenoses, as well as intragraft accumulations of hyperplastic pseudointima. After systemic heparinization, a Simpson Atherocath of appropriate size (usually No. 9 Fr) is then inserted into the graft and guided fluoroscopically to the area to be treated. All pseudointima is carefully removed until fluoroangiography shows a smooth lumen of normal caliber. The process is repeated as necessary until the entire graft, including both anastomoses, is clean. Noncontiguous stenoses of the inflow artery or outflow vein can be treated similarly or dilated with a balloon of appropriate diameter. Completion fluoroangiography then documents the desired result, and the graft arteriotomy and skin incisions are closed as usual. Patients are not anticoagulated postoperatively and are usually discharged the same day. Hemodialysis on the day of procedure is permitted.

Clinical Application

We examined 22 patients in our practice with repeated PTFE graft failures. As shown in table 17-1, the grafts had been in place for an average of nearly three years and had undergone three to four previous thrombectomies prior to endovascular reconstruction. Of interest is that thrombectomy alone was able to maintain graft patency for less than four months on average before failure recurred. In our series, intragraft stenosis due to pseudointimal deposits was by far the most common lesion seen.

Directional atherectomy was done as described in the preceding section. Patients were evaluated weekly after discharge, and any apparent dysfunction was evaluated by the operating surgeon by direct examination, duplex ultrasound, or angiography, as appropriate. Since reocclusion for any reason precludes use of the graft, efforts at graft salvage were considered successful only if no rethrombosis occurred during the follow-up period.

Results

The results of this approach in our patients are shown graphically in figure 17-1. One-month patency was 95.5% and had dropped to 85.4% by the sixth month. One graft developed sustained venous hypertension two weeks after

Table 17-1. Series Summary

Age of graft	All grafts	32.5 mo (range: 11–78 mo)
	Loop grafts	38.7 mo
	Straight grafts	29.6 mo
Time to first thrombosis		10.6 mo (range: 1–46 mo)
Number of thrombectomies		3.7 (range 1–7)
Interval between thrombectomies		3.7 mo (range: 0.5–15 mo)
Length of follow-up		11.8 mo (range: 4–24 mo)
Cause of failure	Intragraft stenosis	18
	Intragraft stenosis + venous stenosis	3
	Intragraft stenosis + arterial stenosis	1

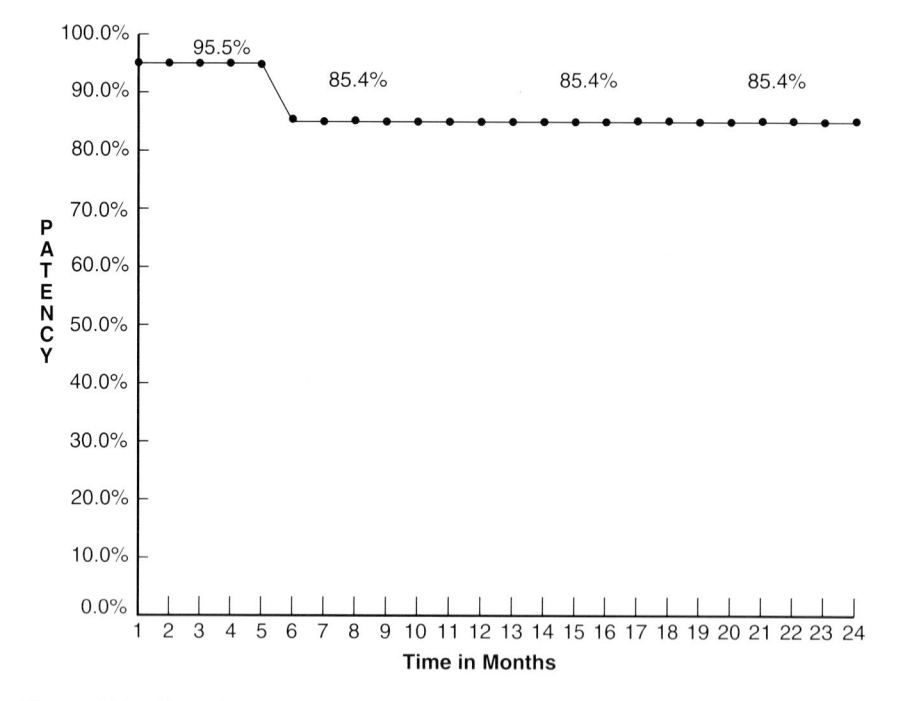

Figure 17-1. Cumulative patency.

atherectomy and failed completely two weeks after that. Reoperation showed a long segment stenosis of the outflow vein beyond the anastomosis. This was corrected by PTFE patch angioplasty of the stenotic segment. Two other grafts failed at six months, and reoperation showed complete obliteration of the outflow vein at a site of previous balloon angioplasty. In both of these cases, extension of the graft to a new outflow site restored function. No other failures occurred during the follow-up period.

Others who have used directional atherectomy for salvage of failing access grafts have reported similar experiences. Zemel et al. reported an 86% patency at six months in their small group of PTFE grafts, although only one graft rethrombosed.[10] Similarly, Gaylord reported an 87.5% patency in 17 patients followed for 60 days or more; only one failure was due to reaccumulation of hyperplastic pseudointima.[16] Gary and Dolmatch reported a 75% patency at five months in their patients with intragraft stenoses due to neointimal fibromuscular hyperplasia.[9] Finally, Brady et al. reported a 60% salvage rate at six months.[17]

Discussion

The volume of literature addressing the problem of maintaining function in arteriovenous access grafts attests to the fact that these difficulties are widespread. More disquieting is the striking similarity in the results of efforts at graft salvage, particularly when percutaneous transluminal angioplasty (PTA) is compared to direct reconstruction. This is rather easily explained when one recalls that hyperplastic neointima is dense, fibrous, and highly noncompressible. Furthermore, PTFE grafts are by design not distensible; therefore, a technique that relies upon intimal compression and vessel distensions is doomed to failure in access grafts.

The experience with directional atherectomy has been somewhat better than that with PTA; this appears to be a result of actual physical removal of hyperplastic neointima and restoration of a normal lumen without vessel wall trauma. One must necessarily be cautious about recommending this technique, inasmuch as there are no long-term studies to document its effectiveness in maintaining long-term patency. Nevertheless, directional atherectomy is simple to perform, requires no anticoagulation, has excellent short-term results, and can be done repeatedly. On this basis, it can and should be employed as a primary treatment method for the acutely failed dialysis access graft.

References

1. Baker LD, Johnson JM, Goldfarb D. Expanded polytetrafluoroethylene (PTFE) subcutaneous arteriovenous conduit: An improved vascular access for chronic hemodialysis. Trans Am Soc Artif Intern Organs 1976; 22:382–87.
2. Butler HG, Baker LD, Johnson JM. Vascular access for chronic hemodialysis: Polytetrafluoroethylene (PTFE) versus bovine heterograft. Am J Surg 1977: 134:791–93.
3. Jenkins AM, Buist TAS, Glover SD. Medium-term follow-up of forty autogenous vein and forty polytetrafluoroethylene (Gore-tex) grafts for vascular access. Surgery 1980; 88:667–72.
4. Palder SB, Kirkman RL, Whittemore AD, Hakim RM, Lazarus JM, Tilney NL. Vascular access for hemodialysis: Patency rates and results of revision. Ann Surg 1985; 202:235–39.
5. Sabanaygam P, Schwartz AB, Soricelli RR, Chinitz JL, Lyons P. Experience with one hundred reinforced expanded PTFE grafts for angioaccess in hemodialysis. Trans Am Soc Artif Intern Organs 1980; 26:582–83.
6. Giacchino JL, Geis WP, Buckingham JM, et al. Vascular access: Long-term results, new techniques. Arch Surg 1979; 114:403–09.
7. Etheredge EE, Haid SD, Maeser MN, Sicard GA, Anderson CB. Salvage operations for malfunctioning polytetrafluoroethylene hemodialysis access grafts. Surgery 1983; 94:464–70.

8. Tortolani EC, Tan AHS, Butchart S. Percutaneous transluminal angioplasty: An ineffective approach to the failing vascular access. Arch Surg 1984; 119:221–23.
9. Gray RJ, Dolmatch BL. Early results of atherectomy treatment for hemodialysis access. Abstr, SCVIR annual mtg, Feb 1991.
10. Zemel G, Katzen BT, Dake MD, Benenati JF, Lempert TE, Moskowitz L. Directional atherectomy in the treatment of stenotic dialysis access failure. JVIR 1990; 1:35–37.
11. Brooks JL, Sigley RD, May KJ Jr., Mack RM. Transluminal angioplasty versus surgical repair for stenosis of hemodialysis grafts. Am J Surg 1987; 153:530–31.
12. Gmelin E, Winterhoff R, Rinast E. Insufficient hemodialysis access fistulas: Late results of treatment with percutaneous balloon angioplasty. Radiology 1989; 171:657–60.
13. Saeed M, Newman GE, McCann RL, Sussman SK, Braun SD, Dunnick NR. Stenoses in dialysis fistulas: Treatment with percutaneous angioplasty. Radiology 1987; 164:693–97.
14. Smith TP, Cragg AH, Castanede F, Hunter DW. Thrombosed polytetrafluoroethylene hemodialysis fistulas: Salvage with combined thrombectomy and angioplasty. Radiology 1989; 171:507–08.
15. Ahn SS. Endovascular surgery. In: Moore WS, ed. Vascular surgery: a comprehensive review. Philadelphia: WB Saunders, 1991.
16. Gaylord GM. Balloon angioplasty (PTA) vs. Simpson atherectomy for treatment of dialysis grafts. Abstr, SCVIR annu mtg, Feb 1991.
17. Brady T, Castaneda F, Bertino R, Smith T, Cragg A. Salvage of failing arteriovenous dialysis fistulas with the Simpson atherectomy catheter. Abstr, SCVIR annual mtg, Feb 1991.

18

THE ROLE OF ENDOVASCULAR STENTS IN HEMODIALYSIS ACCESS

Jeffrey H. Fair, M.D., and Scott O. Trerotola, M.D.

END-STAGE RENAL DISEASE (ESRD) affects about 100 patients per million population, and hemodialysis remains the most common treatment modality.[1] The Brescia-Cimino arteriovenous (A-V) fistula remains the most trouble-free means of establishing long-term hemodialysis access.[2] Numerous reports demonstrate that successful native fistula formation is possible in only 15% of cases. Thus, various configurations of polytetrafluoroethylene (PTFE) A-V fistulas are most frequently used in hemodialysis access. Reported patency rates for PTFE shunts vary greatly in the literature (40–85% at three years), but graft failure precipitated by venous outflow insufficiency is the cause in about 80% of cases.[3,4]

Venous insufficiency in hemodialysis shunts is characterized by progressive neointimal hyperplasia leading to stenosis and thrombosis. The biology of this hyperplasia is unclear and beyond the scope of this article, but mechanical shear stresses and turbulence appear to play a prominent role.[5]

Surgical and percutaneous techniques have been developed to approach access stenosis. Surgical maneuvers include endarterectomy, patch angioplasty, and revision. Revision of the venous outflow on the vein beyond the current structure or to another vein is the most definitive and yields the best results.[6] All surgical approaches carry the inherent risks of vascular reexploration; further, they may "burn bridges," limiting future access placement.

Recent therapeutic percutaneous approaches have developed as logical extensions of diagnostic angiography. Immediate technical success of percutaneous transluminal angioplasty (PTA) of 80–90% has been reported; however, follow-up results reveal only 57% and 24% patency rates at six months and two years, respectively, for stenotic lesions. Occlusive lesions fare even worse, with 14% two-year patency rates.[7]

Because PTA of stenotic lesions in these high-flow venous systems leads to early recurrence and failure, endovascular stenting would appear to be a logical approach. Such a stent must have characteristics of good flexibility and sufficient radial force to expand and/or retain patency after angioplasty. Experimental canine work by Dotter outlined the potential benefits of metallic endovascular stents.[8] Animal studies also show that the stents readily endothelialize.

Experience with endovascular stents in the venous system has been limited to several small clinical series. The Gianturco-Wallace stent (Cook Inc., Bloomington, IL) and the Wallstent (Schneider, Minneapolis, MN) are two stent designs of significantly different configurations that have been used in dialysis access grafts and fistulas. These have been available only on a compassionate need basis. The Gianturco stent consists of relatively coarse stainless steel wire in a zig-zag pattern, whereas the Wallstent is manufactured of much finer stainless steel alloy in a woven pattern. Both are made in different lengths and unconstrained diameters. The Wallstent is more flexible but presents a larger exposed metallic surface area. In one series by Vorwerk et al., Wallstents were used in seven Brescia fistulas and nine PTFE shunts that had failed angioplasty alone, and it was proved that these shunts are useful in extending graft life in refractory cases.[9] Another series recently reported early success in 100% of 25 venous anastomoses of grafts, eight brachiocephalic veins, nine upper limb veins, and six subclavian veins with no complications.[10]

At our institution, we have employed six Wallstents for dialysis shunt problems—two in venous outflow stenoses that were PTA-resistant and four in central venous stenosis. Five out of six are patent after mean follow-up of 10 months. However, three of these have required ancillary procedures such as angioplasty or atherectomy for assisted patency. One upper-arm PTFE graft with a stent in the venous outflow thrombosed at 11 months and was not reopened because of intragraft stenoses, even though the stent was still functional.

Although the experience with endovascular stents in dialysis access so far is small, some observations can be made:

- Stents are effective in increasing the life of grafts with PTA resistant venous stenosis
- The stent does not prevent recurrent neointimal hyperplasia
- Complications related specifically to stent placement are uncommon
- Stent placement does not interfere with future surgical interventions.

Although the stents appear to be an adjunct in the treatment of hemodialysis graft dysfunction, many questions remain unanswered, and the answers are difficult to extract from clinical experiences because of the lack of controlled conditions. This has motivated us to employ a model of PTFE grafts in the canine hindlimb as described by Fillinger.[11] The model allows a standardization of graft size and configuration. Thus, we have begun to study the natural history of different stents and their comparative effects on neointimal hyperplasia.

Our preliminary results consist of 18 of 19 grafts patent in 10 animals. Six grafts were stented with the Gianturco stent and six with Wallstents; as controls, six were not stented. Two of the Gianturco stents developed strut fractures with risk of dislodgement or embolization. One of the Wallstents has migrated moderately from its initial placement position. Data on the rates of incorporation and development of neointimal hyperplasia require further follow-up.

In conclusion, we believe that metallic endovascular stents will be compatible with high-flow venous systems. They should be useful adjuncts for maintaining patency and function of hemodialysis shunts.

References

1. Morris PJ. Kidney transplantation: Principles and practice. 2nd ed. Orlando, FL: Grune & Stratton, 1984.
2. Brescia MJ, Cimino JE, Appel K, et al. Chronic hemodialysis using venipuncture and a surgically created arteriovenous fistula. N Engl J Med 1966; 275:1089–92.
3. Bell DD, Rosenthal JJ. Arteriovenous graft life in chronic hemodialysis. Arch Surg 123: Sept 1988.
4. Rajo S. PTFE grafts for hemodialysis access. Ann Surg 1987; 206:666–72.
5. Sottiura vs. Biogenisis and etiology of distal anastomotic intimal hyperplasia. Int Angiology 1990; 9(2):59–69.
6. Palder SB, Kirkman RL, Whittemore AD, et al. Vascular access for hemodialysis: Patency rates and results of revision. Ann Surg 1985; 202:235–39.
7. Glanz S, Gordon DH, Butt KMH, et al. The role of percutaneous angioplasty in the management of chronic hemodialysis fistulas. Ann Surg 1987; 206(6):777–781.
8. Dotter C. Transluminally-placed coil spring endoarterial tube grafts: long term patency in canine popliteal artery. Invest Radiol 1969; 57:5–10.
9. Vorwerk D, Gunther RW, Bohndorf K, et al. Follow-up results after stent placement in failing arteriovenous shunts: A three-year experience. Cardiovasc Intervent Radiol 1991; 14:285–89.
10. Raynaud HC, et al. Endovascular stents in angio-access for hemodialysis. Abstract. Radiol Soc N Am annu. mtg. 1991.
11. Fillinger MF, Reinitz ER, Schwartz RA, et al. Beneficial effects of banding on venous intimal medial hyplasia in arteriovenous loop grafts. Am J Surg 1989; 158:87–94.

19

THE ROLE OF ANGIOSCOPY IN VASCULAR ACCESS SURGERY

*Arnold Miller, M.B., Ch.B., F.R.C.S., F.R.C.S.C., F.A.C.S.,
Edward J. Marcaccio, M.D., William S. Goodman, M.D., and
Michael N. Gottlieb, M.D.*

ANGIOSCOPY HAS AN IMPORTANT ROLE in vascular surgery performed for revascularization of the lower extremity.[1,4] It is especially useful in the preparation of the venous conduit and detecting unsuspected intraluminal abnormalities such as fresh or organized thrombus, segmental stenosis, or regions of thrombosis and recanalization. In addition, it allows for preparation of the *in situ* and *nonreversed* vein, cutting valves, and identifying unligated tributaries.[5-7] It is also useful as a completion study in monitoring the bypass graft, allowing the detection and immediate correction of technical deficits within the graft, anastomosis, and native vessels that may cause graft failure.[7]

Routine completion angioscopy during infrainguinal bypass grafting has resulted in improved early graft patency. After thrombectomy (for acute occlusions of either the primary artery or graft), angioscopy allows assessment of efficacy of the thrombectomy and provides a means of evaluating the endoluminal pathology so that rational management decisions can be made.[8,9]

In this chapter, we outline the essentials for successful angioscopy for vascular access surgery with regard to the principles of irrigation and angioscopic equipment and technique. Our early experience with the application of routine angioscopy during the establishment of native and synthetic graft hemodialysis fistulas, as well as the management of the failing and occluded fistula, will be discussed. Angioscopic techniques will be illustrated by case descriptions.

Basic Angioscopy Equipment and Technique

Irrigation

Blood is opaque to all light waves. Successful angioscopic examination requires that all blood in the vessel be cleared prior to vessel examination. Even a small volume of blood obscures the image and makes it appear "out of focus." Any blood in the visual field makes meaningful visualization impossible. This is unlike the standard angiogram, where good studies may be obtained when even a small volume of x-ray contrast media mixes with the column of blood. In the clinical situation, saline irrigation is most commonly used to replace the blood in the vessel being examined.

The principles of establishing a clear column of a salt solution in the vessel to be examined, as well as the use of a dedicated irrigation pump, have been previously described in detail.[10] In brief, all antegrade blood flow, from the main vessel and collaterals, must be interrupted. The clear fluid column is established by using a rapid bolus of large volume and high flow rate of saline solution that clears the blood from the region of interest. Once the clear fluid column is established, a lower flow rate maintains the column and prolongs the angioscopic examination. It also minimizes the total volume of fluid necessary for a complete and successful examination. Variable flow rates are preset on the irrigation pump and are controlled by a foot pedal. A monitoring device allows continuous and accurate measurement of the volume of fluid being infused. This has made the use of other fluid delivery systems, such as the venous pressure cuff, obsolete.

In previous studies conducted during angioscopy for infrainguinal bypass grafting, we determined the volume of saline irrigation required for successful and consistent angioscopic examinations,[3,4] whether abnormally high intraluminal pressures were induced in the vein grafts, and whether the irrigation caused any significant injury of the vessel wall that resulted in early graft occlusion. We also looked into whether this necessary saline load increased morbidity and mortality in the high-risk patient group undergoing infrainguinal revascularization procedures.[11]

Our studies showed that if the principles of irrigation for angioscopy were applied and careful technique was used, the volume of fluid necessary for satisfactory angioscopy is usually less than 500 ml per study. This fluid load did not result in any significant hemodynamic changes or increase the mortality or morbidity in our patient group undergoing infrainguinal bypasses. Direct measurement of intraluminal pressures in infrainguinal vein grafts during angioscopy has shown that if the outflow vessel is not obstructed and irrigation is stopped immediately when the visual field has cleared, abnormally high pressures (>300 mm Hg) generated within the vein grafts are rare.

Methods of Antegrade Occlusion

Our standard technique of angioscopy has been described in detail.[12] In the upper extremity, inflow occlusion can be achieved by various means, depending on the circumstances. Direct application of vascular clamps to the exposed inflow vessel is the most efficient technique, but often this is not feasible. Using an occlusion balloon catheter is helpful for control of the unexposed inflow vessel. The only disadvantage with the catheter is that it occupies a portion of the lumen of the vessel, possibly interfering with the thrombectomy or other therapeutic manipulations being performed. Placing a tourniquet around the upper limb preoperatively or even intraoperatively (using a sterile tourniquet) has proven to be a most expeditious and efficient technique. This should be a standard and automated limb tourniquet that allows rapid inflation and deflation with narrow cuffs (2–4 in. wide). Application of an Esmarch's bandage to exsanguinate the extremity is unnecessary. The residual blood is removed from the vessel of interest by irrigation. In our experience, makeshift tourniquets with rubber tubing, such as Penrose drains, have proven unreliable. Their use often occludes only the venous system, resulting in venous congestion and delaying the establishment of an adequate clear saline fluid column.

Instrumentation

Instrumentation for angioscopic examination of vascular access grafts or native fistulas is no different from that used in other areas of vascular surgery. Angioscopes with an outer diameter of 0.5 to 2.8 mm are used. We rarely use angioscopes with built-in irrigation channels. Angioscopes with these channels have the disadvantage of increasing the outer diameter of the angioscope. Also, the irrigating channels are so narrow that the high-volume, high-flow rates necessary for the rapid clearing of the vasculature are inadequate, resulting in the infusion of unnecessarily large volumes of saline.[10] Irrigation is provided by either a collateral catheter, such as an Angiocath gauge 14-20, an Intracath (both Deseret Medical, Sandy, UT), medium and large, or an irrigation sheath with a hemostatic valve through which the angioscope passes.

The angioscope is attached to a light source (xenon) and to a CCD chip video camera. This is done under sterile conditions, using a covering sterile plastic drape. With the newer systems, the angioscope is connected directly to a camera in the base unit. The video camera is connected to a high-resolution color monitor and also to a VCR of comparable quality so that the whole study can be recorded. Review of each procedure plays an important role in becoming proficient in the interpretation of the angioscopic findings. A video-typewriter and a microphone to record the operating room discussion allows for easy patient identification and improves the quality of the videotape review process.

Operating Room Setup

It is best to prepare for angioscopy at the beginning of the procedure. A separate sterile table is prepared on which the angioscope and irrigation fluid tubing is prepared and all connections made. The angioscope and irrigation tubing are secured to the drapes. The camera is "white-balanced" and focused. The table is placed next to the surgeon so that the angioscope and irrigation tubing can be repeatedly moved to and from the operative field by the seated surgeon, maintaining sterility at all times. The foot pedal of the irrigation pump is placed at the surgeon's convenience.

Case Illustrations

The following case reports illustrate our use of angioscopy in the establishment of primary fistulas and autogenous and graft bridge fistulas, as well as in failed and occluded graft fistulas.

Case 1

C.M. is a 73-year-old female in chronic renal failure due to atheroembolic renal disease following an angiogram for bilateral carotid artery stenosis. Dialysis was initiated with a right internal jugular vein Quinton double-lumen catheter. Clinical examination showed thrombosis and absence of all the superficial veins of both upper extremities except for a prominent right cephalic vein at the elbow that appeared to fill out in continuity up the arm.

In the operating room, the patient was continuously monitored by the anesthetist, and sedation was administered as needed. With the right arm extended, a standard nonsterile tourniquet was applied as high as possible to the upper arm. A sterile field, excluding the tourniquet, was prepared. Local anesthetic was infiltrated just below the elbow crease, and the cephalic vein and radial artery just distal to the brachial bifurcation were exposed. The vein was divided at the appropriate length for the end-to-side anastomosis and was gently irrigated and distended with papaverine-heparin solution. No obstruction to flow was noted.

A 1.4 mm angioscope (Olympus Corp., Lake Success, NY) was inserted and passed up the cephalic vein; the monitor was watched for flowing blood. About 10 cm up the arm, a "whiteout" on the video monitor was noted. The angioscope was immediately withdrawn a few centimeters and a 16-gauge Angiocath introduced alongside the angioscope. A Silastic vessel loop was doubly passed around the vein at the entry site of the angioscope to control any leakage of the irrigation fluid. The upper-arm tourniquet was inflated to 200 mm Hg and irrigation begun. At the point of obstruction, an area of dense "webs" obstructing the vein was seen. Withdrawing the angioscope demonstrated that the caudad vein was normal, with normal valves. Total saline irrigation fluid used for this angioscopic examination was 100 cc.

A plan for an autogenous fistula was abandoned. A large deep brachial vein alongside the brachial artery was identified and a polytetrafluoroethylene (PTFE) loop graft, radial artery to the deep brachial vein, was inserted. The PTFE graft was tunneled and the end-to-side venous anastomosis performed. After completion of the venous anastomosis, a 1.4 mm angioscope was inserted through a No. 8 French irrigation sheath with a hemostatic valve and inserted into the open arterial limb of the graft. The angioscope was passed through the graft, beyond the distal anastomosis and into the brachial vein. During insertion, the monitor was observed to be sure the angioscope was not obstructed, and flowing blood was visible on the monitor at all times.

The tourniquet was again inflated to 200 mm Hg and irrigation was begun. Leakage of irrigation fluid was prevented by holding the graft firmly around the sheath. Inspection of the brachial vein showed it to be patent well up into the arm with normal valves and no intraluminal pathology. On examination, the anastomosis showed no technical deficits. The volume of saline irrigation was 200 ml for this study, giving a total of 300 ml for both angioscopic examinations. The patient tolerated this fluid load without any problems. Dialysis with this access graft was begun after three weeks. The vascular access continues to function well four months after surgery.

COMMENT

Intraluminal pathology in the veins of the upper extremity is common. Preoperative examination of the arm, with or without tourniquet, as well as direct surgical exposure and inspection of the veins at operation, frequently fails to detect its occurrence. In a study of 66 arm veins used for infrainguinal bypass grafts, 20 of 27 (74%) vein grafts prepared with angioscopy had intraluminal pathology detected with the angioscope, resulting in various surgical interventions.[13] In none of the remaining 39 arm vein bypasses monitored only by intraoperative angiogram or continuous wave (CW) Doppler was any intraluminal pathology detected or any intervention performed. All angioscopically prepared grafts were patent at 30 days, while 7 of 39 (18%) monitored by angiogram or CW Doppler failed within 30 days.

The most common pathologies shown to cause graft failure include regions of previous thrombosis and recanalization. On angioscopic examination, these are seen as webs, bands, and strands. Segmental stenosis or occlusion, or thrombus in varying amounts and degrees of organization, from fresh to completely organized, are also found. Areas of sclerosis are identified as a thickened intimal surface, thickened valve leaflets, or nondistensible segments of vein. Much of this pathology probably results from the repeated venesections and I.V. infusions so common in the chronically ill, diabetic, or in the elderly, who form such a large part of the patient population.

The role of angioscopy for primary hemodialysis access surgery is similar to that in infrainguinal bypass, where angioscopy allows evaluation and optimization of the conduit. In vascular access surgery, the quality of the runoff vein is critical to long-term patency. Angioscopy also provides a simple and accurate method for detection and immediate correction of any technical flaws in the anastomosis.

Case 2

M.C., a 68-year-old female patient requiring dialysis secondary to end-stage renal disease (ESRD) with chronic renal failure secondary of diabetes mellitus presented with an occluded left forearm shunt. This was a 6 mm PTFE loop bridge graft between the brachial artery and cephalic vein performed at another institution six months before. One month after placement, the graft occluded and was salvaged with a simple thrombectomy performed through an incision at the venous anastomosis. Since that time, dialysis had proceeded without any difficulty or complications. The last dialysis, two days prior to occlusion, had been uneventful, with normal flow rates and venous pressures. Clinical examination confirmed the occluded loop-graft fistula with a palpable proximal brachial artery pulse.

In the operating room, the patient was monitored by the anesthetist, who administered sedation as necessary. With the left arm extended, a standard nonsterile tourniquet was applied as high as possible on the upper arm. A sterile field, excluding the tourniquet, was prepared. Local anesthetic was infiltrated just on the venous side of the U-bend of the graft, extending onto the forearm. A 2 cm incision was made perpendicular to the graft, extending over the lateral aspect of the graft. About 2–3 cm of graft was exposed and encircled proximally and distally with vessel loops. Heparin (3,000 U) was given I.V. The graft was incised with a transverse incision in its anterior aspect. The graft was filled with fresh occluding thrombus and no flowing blood.

A No. 4 French balloon embolectomy catheter was introduced and passed up the venous limb, through the anastomosis and into the upper arm. It was withdrawn so that it was positioned just proximal to the venous anastomosis; the balloon was inflated and a thrombectomy performed. Large volumes of thrombus were removed and brisk venous backbleeding established. The 2.2 mm Olympus angioscope was now introduced beyond the graft opening into the venous limb of the graft, through the venous anastomosis and into the cephalic vein in the upper arm.

The monitor was closely observed to ensure that there was flowing blood at all times as the angioscope was passed up into the arm. With the operating room lights dimmed, progress of the angioscope up the arm was monitored by the light shining through the skin. A 5-in. 16-gauge Angiocath was now inserted collateral to the catheter. The tourniquet was inflated to 200 mm Hg and irrigation begun. The cephalic vein distal to the anastomosis was well visualized. Its endoluminal appearance was normal, with normal valve leaflets and no residual thrombus or other intraluminal pathology. The venous anastomosis, although patent, appeared somewhat narrowed with irregular, circumferential, thickened whitish material. However, the 2.2 mm angioscope appeared to pass easily through the anastomosis.

Withdrawal of the angioscope into the graft showed the walls of the graft to be covered by a somewhat irregular pseudointima, with minimal nonoccluding thrombus scattered over the surface. At the needle puncture sites, more irregularity of the luminal surface was seen, but no significant luminal narrowing was noted. The tourniquet was deflated and the venous limb of the graft was liberally irrigated with heparinized saline. An occluding vascular clamp was placed on the venous side of the graft incision. The volume of irrigation fluid infused for the angioscopic study was 220 ml.

The balloon embolectomy catheter was now inserted into the arterial limb of the graft and thrombectomy was performed, with immediate good arterial flow and graft pulsation. The tourniquet was inflated. The angioscope was introduced up the arterial limb of the PTFE graft, through the arterial anastomosis and into the brachial artery. A 5-in. 16-gauge Angiocath was now inserted collateral to the angioscope and irrigation begun. The brachial artery appeared normal, with no atherosclerotic occlusive disease. The anastomosis was widely patent, and the graft showed minimal residual thrombus with surface irregularity but no significant narrowing at the site of the needle sticks. The tourniquet was deflated. A vascular clamp was placed on the arterial limb and the graft incision closed with continuous 6-0 Prolene suture. Immediately, a pulse could be palpated throughout the graft, with a good thrill at the venous end extending up the arm. Another 250 ml of irrigation fluid was infused, making a total of 470 ml for the entire angioscopic procedure. Two hours postoperatively, the patient underwent successful dialysis. The patient did well for 10 days and three dialyses, where upon the graft spontaneously reoccluded.

The patient was again taken to the operating room with all the preparations as above. Under local anesthetic, the previous incision site (and graft incision) was opened. A thrombectomy of the venous limb was performed, followed by angioscopy. The findings were unchanged from the previous angioscopic examination, except that the anastomosis appeared more stenotic and irregular. A Kevorkian-Younge endometrial biopsy curette, with a 3.5 mm "head" was passed into the graft. Initial passage through the anastomosis was difficult, confirming a tight stenosis of the anastomosis. In a systematic fashion, the entire 360° surface of the anastomosis and venous limb of the graft underwent curettage. Each pass of the curette was followed by an angioscopic examination until the anastomosis appeared widely patent and the surface of the venous limb of the graft showed no residual obstructive intimal flaps. The arterial limb was thrombectomized without angioscopic examination and the graft incision closed. Immediately, pulsations were felt over the entire graft and a thrill was palpable at the venous end. The patient was maintained on continuous I.V. heparin overnight, keeping the partial thromboplastin time between 40 and 60 seconds. Over the succeeding 11 months, the vascular access has remained functional without any further occlusions or other problems.

COMMENT

Interpretation of angioscopic findings remains a challenge to the surgeon. The images produced by the angioscope are qualitative. The size of an object varies according to the distance the lens is from the object—the closer the lens, the larger the object. In this case, one from our early experience, the degree of stenosis of the venous anastomosis due to intimal hyperplasia was underestimated. Only when the graft reoccluded was the significance and degree of the stenosis at the venous anastomosis appreciated.

In occluded bypass grafts, angioscopy has been shown to be an extremely useful technique for determining the adequacy of thrombectomy. It also allows accurate differentiation of residual thrombus from atherosclerotic disease of the native vessels and often detects unsuspected underlying intraluminal pathology.[8,9] Although it has not yet been systematically investigated, the same advantages of angioscopy would seem to apply to vascular access grafts. Not only is the completeness of thrombectomy important, but the detection of anastomotic or needle stick site stenosis provides crucial information that may change the surgical approach as well as improve the salvage rate and long-term patency of these grafts.

Puckett and Lindsay have described the midgraft region (needle sticks) of occluded PTFE vascular access grafts as a site of frequently unrecognized stenosis that may contribute to graft occlusion.[14] They have shown that routine "blind" curettage of these regions of the grafts appears to reduce the incidence of early (<30-day) reocclusion of these grafts. With angioscopic visualization of endoluminal surface of the graft, this technique can be applied in a selected fashion, and only when the midgraft stenosis is present. Curettage of the PTFE graft venous anastomosis directed by the angioscope has not been previously described, and our early results are encouraging (unpublished data). The angioscope provides a method for determining the completeness of anastomotic or graft curettage and avoids leaving large, obstructing intimal flaps. If unrecognized, these flaps may cause intraluminal obstruction and early reocclusion. However, the long-term benefits over conventional patch angioplasty of graft or anastomotic stenoses or distal jump grafts remains to be determined. This case illustrates a new—but still unevaluated—approach to the occluded synthetic access graft whose success depends on visualization of the endoluminal aspects of the vascular access graft. The aim of such an approach is to use the angioscope to characterize the underlying pathology causing vascular access failure and to simplify and minimize the extent of the corrective surgery, thereby preserving as much runoff vein as possible for future revisions.

Conclusion

As in all endoscopy, there is a fairly steep initial learning curve in both the technical aspects and the interpretation of the findings. Achieving consistently high-quality angioscopic studies requires knowledge, skill, attention to detail, and a great deal of practice. Instrumentation and angioscopic systems have become less cumbersome and more "user friendly." The use of intraoperative endoscopy in the operating room and minimally invasive procedures is now an integral part of modern surgical practice.

Angioscopy provides the surgeon with the ability to see inside the graft, anastomosis, and native vessels. This allows one to make "informed" surgical decisions rather than rely solely on acquired "experience." The systematic characterization of the findings associated with failure of the vascular access graft or fistula may also provide new insights into the pathogenesis and mechanisms of the underlying causes of this failure.[15] Although the true value and role of the technique in its routine application to vascular access surgery has yet to be fully defined, the usefulness and varied applications of angioscopy are limited only by the ingenuity and creativity of the individual surgeon.

References

1. Grundfest W, Litvack F, Glick D, et al. Intraoperative decisions based on angioscopy in peripheral vascular surgery. Circulation 1985; 78 (suppl I):I-13-I-17.
2. Mehigan J, Olcott C. Videoangioscopy as an alternative to intraoperative arteriography. Am J Surg 1986; 152:139-45.
3. Miller A, Campbell D, Gibbons G, et al. Routine intraoperative angioscopy in lower extremity revascularization. Arch Surg 1989; 124:604-08.
4. Miller A, Stonebridge P, Jepsen S, et al. Continued experience with intraoperative angioscopy for monitoring infrainguinal bypass grafting. Surgery 1991; 109:286-93.
5. Matsumoto T, Yang Y, Hashizume M. Direct vision valvulotomy for nonreversed vein graft. Surg Gynecol Obstet 1987; 165:181-83.
6. Mehigan J. Angioscopic preparation of *in situ* saphenous vein for arterial bypass: technical considerations. In: White G, White R, eds. Angioscopy: vascular and coronary applications. Chicago: Year Book Medical, 1989; 72-5.
7. Miller A, Stonebridge P, Tsoukas A, et al. Angioscopically directed valvulotomy: A new valvulotome and technique. J Vasc Surg 1991; 13(6):813-21.
8. White G, White R, Kopchok B, Wilson S. Angioscopic thrombectomy: Preliminary observations in a recent technique. J Vasc Surg 1988; 7:318-25.
9. Segalowitz J, Grundfest W, Treiman R, et al. Angioscopy for intraoperative management of thromboembolectomy. Arch Surg 1990; 125:1357-62.
10. Miller A, Lipson W, Isaacsohn J, Schoen F, Lees R. Intraoperative angioscopy: Principles of irrigation and description of a new dedicated irrigation pump. Am Heart J 1989; 118:391-99.
11. Kwolek C, Miller A, Stonebridge P, et al. Safety of saline irrigation for angioscopy: results of a prospective randomized trial. Ann Vasc Surg 1992; 6:62-68.
12. Miller A, Jepsen S. Angioscopy in arterial surgery. Bergan J, Yao J, eds. Techniques in arterial surgery. Philadelphia: WB Saunders, 1990; 409-16.
13. Stonebridge P, Miller A, Tsoukas A, et al. Angioscopy of arm vein infrainguinal bypass grafts. Ann Vasc Surg 1991; 5:170-75.
14. Puckett J, Lindsay S. Midgraft curettage as a routine adjunct to salvage operations for thrombosed polytetrafluoroethylene hemodialysis access grafts. Am J Surg 1988; 156:139-43.
15. Koga N, Sato T, Baba T, et al. Angioscopy in transluminal balloon and laser angioplasty in the management of chronic hemodialysis fistulae. Trans Am Soc Artif Intern Organs 1989; 35:193-96.

20

VENOUS HYPERTENSION

Mark B. Adams, M.D.

VENOUS HYPTERTENSION OF THE UPPER EXTREMITY is an increasingly common complication of vascular access for hemodialysis. It manifests mainly with edema and erythema, but may progress to pain and tissue necrosis and often is associated with considerable morbidity. Venous hyptertension is usually preventable; however, once it occurs, the best treatment is usually to take down the original procedure and create a new one at a different anatomic position, i.e., resite the arteriovenous (A-V) fistula. Fistulas associated with venous hypertension are also a problem for dialysis personnel because of the edema present, which makes cannulation difficult; high venous pressures, which may limit flow or result in excessive weight loss during the dialysis treatment; and/ or prolonged bleeding following decannulation.

Causes of Venous Hypertension

Causes of venous hypertension in vascular access patients are several. An increasing number of patients presenting with end-stage renal disease (ESRD) are currently initiated on hemodialysis using temporary percutaneous subclavian dialysis catheters. These catheters have largely replaced Scribner shunts for acute and early chronic hemodialysis because of their convenience. Although such catheters were originally viewed as temporary and it was recommended that they not be used more than one or two weeks, many are now left in place for many months. Because of the need for high blood flow during dialysis, these catheters are large and are made of stiff material (such as polyurethane) to prevent collapse from negative pressures generated during hemodialysis.

Both size and stiffness are felt to be major contributing factors in the 30–50% subclavian stenosis or thrombosis rate associated with their use. Unfortunately, stenosis of these central veins can result from use of the catheters. It is therefore important to check for patency or proximal venous runoff before constructing A-V fistulas in patients with a prior history of subclavian dialysis catheter placement.

An additional cause of venous hypertension that presents immediately or soon after A-V fistula formation is failure to ligate venous outflow that provides flow into the deep venous system distal to the fistula site. This is most often a problem when the A-V fistula is placed in the antecubital fossa, making the upper arm cephalic vein the main venous outflow. In this situation, it is often convenient to use the median antecubital vein as a short conduit into the cephalic system. Doing so minimizes the size of the required incision and allows preservation of some flow distally into the cephalic system. At the point where the median antecubital vein meets the cephalic system are usually found one or more deep branches that must be ligated to prevent venous hypertension. Superficial branches may be left, and may provide sites for cannulation as they dilate, but they may also become problematic as valves become incompetent and allow arterial flow distally into the superficial venous system. Similar problems of venous hypertension may result when constructing a polytetrafluoroethylene (PTFE) loop A-V fistula in the forearm or upper arm. In either situation, ligation of distal venous outflow will prevent subsequent development of venous hypertension.

Venous hypertension occurring in the hand after a wrist A-V fistula is usually due to failure to ligate the distal venous limb at the time of fistula placement. As the cephalic vein dilates and valves become incompetent, arterial flow courses into the cephalic system distal to the A-V fistula. Approximately 20% of patients with a wrist A-V fistula in a side-to-side configuration and an unligated distal venous limb eventually will develop this problem. However, because the cephalic vein distal to the A-V fistula may provide additional sites for cannulation, some surgeons believe that the distal venous limb should not be ligated at the time of fistula formation. If significant venous hypertension subsequently develops, ligation of this venous limb is a simple measure under local anesthesia.

Venous hypertension of the hand may also occur as a result of occlusion of the main proximal cephalic outflow to a wrist A-V fistula when it occurs proximal to the lateral ulnar branch of the forearm cephalic vein. The main cephalic occlusion redirects flow distally to the hand through this lateral ulnar branch and may cause venous hypertension. Correction requires reestablishment of proximal venous outflow, usually by means of a prosthetic graft.

Prevention

Venous hypertension can usually be prevented by attention to venous anatomy proximal to the A-V fistula both prior to and at the time of fistula formation.

Patients presenting for fistula placement should be questioned about prior placement of subclavian lines, especially subclavian dialysis catheters. The subclavian areas should be examined for the presence of scars typical of such catheter placement. If either is present, a study of the venous system should be undertaken either with color flow Doppler or venography prior to fistula placement. Whereas the veins immediately proximal can be checked by visualization, probing, or use of irrigation during operation, those more proximal beyond the reach of these techniques are also important in the eventual outcome of the A-V fistula. Current Doppler technology (color dynography) allows accurate visualization of the veins and documentation of flow within them. When either the instrumentation or expertise is not available to perform color dynography, venography should be performed to exclude a proximal large-vein occlusion. Although it may be relatively unlikely that a proximal venous stenosis or thrombosis would be present in a subclavian vein that has not been cannulated, we have seen at least one case in which this apparently occurred because the catheter tip crossed over into the contralateral side instead of directly inferior into the superior vena cava. If the patient has never had a subclavian catheter by history and/or examination, study of the venous system probably is not indicated.

When using color dynography, it is important to ask the examiner also to study the axillary and brachial veins, as these may contain occlusions or stenoses that would be missed if the examination were limited to the subclavian veins.

Intraoperative testing of proximal venous patency also is an important part of fistula formation. It is best done by use of vascular probes. If a probe of reasonable size (e.g., 3–4.5 mm) easily passes proximally, one can be assured that the immediately proximal venous runoff will be adequate. Powerful irrigation with heparinized saline is less reliable, because a high-grade stenosis must be present before any resistance to injection is felt. Visual inspection of the vein is also a useful guide. If the vein is of adequate caliber (3–4 mm) and not sclerotic, it most likely has adequate proximal outflow. Visual inspection alone, however, is not sufficient in the current population of patients with ESRD, inasmuch as the majority have had previous admissions and indwelling venous catheters.

If a proximal obstruction is encountered during the course of fistula formation, intraoperative venography can be useful in deciding whether an alternative method of fistula formation, e.g., PTFE jump graft, might salvage the situation at that site. Unfortunately, when a proximal venous stenosis is encountered during the course of fistula placement, the long-term patency of the fistula at the site is usually poor.

Correction

When venous hypertension complicates a fistula placed for dialysis, correction is necessary if the patient is to regain use of an extremity that is the site of massive edema and/or pain. This will allow continued use of a fistula that has become problematic. These fistulas are problems for both the dialysis personnel and the patient. The edema can cause difficult cannulation, elevated venous pressures that limit flow rates, and/or prolonged bleeding after decannulation.

The site of venous obstruction must be identified and its nature determined. Often, physical examination is sufficient, especially in more distal (e.g., wrist and elbow) A-V fistulas. As in lower extremity venous hypertension, the proximal extent of the edema usually extends to the level where the problem lies. For example, when edema is limited to the hand and a wrist fistula is present, a patent distal venous limb is often the problem. However, edema to the level of the shoulder can occur due to a wrist A-V fistula with ipsilateral subclavian stenosis or occlusion. In such cases, the edema may be somewhat slow in onset compared to what occurs with a higher flow, more proximal fistula, such as those at the elbow.

In general, venous hypertension can be easily corrected if it results from high flow into an unintended distal venous outflow. It is more difficult to remedy if it is due to proximal venous obstruction.

If edema of the entire arm up to and/or including the shoulder occurs after fistula placement, the problem usually is subclavian or axillary venous stenosis or occlusion. Color flow Doppler imaging is a useful first test to evaluate the situation. If the vein is shown to be occluded, the best solution usually is to take the fistula down. Doing so will typically result in prompt resolution of the edema. More heroic solutions, such as venous bypass into the central thoracic veins (e.g., superior vena cava), have been reported, but are usually not indicated in most patients. In patients for whom few or no other access options exist, whether or not to take the fistula down must be decided. Reasonable control of the edema can sometimes be attained using elevation and compression sleeves such as those made for patients with postmastectomy arm edema. The use of these devices in conjunction with arm elevation often makes the edema manageable and may allow continued use of the fistula.

If the Doppler and/or venogram evaluation shows evidence of a stenotic area, percutaneous angioplasty should be considered. Using this technique, we have had success in correcting these areas of stenosis in several patients. Many of these lesions are too long and/or complex to correct with angioplasty, however.

When the pattern of edema extends mostly below the level of the A-V fistula, distal arterial flow into the venous system due to a patent distal venous limb, or unrecognized and unligated deep venous limb, is suggested. In an autogenous A-V fistula in the antecubital space, venous hypertension is often the result of a patent deep venous branch into the forearm. Although a fistulogram can be helpful in visualizing this branch, it usually is not necessary. Exploration of the fistula and ligation of the branch will correct the problem. Proximal tourniquet control is helpful and minimizes blood loss in case of any operative difficulty.

Venous hypertension in PTFE fistulas that occurs roughly in the distribution distal to the level of the venous end of the fistula suggests failure to ligate the distal (toward the hand) venous outflow of the fistula. PTFE shunts are often anastomosed to a deep vein such as the branchial vein. If the anastomosis is made end-to-side, arterialized blood can flow distally, causing venous hypertension. This can be prevented by ligating this limb at the time of fistula formation. When it occurs postoperatively, ligation will likewise solve the problem. Alternate solutions, such as thrombosis by means of percutaneous coil placement, may be considered, but are not as reliable and may risk the fistula itself.

When venous hypertension of the hand occurs as a result of wrist fistula, the usual causes are either a patent distal venous limb supplying arterialized blood to the hand or proximal venous occlusion due to thrombosis. In the first case, ligation of the distal venous limb will solve the problem. In the second case, the decision must be made either to take down the fistula and resite it, or to attempt correction of the proximal stenosis/occlusion. This is usually best accomplished by use of prosthetic material as a jump graft to a more proximal patent venous outflow vessel.

An unusual cause of venous hypertension is proximal venous occlusion occurring in a fistula that has been functioning well for some time. The usual cause is a proximal venous occlusion or stenosis that has been unrecognized by dialysis personnel. This has redirected arterialized flow into a side branch, resulting in distal venous flow and hypertension. This situation is dealt with either by fistula takedown and resiting, venoplasty, or bypass of the occluded segment, usually with PTFE.

Summary

Venous hypertension has increased in frequency because of the recent higher use of temporary percutaneous dialysis catheters. These catheters are associated with a 30–50% incidence of subclavian stenosis or occlusion. Careful preoperative assessment of the patency of these proximal vessels is mandatory in any patient with a prior history of subclavian catheter placement. Avoiding the placement of A-V fistulas ipsilateral to problematic subclavian and axillary veins will prevent subsequent venous hypertension. Correction of venous hypertension in this setting usually requires ligation of the A-V fistula. Most other cases of venous hypertension result from failure to ligate distal venous outflow during fistula formation. Diagnosis often requires only physical examination, and correction is accomplished by ligation of the offending vein or veins. Rarely, venous hypertension occurs long after fistula formation and is due to occlusion of the main proximal venous outflow vessel, with patency of the fistula maintained through some other collateral vessel supplying a distal venous bed. Correction requires fistula takedown or bypass of the occluded vessel.

References

1. Glanz S, Gordon D, Butt KMH, Hong J, Adamson R, Sclafani SJA. Dialysis access fistulas: Treatment of stenoses by transluminal angioplasty. Radiology 1984; 152:637–42.

2. Suratt RJ, Picus D, Hicks ME, Darcy MD, Kleinhoffer M, Jendrisak M. The importance of preoperative evaluation of the subclavian vein in dialysis access planning. Am J Roentgenol 1991; 156:623-25.
3. Glanz S, Gordon DH, Lipkowitz GS, Butt KMH, Hong J, Sclafani SJA. Axillary and subclavian vein stenosis: Percutaneous angioplasty. Radiology 1988; 168:371-73.
4. Spinowitz BS, Galler M, Golden RA, et al. Subclavian vein stenosis as a complication of subclavian catheterization for hemodialysis. Arch Intern Med 1987; 147:305-07.
5. Surratt RS, Picus D, Hicks ME, et al. The importance of preoperative evaluation of the subclavian vein in dialysis access planning. Am J Roentgenol 1991; 156:623-25.

PANEL DISCUSSION

Moderator:
  Mitchell L. Henry, M.D.
Panelists:
  Mark B. Adams, M.D.
  Jeffrey H. Fair, M.D.
  Arnold Miller, M.B., Ch.B., F.R.C.S., F.R.C.S.C., F.A.C.S.
  Michael J. Verta Jr., M.D.

Discussant: Has anybody had any experience with urokinase with these grafts?
Panelist: Yes, we have tried urokinase on a couple of them. It does work, but the problem is that you have to correct whatever caused the graft to go down if you want it to stay. We have tried once or twice to open an occluded subclavian vein with urokinase, but we haven't been able to maintain any of them for very long.
Moderator: In the literature, it has been held that the most effective way is to install dual catheters, one from each end, and lyse the lumen graft completely with urokinase. Unfortunately, hundreds of thousands of units of urokinase are used to open it up, with the attendant problem of systemic administration. Also, this is a very expensive technique. It almost always needs an adjunctive procedure, and in that setting it is usually percutaneous transluminal angioplasty. When all is considered, it is probably best to approach it directly from a surgical standpoint. That is my prejudice, anyway.
Dr. Miller: I agree with Dr. Henry. We have done a few thrombolyses, but it is just so expensive, and it is so simple to do a surgical thrombectomy. Using the angioscope, you can define the pathology, so it really doesn't make too much sense.
Discussant: I have had some limited success with angioplasty and a few situations using the technique advocated by Samuel Long and Wesley Moore of extremely high pressures using a high-pressure balloon at 15–17 atmospheres for 15–20 minutes with the patient heparinized. I was just wondering if that was the angioplasty technique used by the presenters.
Panelist: The angioplasty technique I use doesn't call for 15 atmospheres; we usually go only to 10 or 12. But it has been my experience that with intimal hyperplasia in the vein, you end up disrupting the vein or see an early recurrence. It is usually easier to surgically attack the problem. As for intragraft stenoses, I don't know that you really want to distend the GORE-TEX Graft.
Discussant: No. Not with intragraft and not even with graft venous anastomosis, but for more proximal lesions at higher pressures for longer periods of

time. In about 10 cases I have had a secondary patency rate of anywhere from three to 14 months.

Moderator: Balloon angioplasty with low-pressure balloons has miserable outcomes. The only ones that have reasonable results are with high-pressure applications.

Discussant: Is there any difference with subclavian vein stenosis with particular accesses or PermCaths? Do jugular vein catheters cause less morbidity?

Panelist: I think that a PermCath is probably a better choice for many of these patients. This allows enough time for the access that you have formed to mature completely before you are compelled to use it.

Panelist: You should be aware that even the soft Silastic PermCaths placed through the right internal jugular will still develop problems with central venous stenoses, and we have seen that time and again over a period of many months.

Moderator: The stenosis is usually more proximal when it occurs after surgical placement directly in the vein rather than percutaneous placement. With percutaneous placement, the stenosis usually occurs at the site of the entry of the catheter into the vessel wall. If an internal or external jugular approach is used, the stenotic portion, if it occurs, is usually more central.

Discussant: Dr. Verta, what is the experience with atherectomy devices or curetting devices across the anastomosis? What kinds of problems can be expected?

Dr. Verta: I have used them at the anastomotic site. Particularly since the blade is shielded, I have had no problems at all. We don't seem to disrupt the suture line or divide the suture. After a while, even with the GORE-TEX Graft, the external fibrosis usually tends to hold the graft in place. That's the reason for adopting the Simpson catheter, because the blade is shielded and the surgeon is less likely to get hooked or caught on something, or leave a flap behind. It's particularly difficult with an anastomosis to avoid a flap with an open curette.

Discussant: Don't you think it is easier to use the Simpson catheter percutaneously rather than intraoperatively because of the way it is designed?

Dr. Verta: There is no question that the Simpson catheter is easier to use percutaneously, but I have a little problem with a No. 9 French hole in a percutaneous dialysis graft. I prefer to make a small incision and use a hemostatic sheath so I don't get much bleeding. Also, irrigation volumes can be reduced.

Moderator: I was glad to hear Dr. Miller talk about using a curette across the anastomosis, because we do that routinely. Not only intragraft, but across the anastomosis. Following standard Fogarty thrombectomy, we use a pituitary curette and go up proximally through the anastomosis. You can always get more clot than you did, and this is fresh clot. You almost always get intimal hyperplastic material. Although I worry about the flaps that you can see through the angioscope, they have not been a real problem.

Discussant: I would like to commit surgical heresy here and say that we do use the stents placed through Nos. 7 and 8.5 French sheaths. We have had very few problems with the big holes.

Discussant: The Simpson catheter does have a lot of appeal. How much does it cost, and can you give us a few more details about its use?

Dr. Verta: It is disposable, and unfortunately, it is not cheap—it costs about $700 to $800 per unit. The battery pack with the handle, the motor drive, and the catheter are all disposable, as it is a single-use item. It is expensive, but if you pick the right size you use only one. In the tapered dialysis grafts, using a No. 9 French catheter, you can go from a 4 mm size to a 7 mm within the working range of that particular unit. In addition, you can empty the collecting chamber if necessary. You just remove it, empty it and reuse it until you're finished.

Discussant: There have been incidental reports of bypassing the subclavian by bringing down the external jugular. Have you had any experience with that?

Dr. Adams: No, I have not. My basic philosophy is that I wouldn't subject the patient to something like that unless I had exhausted all other possibilities. Obviously, you could theoretically do that. It is just another route of plumbing, but I assume that this would require taking out at least part of the clavicle, and that is a big operation.

Discussant: Subclavian stenosis is a very big problem, and we are relying a lot on the angiographers to dilate them. I have been reluctant to have them put in stents. Understandably, these things last only a couple of months. But what is the experience with migration of those stents?

Dr. Fair: As I mentioned, the one stent that moved a bit went up into one of the collaterals. That has been the only human experience we have had with migration. In literature that I have reviewed, it was reported that one out of about 100 patients experienced local migration, so it really has not been a big problem. Distal migration has not been reported. Clearly, it is a potential problem that you can't ignore.

Discussant: One could argue that the stent device might absorb some of the kinetic energy that you are seeing as vibration about your anastomosis. Is there any evidence to that effect by color flow Doppler or anything else?

Discussant: Actually, I don't think anyone has really looked at that. Based on our experience, neointimal hyperplasia occurs at the end of the stent, so we seem to transmit the problem from the end of the graft to the end of the stent.

INDEX

Access volume flow, 103
  criteria, 94
  equation, 94
  form, 85
Adhesion. *See* Cell
  adhesion
Air-plethysmography,
  139-40
Amplitude, 94
Amyloid, 188
Analgesia overuse, 188
Anemia, 115, 120
Aneurysm, 200
  complications of, 160
  occurrence of, 162
Angina, 52
Angioaccess ischemic steal,
  123-27, 137-38. *See
  also* Steal
Angiocath, 212
Angiography, 95-101
Angioplasty, 226-27
  patch, 171
  of stenotic lesion, 96
Angioscopes, 212
Angioscopy
  thrombectomy assist,
    128-31, 139
  in vascular access
    surgery, 210-17
Angiotensin-converting
  enzyme (ACE),
  29-31
  inhibitors, 54, 62-63
Angiotensin II, 29-31
Antecubital incision, 199
Antegrade occlusion
  methods, 211-12
Antimigratory agents,
  59-62
Antiplatelet agents, 49-53
Antiproliferative drugs,
  62-64

Antithrombin-III, 49
Area reduction,
  cross-sectional, 110
Arm grafts, lower, 76
Artemisia rubrites naki, 61
Arterial anastomosis, 100
Arterial size, 138
Arteriovenous (A-V)
  fistula, 41
  angioaccess ischemic
    steal and, 123-27,
    137-38
  See also Brescia-Cimino
    fistula
Arteriovenous grafts,
  intimal hyperplasia
  and, 14
Arteriovenous shunt,
  development of, 3
Artifact, 86-90
Aspirin, 41-43, 45, 47, 49,
  51, 53, 99, 101
Atherosclerosis, 14-15, 25,
  28, 43, 54, 147
Atrium, 153

Balloon angioplasty,
  226-27
Balloon catheter
  occlusion, 212
  embolectomy, 190
Barrett, N., 152
Bauer, R., 146
Biologic mediators
  hemodynamic response
    theory, 28-30
  immune/inflammatory
    response theory,
    22-28
  injury-response theory,
    17-22
  interventions for, 30-34

intimal hyperplasia,
  14-17
list of potential, 18
Blood, 116-17
  flow rates, 109-10, 140
  flow turbulence, 28, 30,
    34, 74-75, 76-77, 89,
    90
  flow velocity, 86
  platelet
    aggregometry, 75
    count, EPO and, 12
    function, 75
  pressure cuff, 197-98
  volume flow
    criteria, 94
    equation, 94
    wave form, 85
  white cell count, EPO
    and, 12
B-mode, 94
Boehringer-Ingelheim, 45
Bone shadowing, 87
Bovine grafts, 49, 157-61,
  166
  salvage surgery, 170,
    171-73
Brady, T., 204
Brems, J., 161
Brescia, M. J., 152
Brescia-Cimino fistula, 95,
  97-98, 115-16, 169,
  175, 182, 208
  See also Arteriovenous
    fistula
Bridge fistula, 125-26
Brooks, J. L. 202
Bruit, 89
Butler, H. G., 174

Caffeic acid, 61
Caffeine, 51

Calcium channel blockers, 55, 61
Canadian Cooperative Study Group, 41
Cannulation, 199-200
  incidence with expanded PTFE graft, 134-36, 144
  plasma TFE, 147
Cardiac disease, 179
Casati, S., 120
Case illustrations, angioscopy, 213-16
Catheters
  atherectomy, 202-5
  balloon, 190, 212
  central venous dialysis, 77
  Dow study, 77
  Fogarty, 129, 186, 190
  Simpson, 202-4, 226-27
CCD chip video camera, 212
Cefazolin, 188
Cell adhesion, 47
  assays, 75
  mediators associated with, 26-27
  molecules, 23-24
  phenomena, 22, 24-28
Central venous dialysis catheter, 77
Cephalosporin, 158
Clotting. See Thrombosis
Clowes, A. W., 20, 31, 32
Cochran (John) Veterans Administration Medical Center, 158
Colburn, M. D., 32
Colchicine, 58, 61
Color
  aliasing, 89, 90
  flashing, 89, 90
Color flow Doppler, 75, 84, 221, 222, 227
  angiography and, 95-101
  clinical application, 81-94, 102-7
  intervention and, 110

6-mm stretch PTFE graft assessment, 143, 144, 164
PTFE graft monitoring cost, 111
Continuous-wave Doppler, 83, 84
Cook, Inc., 208
Corticoids, 64
Cox, D. R., 148
Curettage, 217
  graft, 186-94
Curette, 198
Cyclic nucleotide promotors, 53
Cyclooxygenase inhibitors, 42-45, 53
Cyclosporine A, 32-33
Cystic disease, morbidity, 11
Cytokines, 22-24, 26-27

Dacron, 153, 182
Daemen, M. J., 31
Danacrine (danzol), 55-56
Defibrotide, 54
Desert Medical, 212
Devices for Vascular Intervention, 202
Dexamethasone, 32
Diabetes, 147, 179, 188, 198
  hospitalization predictors, 10-11
  presence of, 158-59
  revascularization and, 137-38
Dialysis
  high-flux, 77
  patients, 5
Digital subtraction angiography, 95
Dimethyl sulfoxide, 58-59
Dinarello, C. A., 47-49
Dipyridamole, 41-42, 50, 51
Dolmatch, 205
Doppler shift, 94
Doppler study, 96
Dousset, V., 97

Drugs, summary of, 65. See also Pharmacologic intervention
Duplex scanner, 83-84, 93, 198
Du Pont, 153

Edema, 221-22
Eicosapentanoic acid (EPA), 43-45, 47, 49, 61, 62. See also Fish oil
End-stage renal disease (ESRD), 48
  morbidity, 3-5
  pharmacologic intervention, 52-53
  plasma TFE, 146
  prevalence of, 207
  severe anemia in, 115
  thrombosis, 118, 120
Endothelial cells (ECs), PDGF and, 17
Endothelial leukocyte adhesion molecules (ELAM-1), 47
Endothelial-derived relaxing factor (EDRF), 29
Endothelial-seeded grafts, 53
Endothelin, 47
Endothelium-dependent relaxation factor (EDRF), 47
Endovascular stents, 207-9
Erythropoietin (EPO), 74, 75
  dose, 9
  hematocrit, 137
  hospitalization predictions, 10
  morbidity, 4-12
  patient comparison, 8
  thrombosis and, 115-21
Esmarch's bandage, 212
Etheredge, E. E., 173, 201

Event-free patency, 147-48, 154. *See also* Patency
Expanded PTFE graft, 133-36, 140-41, 153
  cannulation of, 147
  compared to plasma TFE, 148-55
  4-7 mm tapered, 175-84

Ferns, G., 33
Fibroblast growth factor (FGF), 19, 33
Fibronectin, 59
Fibrous tissue ingrowth, 193
Fillinger, M. F., 183, 208
Fish oil, 32, 53, 59
  as drug base, 65
  fatty acid profile and, 47-49
Fisher exact test, 147
Fistulagram, 96, 97, 158
Flow turbulence, 28, 30, 34, 74-75, 76-77, 89, 90
Flow velocity, 86
Fogarty catheter, 129, 186, 190
Forearm loop graft, 76

Gamma interferon, 28
Gangreous lesions, 124-25
Gaylord, G. M., 202, 204
Genetic therapy, 33
Gianturco-Wallace stent, 208, 209
Glomerulonephritis, 188
  morbidity, 11
Glucocorticoids, 64
Glycyrrhetinic acid (GRHA), 61-62
Glylocalyx regulation, 56-58
GORE-TEX grafts, 49, 146, 188
  stretch, 133-36, 140-41

tapered, 175-84
Gore tunneler, 147, 165, 176-78
Graft
  complications, 4
  configuration, 75-76
  curettage, 186-94
  failure, 74, 110
    color flow Doppler and, 99
    hospitalization and, 102
    managing, 201-5
  infections, 160
  interposition, 197
  PTFE use after installation, 141
  reinforced, 141
  revision, 161, 172, 180. *See also* Salvage
  survival, 160
  variety of, 182
Graftotomy, 186-93
Gray, R. J., 205

Harter, H. R., 41
Hegar dilators, 189
Hematocrit, 4, 8-11, 99, 101
  values, 116-17, 120
Hematoma, 92
Hemodynamic intervention, 33-34
Hemodynamic response theory, 28-30
  potential mediators of, 29
Hemoglobin, 116-17. *See also* Blood
Heparan sulfate, 31, 58, 59
Heparin, 20, 31, 56, 58, 63, 177, 189
  saline flush, 190
Heparin-binding endothelial cell growth factorlike growth factor mitogens, 19, 31

Herring, Constantine, 52
Hertz (Hz), 93-94
Hoffman, A. S., 146, 153
Hospitalization, 75
  leading causes of, 6
  morbidity and, 4-12
Hurt, A. V., 161
Hypertension, 179
Hypotension, 52

Ibuprofen, 51
Ig class integrin ligands, 26-27
Immune/inflammatory response theory, 22-28
  cell adhesion phenomena and, 22, 24-28
Implant complications, 4
Impra grafts, 199. *See also* PTFE grafts.
Indiana University Medical Center, 170
Infection
  4-7 mm tapered expanded PTFE grafts, 180
  rate, 159
Injury-response theory, 17-22, 32
Integrin, 22-23, 26
Intercellular adhesion molecules (ICAM-1), 47
Interleukin-8, 24
Interleukin-1, 46, 47
Interposition grafting, 171
Intervention
  color flow Doppler and, 110
  hemodynamic, 33-34
  pharmacologic. *See* Pharmacologic intervention
  potential areas of biologic mediators, 30-33
  secondary, 75

Intimal hyperplasia
  background on, 14-17
  hemodynamic response theory, 28-30
  immune/inflammatory response theory, 22-28
  injury-response theory, 17-22
  interventions for, 30-34
  outflow vein, 91
  pharmacologic intervention. *See* Pharmacologic intervention
  thickening of, 60
Intimal-medial hyperplasia, 17
Intracath, 212
Irrigation, 227
  saline, 211
  sheath, 212
Ischemia, 123-27

Jendrisak, M., 146, 153

Kaplan, E. L., 148
Kaplan-Meier life table analysis, 171
Ketanserin, 64
Kevorkian-Younge curette, 186-87, 188, 190, 191, 193-94
Koga, N., 130
Kolff, Willem, 181

Langille, B. L., 29
Leg grafts, 76
Leukocyte, 24
  attachment to vein graft, 21
Leukotriennes, 47
Licorice, 61
Lilly, L., 173-74
Lindsay, S., 217
Loop graft, 106, 137, 139, 147, 150, 154, 177-78, 198
  configuration of, 196-97
  patency rate, 183-84
  placement of, 199
Lovastatin, 63
Low-flow grafts, 109
Lowrie, E. G., 95

Macrophages (MΦs), 15
  PDGF and, 17
Mechanical complications, 4
Medtronics, 146, 153
Meier, P., 148
Microscopic examination, 192
Middleton, W., 97
Midgraft stenosis, 186, 193
Mills, Lee Ann, 45
Misoprostol, 64
Monoclonal antibodies, 33
Morbidity
  A-V fistula and, 1-12
  graft location and, 76
  vascular access research methods, 4-5
  results, 5-12
Myeloma, multiple, 188

Nabel, E. G., 33
National Medical Care (NMC), 3-12, 95
Neointimal hyperplasia, 180, 227
Nephrosclerosis, 188
Nifedipine, 51
Nitrate effect, 46
Nitrates, nitrites, 52, 56
Nitroprusside, 52
Nonnast-Daniel, B., 98
Nursing technique, 76
Nyquist limit, 88, 90

O'Donnell, F., 29
Ohio State University Hospitals, 95, 98
Omega-3 fatty acids, 32, 47-49. *See also* Fish oils
Outflow stenosis, 131
Outflow veins, 110
Oxpentifylline, 51

Paganini, E. P., 120
Palder, S., 193
Parke-Davis, 147
Patency, 166, 169
  atherectomy catheter, 203-5
  curettage, 188
  event-free, 147-48, 154
  expanded PTFE grafts, 182
Patency rate, 161, 162
  curettage, 190-94
  4-7 mm tapered PTFE grafts, 180-81
  salvage surgery, 171
Patient statistical profile (PSP), 3
Penrose drains, 212
Pentoxiflylline, 51-52
Percutaneous transluminal angioplasty, 207-8
PermCaths, 226
PET, 153
Pharmacologic intervention
  drugs summary, 65
  future therapy implications, 64-66
  historical attempts, 41-48
  other possibilities, 48-64
Phenylbutazone, 49, 50
Plasma-TFE grafts, 146-55
Platelet
  aggregometry, 75
  count, EPO and, 12
  function, 75
Platelet-derived growth factor (PDGF), 17, 19, 43, 47
Platelet-SMC interactions, 32
Polo, J. R., 174

Polycystic renal disease, 188
Polytetrafluorethylene grafts. *See* PTFE grafts
Procoagulant effect, 46
Proendothelial agents, 53-56
Prostacyclin, 29, 42, 54
 -thromboxane balance, 42
Protein C, 55-56
Pseudoanyuerism, 92-93, 200
Pseudointimal hyperplasia, 202-3
PTFE bridge, 123
PTFE graft, 41, 75-76, 95-96
 angioscopy-assisted thrombectomy experience, 128-31, 139
 -coated, woven, 146-55, 165-66
 color flow Doppler, 102-7
 cost, 111
 sensitivity, 98-99
 compared to bovine, 157-61
 curettage, 186-94
 EPA and, 43
 erythropoietin and, 115-21
 salvage surgery for, 170, 171-73
 expanded, 133-36, 140-41
 screening and, 109
 Simpson catheter treatment, 202-4
 6-mm stretch, 142-44, 164-65
Puckett, J., 217
Pulsed-wave Doppler, 83, 84-86, 90

Quantum Medical Systems, 103

Radial-cephalic fistulas, color flow Doppler and, 102-7
Real time, 94
Recirculation, 109-10
 abnormal, 102-3, 105
Recombinant human erythropoietin, 115-21. *See also* Erythropoietin
Renovascular hypertension, 188
Revascularization, 123-27
Reverberation artifact, 88, 90
Rizzuti, R. P., 183-84
Rolling, on cell surface, 22-25
Ross, R., 17, 22
Roudebush Veterans Medical Center, 170

Sabanayagam, P., 161, 173
Safflower oil, as drug base, 65
Saginaw (Michigan) General Hospitals, 116
Saint Louis University Hospital, 158
Salvage methods
 curettage, 186-94
 failing PTFE grafts, 201-5
Salvage surgery, 169-74
Saphenous vein grafts, 170, 171-73
Schneider, 208
Schwab, S. J., 152
Scribner shunts, 41, 49, 52, 181, 219
Selectins, 24, 26
Seromas, recurrent, 200
Shadowing, 86-87
Shear stress, 28-29
Siemens Quantum, 83-84
Silastic shunts, 169, 226

Simpson catheter, 202-4, 226-27
Smooth muscle cells (SMCs)
 biologic mediators, 14-20, 24, 28, 31-33
 PDGF and, 47
Soybean oil, as drug base, 65
Spinowitz, B. S., 152
Steal, 144, 173, 177, 183
 angioaccess ischemic, 123-27, 137-38
 in 4-7 mm tapered graft, 198-99
Stenosis, 110, 201
Stents, endovascular, 207-9
Sticking, 25, 46
Straight graft, 106, 137, 139, 147, 150, 154
 forearm, 158-59
 patency rate, 183-84
Subclavian vein
 color flow Doppler and, 99
 stenosis, 152-53, 227
Sulfinpyrazone, 49-50, 120
Surgical technique, 76
Survival curve, 148-49
Systemic lupus, 188

Tapered grafts, 76-77, 175-84, 197-99
Target cell, 24
Theophylline, 51, 52
Thrill, 89
Thrombectomy, 171
 adjunctive angioscopy in, 128-31
 expanded PTFE grafts, 182
 plasma TFE grafts and, 155
 6-mm stretch PTFE grafts and, 143-44, 164-65
 timing of, 196

Thrombin, 19
  liquid, 147
Thrombocytopenia, 42
Thrombosis, 34, 102, 103-7, 109
  access, 41
  annual access, 119
  annualized risk of vascular access, 119
  aspirin in, 43
  curettage, 186-93
  early grafts and, 193
  erythropoietin and, 115-21
  in EPO and non-EPO groups, 118
  4-7 mm tapered expanded PTFE grafts, 179-80
  incidence with expanded PTFE graft, 134-36, 143-44
  late, 193
  plasma TFE graft, 154
  using PTFE-coated woven grafts, 151-52
Thrombospondin, 19
Thrombostat, 147
Thromboxane A2, 42
Ticlopidine, 52-53
Time trend curve
  for access-related morbidity, 5
  for EPO patients, 8
  for hospitalization days, 5

Tissue plasminogen activator, 20, 56
Tissue vibration, 109
T lymphocytes, 15
Tordoir, J. H. M., 98
Tortolani, E. C., 202
Tourniquet, 212
Transducers, 82-83, 85, 94, 103
Transforming growth factor beta, 19
Triazolopyridine, 62
Tumor necrosis factor (TNF), 46, 47
  alpha, 19
12-L-hydroxy-5,8,10,14 (12HETE), 60, 61

Ultrasound, 82-90
  Doppler, 83-84
Upper-arm fistulas, 139
Urokinase, 225-26

Vancomycin, 188-89
  infection rates, 140
Vascular access
  stenosis, 102
  surgery, angioscopy in, 210-17
Vascular clamps, 212
Vascular probes, 221
Vasorelaxation, 29
Vein stenosis, 91
  midgraft, 92
Venogram, 199

Venography, 221
Venous anastomosis, 44, 49, 100
  hyperplasia, 16
Venous hypertension, 219-23
Venous intimal hyperplasia, 91
Venous stenosis, 77, 202
  PTFE graft outflow, 96
Verapamil, 51
Volume flow
  criteria, 94
  equation, 94
  wave form, 85
Vorwerk, D., 208

Wallstent, 208, 209
Warfarin, 41
White blood cell count, EPO and, 12
Wilcoxon analysis, 192
Winearls, C., 120
Wound healing, 59, 75

Xenon light source, 212

Yeh, Y. S., 146, 153
Yugoslavia test, 52

Zemel, G., 202, 204

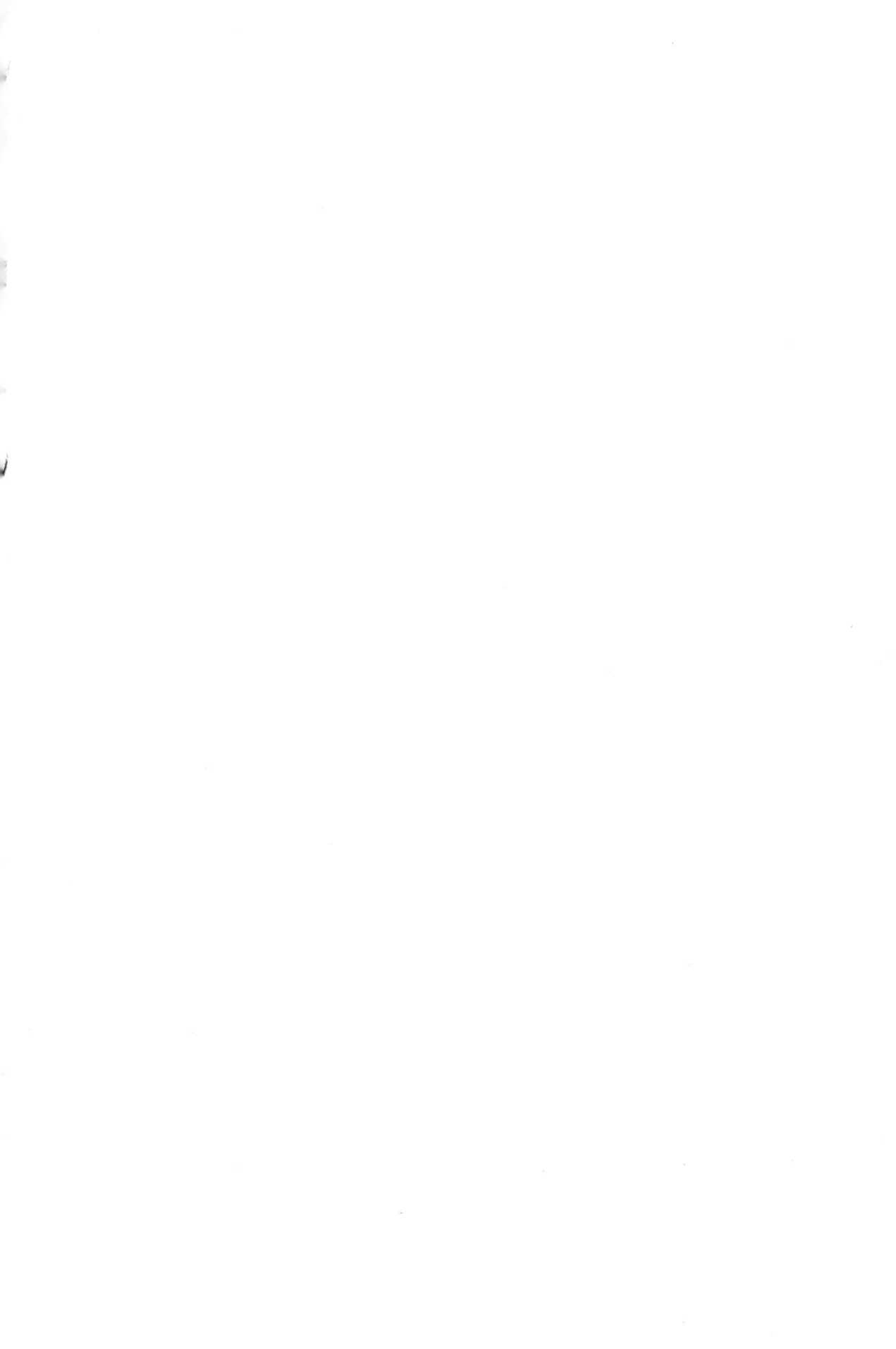

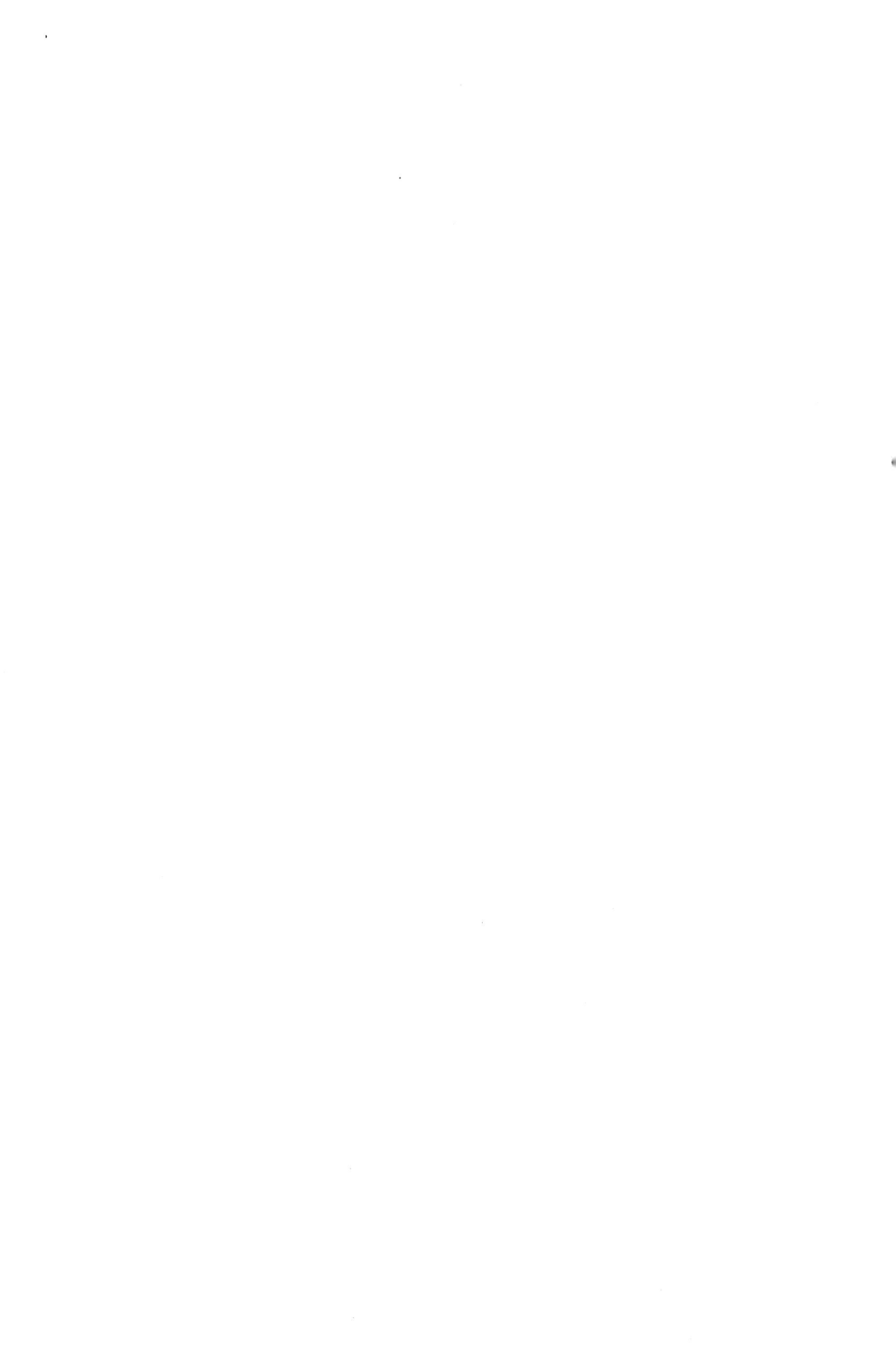